Psychedelics and Individuation

Essays by

Jungian Analysts

Edited by
Leslie Stein and Lionel Corbett

CHIRON PUBLICATIONS • ASHEVILLE, NORTH CAROLINA

www.ChironPublications.com

Cover design by Celeste Stein
Interior design by Danijela Mijailovic
Printed primarily in the United States of America.

ISBN 978-1-68503-201-2 paperback
ISBN 978-1-68503-202-9 hardcover
ISBN 978-1-68503-203-6 electronic
ISBN 978-1-68503-204-3 limited edition paperback

Library of Congress Cataloging-in-Publication Data Pending

Table of Contents

Indigenous Healing Perspectives

Establishing Intentions

The Setting

Integration in Practice

Contributors

Marcel van den Akker, PhD is a Jungian Analyst and registered Psycho-therapist and Clinical Psychologist in private practice in The Netherlands. He is a former Graduate Analyst at the ISAP Zurich. During the last couple of years he has been exploring the benefits of psilocybin use in his clinical work and for his personal process.

Walter Boechat, MD, PhD, is a graduate of the C.G. Jung Institute Zurich (1979), Founding-member of *Jungian Association of Brazil* (AJB-IAAP), Past Representative of AJB at the Executive Committee of IAAP from 2007 to 2013, Past IAAP Co-Regional Organizer (together with Misser Berg) for Latin America from 2011-2013, PhD at the University of the State of Rio de Janeiro. Walter Boechat is part of the staff in charge of the Brazilian edition of the C.G. Jung Books: *The Red Book* and *The Black Books*, as the reviewer of the translation from the original German version to Portuguese. He published extensively in Brazil and abroad including: *The Red Book of C.G. Jung: A Journey to Unknown Depths* (London: Karnac, 2017).

Jerome Braun is a bilingual, Spanish/English-speaking, Jungian analyst in private practice in Northern California. He trained and is certified by the C.G. Jung Institute Zurich and is an active member of the International Association for Analytical Psychology (IAAP). In 2019, Jerome completed his training at the California Institute of Integral Studies at the Center for Psychedelic Therapies and Research. He is a certified psychedelic-assisted psychotherapist who specializes in pre- and post-psychedelic integration psychotherapy from a Jungian perspective. Also, Jerome has over 30 years of providing trauma treatment to adults with histories of incest and sexual abuse. Jerome serves on the Elder

Council of the American Psychedelic Practitioners Association which is developing the Standards of Practice for psychedelic practitioners in the U.S. He has presented on Jungian psychology and psychedelic-assisted therapy in the U.S. and abroad. He contributed the chapter, "Impact of Personal Psychedelic Experiences in Clinical Practice" in the book edited by Tim Read and Maria Papaspyrou, *Psychedelics & Psychotherapy: The Healing Potential of Expanded States*. Since 2017, Jerome is in ongoing training with Indigenous Shipibo healers living in the Peruvian Amazon. In a cultural exchange with the Shipibo healers and their families, he is bridging Jungian psychology and treatments based on ancient Indigenous knowledge and traditions.

Deborah Bryon is a graduate of UCLA and received her doctorate in Counseling Psychology from the University of Denver, before becoming a diplomate Jungian analyst with the Inter-Regional Society of Jungian Analysts. She is the author of two books and several articles on Andean medicine, the mesa, and Andean teachings in magazines and Jungian publications, and is a frequent lecturer in the analytic community. In addition to writing, teaching, and seeing clients in private practice, Deborah is a painter and member of Spark Gallery, Denver, Colorado.

Aurea Afonso M. Caetano is a psychologist and Jungian analyst in private practice in São Paulo, Brazil. She is an active member of the Brazilian Society of Analytical Psychology (SBrPA), working currently with the Teaching Board. While studying for her Master's degree in clinical psychology at PUCSP, she conducted research into the practice of Jungian analysts in Brazil. For the last 10 years, with Dr. Teresa Cristina Machado, she has coordinated a study group exploring interconnections between psychiatry, neurosciences, and analytical psychology. She has published several articles in this area, including in *Junguiana*, the SBrPA's journal.

Linda Carter MSN, CS, IAAP is a nurse/Jungian analyst practicing in Carpinteria, California; graduate of Georgetown, Yale, and the C.G. Jung Institute-Boston; *Journal of Analytical Psychology* Book Review Editor, US Editor-in-Chief, and Arts and Culture Editor; chair/founder of Art and

Psyche Working Group; and winner of two Gradiva Awards (NAAP) with article "Amazing Grace" short-listed for Gradiva.

Lionel Corbett trained in medicine and psychiatry in England and as a Jungian Analyst at the C.G. Jung Institute of Chicago. He is a professor of depth psychology at Pacifica Graduate Institute, in Santa Barbara, California. He is the author of seven books: *Psyche and the Sacred: The Religious Function of the Psyche*; *The Sacred Cauldron: Psychotherapy as a Spiritual Practice*; *The Soul in Anguish: Psychotherapeutic Approaches to Suffering*; *Understanding Evil: A Guide for Psychotherapists;* and *The God-image: From Antiquity to Jung*. He is the co-editor of four volumes of collected papers: *Psyche's Stories*; *Depth Psychology, Meditations in the Field*; *Psychology at the Threshold*; and *Jung and Aging*.

Renée M. Cunningham, MFT, is a Diplomate Jungian Analyst in private practice in Phoenix, Arizona. She is a training analyst in the Inter-Regional Society of Jungian Analysts-Texas Chapter. She is an international speaker, and author. Her current book is *Archetypal Nonviolence: Jung, King, and Culture Through the Eyes of Selma* (Routledge 2020).

James A. Fidelibus, Ph.D., is a licensed psychologist in the State of Ohio and holds a diploma as a Jungian Analyst from the C.G. Jung Institute of Chicago. In addition to psychology, his academic background includes training in philosophy and theology. He holds certificates from the Gottman Institute, the Ottawa Couple & Family Institute, and the Cleveland Center for Cognitive Therapy. Dr. Fidelibus has published articles on psychotherapy outcomes and has presented on Jungian psychology locally, nationally, and internationally. He maintains an active psychology practice in Columbus, Ohio.

Anne Flynn is a Jungian Analyst in private practice in Sarasota, Florida. She is a graduate and member of the Jungian Psychoanalytic Association in New York and a member of the International Association for Analytical Psychology. She completed Naropa University's Psychedelic-Assisted Therapies Certificate and MDMA Training Program, which includes an intensive training through the Multidisciplinary Association for Psychedelic Studies (MAPS). She is a Board Certified art therapist and holds Master's degrees in Art Therapy and in Fine Arts-Painting. She has a special interest in non-ordinary states of consciousness and has explored these through trainings in dreamwork, clinical hypnotherapy, Jungian sand tray, and extensive clinical supervision with Philip Bromberg exploring uncanny, dissociative and non-ordinary states in the consulting room. From an earlier iteration of her consciousness, she holds a JD from Fordham University and worked in New York as an attorney in various capacities.

Nancy Swift Furlotti, Ph.D. is a Jungian Analyst living in Aspen, Colorado. She is a past president of the C.G. Jung Institute of Los Angeles, where she trained, a founding member and past president of the Philemon Foundation, and is on the Mercurius Film Prize Committee. She is a member of the C.G. Jung Institute of Colorado and the Interregional Association of Jungian Analysts. She is on the boards of Pacifica Graduate Institute in Santa Barbara and the Smithsonian National Asian Museum. Dr. Swift Furlotti lectures internationally on Jungian topics such as dreams, mythology, trauma, the feminine, and the environment. Her company, Recollections, LLC, publishes early analysts' unpublished material, such as the manuscripts of Erich Neumann. She has two forthcoming books, *The Continuing Relevance of Erich Neumann: On God, Consciousness, and The Existence of Evil,* and *The Splendor of the Maya: A Journey into the Shadows at the Dawn of Creation.*

I. Joseph McFadden, M.D., NCPsyA (USA), is a Board Certified psychiatrist, anesthesiologist and member of the IAAP. He is a past Book Review Editor of the *Journal of Analytical Psychology* and continues on the Editorial Board. He is a training and supervising analyst with the IRSJA. He maintains a part-time analytic practice in Southport, N.C. His particular clinical interests have been in trauma and dissociative disorders.

Ana Luisa Teixeira de Menezes, PhD (AJB) Psychologist (UFC), PhD in Education and Post-Doctorate in Education (UFRGS). Professor at the Department of Psychology and at the Graduate Program in Education

4

of the University of Santa Cruz do Sul. Vice-leader of the CNPQ research group Amerindian Education and cultural exchange (UFRGS/ UNISC). CNPq productivity scholarship holder. Jungian Analyst (IJRS/ IAAP). Author of the book *The Girl and the Jaguar: Indigenous Ancestral Voices* and co-author of the book *Amerindian Education: Dance and the Guarani School.*

Romano Madera studied philosophy and graduated at the University of Milan (1971) and specialized in sociology at the School for Sociology in Milan (1971-1973). He is professor emeritus of Moral Philosophy and Philosophical Practices at the University of Milano-Bicocca. He is a member of AIPA and IAAP. He is the founder of Philo, School of Philosophical Practices and the Society for Biographic Analysis Philosophically Oriented (SABOF). He is the author of *La filosofia come stile di vita* (2003) translated into English as *Philosophy as Life Path: Introduction to Philosophical Practices* (2007); *Una filosofia per l'anima (2013)* translated into English as *Approaching the Navel of the Darkened Soul: Depth Psychology and Philosophical Practices* (2013); With G. Cappelletty, *Il caos del mondo e il caos degli affetti* (2020), English edition: *Into the Maelstrom: Toward a Theory of Crisis and Chaos* (2022); and many other books and articles.

Felicia Matto-Shepard, M.S. is a Jungian Analyst, artist and a member of the C.G. Jung Institute of San Francisco practicing in Petaluma, CA. She works at the threshold where nonverbal experience is transformed into image and language. She facilitates Alchemical Art workshops utilizing creative processes such as art making, ritual and movement. Felicia holds a Certificate in Psychedelic Therapies and Research from California Institute of Integral Studies and is trained in the use of Ketamine Assisted Psychotherapy, as well as MDMA Assisted Therapy at MAPS. She is a clinician on the MAPS MDMA Expanded Access team at Temenos Center for Integrative Psychotherapy. Felicia is a past faculty member in the Depth Psychology Master's Program at Sonoma State University and offers lectures, workshops and analytic training internationally.

Leslie Stein trained as a Jungian Analyst at the C.G. Jung Institute in New York and is in private practice in Sydney, Australia. Professor Stein's books include *Becoming Whole: Jung's Equation for Realizing God* (Helios); *Working with Mystical Experiences in Psychoanalysis: Opening to the Numinous* (Routledge); *The Self in Jungian Psychology: Theory and Practice* (Chiron) – winner of the IAJS Award for the best book on Jungian theory, 2022; *The Journey of Adam Kadmon: A Novel* (Arcade, New York); Editor, *Eastern Practices and Individuation: Essays by Jungian Analysts* (Chiron); and Editor with D. Rickles of *Varieties of Nothingness* (Chiron, forthcoming). He is also on the Board of Directors of the Philemon Foundation.

Miriam Stein, PhD is a Clinical Psychologist and Jungian analyst in private practice in Sydney. She is a graduate and member of the Jungian Psychoanalytic Association (JPA) in New York, and a member of ANZSJA and IAAP. Her practice as a clinical psychologist and analyst spans over 40 years. She has also provided training and seminars to psychologists seeking a depth approach to incorporating non-verbal methods of working at the threshold between conscious and unconscious experience and knowing in the service of individuation. She has published across these areas and provided clinical and academic supervision. Her earlier research and its application in the community by way of services and social action, was in relation to the experience of and adjustment to breast cancer. She was a lecturer at the University of Western Australia Psychiatry Department and Behavioural Science.

Murray Stein, Ph.D. is a Training and Supervising Analyst at the International School of Analytical Psychology Zurich (ISAP-ZURICH). He has been president of the International Association for Analytical Psychology (IAAP) (2001-2004), president of ISAPZURICH (2009-2013), and lectures internationally. He is the author of *Jung's Map of the Soul, Outside Inside and All Around, The Mystery of Transformation* and many other books and articles. Six volumes of his *Collected Writings* have been published to date. He lives in Switzerland and has a private practice in Zurich and online from his home in Goldiwil.

John R. White, PhD, LPC, is a Jungian psychoanalyst and mental health counselor in private practice in Pittsburgh, Pennsylvania, USA. He received his doctorate in philosophy in 1993 from The International Academy of Philosophy, in the Principality of Liechtenstein, an institution accredited through the Austrian university system. He received his diploma as a Jungian Psychoanalyst from the Interregional Society of Jungian Analysts in 2017. He is currently Coordinator of the C.G. Jung Institute Analyst Training Program of Pittsburgh and President Elect of the Board of the Pittsburgh Psychoanalytic Center. He has more than forty published articles, book chapters, edited volumes, and book reviews in both philosophy and psychoanalysis and is author of the book *Adaptation and Psychotherapy: Langs and Analytical Psychology*, published by Rowman & Littlefield.

Susan Williams, MFT is an Adult and Child Jungian Analyst member of the C.G. Jung Institute of San Francisco. She trained in London, England at the Association of Jungian Analysts. Susan worked for the United Kingdom National Health Service and had an adult and child private practice in London. Susan currently has a private practice in Berkeley, California where she sees adults, adolescents, and children of all ages. She has extensive experience working with children with disabilities in hospitals, clinics and schools and has consulted to many Bay Area school programs for children with autistic spectrum disorders. She has published and taught both in the UK and US on topics including the numinous, 'The Unbearable Weight of Truth,' expanded states of consciousness, psychedelic enhanced psychotherapy, aliveness and deadness, autism, and autistic states of mind. She has completed the MAPS MDMA Therapy Training Program and has trained in Ketamine Assisted Psychotherapy. Susan organized a conference through the San Francisco Jung Institute in 2019 entitled: *Encountering the Numinous: Depth Psychotherapy, Analysis and Psychedelics*, looking at the role of Jungian and Depth psychotherapy in the current renaissance in psychedelic assisted psychotherapy and research.

Note on the Collected Works and the Red Book

As the *Collected Works of C.G. Jung* are cited extensively and repeatedly in this work, for the purpose of convenience, all references are of the Volume and Paragraph number: e.g., CW 7, § 388. The citation of the *Collected Works of C.G. Jung* is:

> Jung, C.G. *Collected Works of C.G. Jung.* R.F.C. Hull, Trans. Bollingen Series XX. Princeton University Press. 19 Volumes + Index + Vol. A. and B.

As *The Red Book* is also cited extensively, all references in the text to Jung (2009) are references to *The Red Book*. The citation of *The Red Book* is:

> Jung (2009). *The Red Book: Liber Novus* (S. Shamdasani, Ed.) (S. Shamdasani, J. Peck, & M. Kyburg, Trans.). W. W. Norton & Co.

Introduction

Editors' Preface

It is accurate to say that every contributor to this book of essays has wrestled with the relationship between Jungian psychoanalysis and the therapeutic use of psychedelics. There are no straightforward answers to this question, perhaps because the Jungian enterprise is over a century old, weighted in intricate theory and praxis, while the appropriate therapeutic use of psychedelics is just emerging.

The Jungian lens is sharply focused on what lies behind the conscious mind, what Jung refers to as the *Spirit of the Depths*. It relies on the fact that unconscious material from the depths can be understood by our conscious mind when we turn to it, find that it is purposeful, and therefore allow it to alter and expand our consciousness. Within that exposition, there are many aspects that require great subtlety, such as being able to understand pathologies and their consequences for analysis, being aware of the transference / counter-transference relationship dialogue that is ever present, opening to and interpretating symbolization of what is presented from the unconscious, and accepting the significance of the Self, the centering process of psyche behind all revelation. It is through this many prismed lens that these essays examine the congruence of psychedelics with a Jungian orientation.

There are certainly ways that psychoanalysis and psychedelics theoretically converge. Jung, arising from his own experiences, concluded that numinous experiences, where the mind is overwhelmed by the presentation of a primal truth, point to the possibility that the conscious position can be altered. In this spirit, psychedelics as a therapeutic tool have an immediate relevance to psychological growth. Jungian psychoanalysis can be useful for psychedelics in establishing a road map into the numinous, showing how to interpret the contents of an experience.

Psychedelics, because of the immediate, direct numinosity they produce, can be of use in breaking through stuck psychological situations, often presented as PTSD, depression, eating disorders, and similar situations where analysis will be slow, and the changes are measured in small increments.

The practical connections and congruence between psychedelics and Jungian psychotherapy are the subject matter of these essays: how can they benefit each other in some coherent, non-speculative manner to open the possibilities that Jungian psychoanalysis may be of use to psychedelic-assisted psychotherapy, and psychedelics can be useful to psychoanalysis in particular situations. Of course, for many jurisdictions this requires changes to laws, as well as acceptance by the Jungian supervisory bodies in terms of ethical considerations and the professional values flowing from Jung's work, all of which are assumed possible for the purpose of these essays. Accordingly, a reason for these essays is that some form of protocol may emerge for Jungian psychoanalysis that offers how psychedelics can be used, where appropriate, in psychoanalytic practice.

The discussion amongst Jungian analysts as to psychedelics is accelerating. We turned to Jungian analysts who had a known interest in this research, a leading-edge view on working with psychedelics, a cultural connection with indigenous psychedelic use, or who had an expert view as to the process of individuation and how that would be impacted. Many were well advanced in these issues long before we sought them out to contribute to this book. As but one example, Susan Williams, Jerome Braun and Felicia Matto-Shepard had a working group to explore the deepest questions behind psychedelics. They write about their collaboration: "What emerged was a creative, sometimes challenging and radically unexpected exploration of what psychedelic plants and medicines are trying to communicate and how we can co-dream with the plants, allies, entities, each other and with the wider community, honoring the dream like nature of reality."

What we as editors find most fascinating is that every author, no matter the title of their essay or their attempts to limit their topic for this book, has had to go far and wide, drawing on personal experiences, theoretical viewpoints, and decades of psychoanalytic practice to grab hold of the possibility that the psychedelic future is upon us. This made narrowing the topics of the essays difficult, except for the few essays on specific topics, such as microdosing and psychedelic assisted therapy training.

These essays will be presented as conversations during a conference to be held at Pacifica Graduate Institute in December 2023. The conference, *Psychedelics and Individuation: Conversations with Jungian* Analysts, co-sponsored by the IAAP (International Association of Analytical Psychology), will also be focused on putting into words how the many thousands of Jungian analysts and Depth Psychologists might incorporate and use psychedelics in their practice.

Leslie Stein
Lionel Corbett

23 September 2023

The Therapeutic Use of Psychedelic Agents: An Overview

Lionel Corbett

Throughout the world and from time immemorial, indigenous people have recognized the spiritual value of the non-ordinary states of consciousness produced by certain plants (Schultes et al., 2010). These plants have long been used within indigenous communities for the purposes of divination and healing in ritual and religious contexts, which provide a safe container. They are considered to be gifts of the gods, and to mediate between the gods and humanity.

The term *psychedelic,* or *mind-revealing,* was coined by Humphrey Osmond in 1961, in an exchange of letters with Aldous Huxley. Later, religious scholars and ethnobotanists coined the term *entheogen,* or *God-creating,* to indicate the important spiritual effects of these plants (Ruck et al., 1979). I prefer the term *entheogen* because the etymology of this word suggests that these plants induce sacred experience, transcendent levels of meaning, and access to otherwise inaccessible levels of truth if used correctly.

A Short History of Psychedelics in the West

In the West, scientific research into psychedelics began in the mid-19th century, reaching a significant level with Louis Lewin's *Phantasticka* in 1924, which describes 28 plants used round the world for their psychological effects. He was the first Western pharmacologist to describe the use and effects of peyote. The active principle in this plant is mescaline, the chemical structure of which was first clarified in 1919.

In 1927, Kurt Beringer published the classical monograph on this subject, *Der Meskalinrausch*. Perhaps the next major step was Albert Hofmann's discovery of LSD in 1938, which he first ingested in 1943. An upsurge of interest began over the next 20 years, but stopped almost completely after that because of government prohibition, despite evidence of these agents' therapeutic value. About 30 years ago, thanks to persistent advocacy, psychotherapeutic and scientific inquiry into the use of entheogens experienced a renaissance across the Western world (Walsh et al., 2018).

Jung's Attitude to Psychedelics

Entheogens expose the subject to the deepest levels of the psyche, far beyond its personal levels. Without the use of such compounds, this material might never reach consciousness. Jungian psychology is of great value in elucidating the meaning of these experiences, and also in their integration into the personality. Paradoxically, Jung did not value and even disapproved of the use of entheogens. Although they confirmed his discovery of the collective unconscious, he highlighted the difficulty of integrating the unconscious contents these agents release. In a letter to Victor White, Jung (1975, p. 172) suggested that "there is no point in getting to know more of the collective unconscious than one gets through dreams and intuitions. The more you know of it the greater and heavier becomes our moral burden" because these contents then become our task and duties to deal with. He was afraid that we pay dearly for the "pure gifts of the Gods," and the use of these agents would create the problem of the sorcerer's apprentice, who knows "how to call the ghosts but did not know how to get rid of them again" (Jung, 1975, p. 173). He believed that such new knowledge incurs "a corresponding development of morality" (1975, p. 173). Jung insisted that one has to know how to deal with unconscious contents, and he was concerned that the individual be mature enough to integrate this material. An artificially induced experience of the unconscious may not accord with the individual's level of psychological development. He saw these agents as a substitute for human effort and spontaneous experience. He saw a possible role for mescalin for people who are otherwise unable to access the unconscious, but he saw it as a "short cut" that yields an "unintegrated experience contributing very little to the development of human personality" (1975, p. 223). Rather than seeing the effects of the drug as a demonstration of the spiritual dimension of reality, for Jung mescalin use is a "demonstration of Marxist materialism" because it manipulates the brain chemically (1975, p. 224), implying that matter somehow invokes spirit. In that letter Jung also noted the danger of triggering a latent psychosis. In a later scathing comment, he described psychedelically induced mental phenomena as "dangerously simple 'Ersatz' and substitute for a true religion" (1975, p. 383). In a somewhat condescending tone, he conceded, "There may be some poor impoverished creatures, perhaps, for whom mescaline would be a heaven-sent gift without a counterpoison" (1975, p. 174). In her biography of Jung, Marie-Louise von Franz (1975, pp. 110-120) wrote of her belief that the medical use of psychedelic agents is "crippled" by the misuse of power, when the therapist is in control of the experience. Picking up on Jung's disapproval, she pointed out that the unconscious "has its own way of revealing what is destined in a human life just at that time when it is ready to be integrated," and she noted that it seemed illegitimate to Jung to "seek the holy secret of the innermost light out of simple vain curiosity."

Probably because of Jung's disapprobation, until recently there was little written about entheogens in the Jungian literature. However, early accounts by Jungian-oriented psychotherapist Ronald Sandison (1954) and analyst Margo Cutner (1959) described the use of LSD to bring unconscious material into consciousness and enhance Jungian oriented therapy. Cutner found that the material that emerged during LSD sessions compensates the patient's conscious attitudes in the same way as images that emerge in dreams. Both Cutner and Sandison stressed the importance of integrating the material that emerged, but Michael Fordham (1963) complained that the use of these agents makes the subject too passive compared to the psychotherapeutic process. He highlighted the difficulties of integrating the experience although he admits it is not impossible. However, he concluded that the lasting effect of the compound is slight. Sandison (1963; 1997) acknowledged that integration may be difficult but insisted that it is possible with the therapist's support. He also noted the risk of psychosis or even suicide in the absence of adequate containment, but his experience suggested that the risk is low. Since these early papers, a few specifically Jungian approaches to the use of entheogens have appeared, beginning in 2013, when Scott Hill published *Confrontation with the Unconscious*, which explores the relationship between Jungian therapy and psychedelic agents. This was followed by a valuable review with case examples by Greg Mahr and Jaime Sweigart (2020), in which they found, "The door to the inner world that psychedelic drugs offer may be more important and valuable now than ever before to challenge the dominance that the conscious ego has acquired" (p. 91). They echoed Jung's concern that easy access to deep psychological material may "cheapen, trivialize, and demystify it" if these agents are not used for personal growth. Other theorists such as Ralph Metzner (1998) and Stanislav Grof (1976) have credited the relevance of Jung's work to their own approach to these compounds.

Entheogens seem to work by producing new insights into reality or into the subject's own personality, rather than by modulating neurotransmitters in the manner of antidepressants or antipsychotic agents. The effects of entheogens depend on the dose used. At low doses, producing *psycholytic* effects, sensory changes predominate with subtle changes in the meaning of perceptions. (The term *psycholysis* was invented by Sandison.) Repressed memories or insights may occur. At high or *psychedelic* doses, major perceptual changes occur, with vivid experiences of alternate realities and profound affective changes. Synesthesia, or the blending of the boundaries of sensory systems, also occur, so that one hears colors and so on. A profound feeling of connection to others and to the world may occur, leading to self-transcendence. Painful experiences of loss and terror may appear.

Grof (1976) showed that the psyche permeates all levels of human existence, and any of these may occur during an LSD session, including prenatal and birth experiences, ancestral and archetypal experiences, precognition, experiences of past incarnations, and a sense of connection to all that is. All this occurs irrespective of the subject's culture, religion, and ethnicity. Experiences of identification with animals and the rest of creation, as well as planetary and even extraplanetary forms of consciousness have also been reported. Grof also described mediumistic experiences and even contact with other universes and the Universal Mind. The possibility of these agents extending our knowledge of the non-egoic levels of the psyche is obviously considerable. Residual effects of psychedelic doses may take weeks to subside.

The Use of Entheogens in Psychotherapy

Clinical trials of entheogens are currently underway for several types of psychological problems. In combination with psychotherapy or at least psychological support, entheogens seem to be helpful for treatment refractory PTSD (Mithoefer et al., 2019), alcoholism (Bogenschuz et al., 2015), emotional distress during treatment for late-stage cancer (Griffiths et al., 2016; Ross et al., 2016), obsessive compulsive disorder (Nagra, 2022); eating disorders (Lafrance et al., 2017), treatment resistant depression (Carhart-Harris et al., 2018a), tobacco dependence (Johnson et al., 2017), and even interpersonal violence (Thiessen et al., 2018). Anecdotal reports suggest that microdosing with LSD and psilocybin produce antidepressant, anxiolytic, or even pro-cognitive effects, but the majority of controlled studies to date do not show much benefit of microdoses compared to placebo. However, my own experience with psilocybin microdosing is that it enhances access to the inferior function. In my case, this means greater ability to focus on details and indeed to become captivated by details that I would otherwise ignore.

The therapeutic entheogen experience can be divided into three chronological stages: the preparatory stage, the administration stage, and the stage of integration after the session. Preparation includes education about the typical effects of the substance. Desires and intention, hopes and fears about the session may be also discussed. Preparation seems to contribute to a more profound experience, but the outcome of the experience is often entirely unpredictable. It may be important to explain to the potential subject that it is necessary to approach rather than resist challenging imagery and sensations such as melting or dissolving. In this context, my own experience with psilocybin made me realize that the level of consciousness produced by this plant *cannot* be integrated into the empirical personality; that would be like trying to empty the ocean into a teacup. For me the problem became finding a way to integrate the ego into the higher level of consciousness produced by the plant.

It is now well understood that not only is psychological preparation for the session and its context important, so is reflection, meaning making, and integration after the experience (Hartogsohn, 2017: Carhart-Harris et al., 2018b). The quality of the therapeutic relationship (Garcia-Romeu et al., 2018), the therapist's (or guide's) ability to be empathic, psychologically present, and to "hold the space" (Tai et al., 2021; Thal et al., 2022), and a shared interpersonal experience with the therapist (Cosimano, 2021) are very important. A sense of safety fosters surrender to the experience. Ideally, an extended period of psychotherapy precedes the use of these compounds.

In the therapeutic context, as these agents are increasingly more broadly used, there is a need for ethical guidelines in their use. Vigilance on the part of the therapist is required because non-ordinary states of consciousness may induce unusually intense feelings of open-heartedness and sexuality; unfortunately, sexual abuse has been reported during Ayahuasca rituals (Peluso et al., 2020). A further problem for therapists is the time it takes to sit with a person undergoing this experience, which lasts several hours. Clearly, the usual frame constraints do not apply. Therapists should be sensitive to spontaneous shifts in the subject's mental state, which may require considerable clinical experience, since an intensification of the transference, such as unexpected hostility or overt sexuality, may suddenly emerge. Sandison (1959) also noted that the transference in psychedelic psychotherapy becomes more complicated and intense in LSD treatment, compared to conventional analysis, partly because of the perceptual changes that occur and partly because of paranoid feelings directed at the therapist. However, he believed that the transference remains analyzable.

A psychologically supportive context is very important in determining the outcome of the experience (Carhart-Harris et al., 2016). Comfort with a trusted therapist and a feeling of safety are linked to higher long-term benefits (Tennant et al., 2007; Vizeli et al., 2017). At times the therapist's role goes further than usual, becoming a spiritual companion. Phelps (2017; 2019) has outlined six core competencies for therapists who work with entheogens as adjuncts for therapy: empathetic abiding presence, trust enhancement, spiritual intelligence, knowledge of the physical and psychological effects of psychedelics, therapist self-awareness, ethical integrity, and proficiency in complementary techniques such as body work or Gestalt therapy. These criteria are not dissimilar to the kind of analytic attitude to which we are accustomed, with some additions. Spiritual intelligence in this context refers to familiarity with altered states of consciousness and some knowledge of a range of spiritual traditions. It is also important to know something of the global use of entheogens in different cultures. Knowledge of the range of effects of these agents in relation to dose is also valuable (Fadima, 2011; Metzner, 2015). Many practitioners believe that personal experience with these agents is essential in order to function as an effective therapist (Nielson et al., 2018). The formal qualifications of the therapist are less important than his or her capacity for empathy (Johnson et al., 2008). A range of institutions and organizations are now offering specific training for the use of entheogens (Tai et al., 2021), for example the California Institute of Integral Studies and the Multidisciplinary Association for Psychedelic Studies. Ultimately the outcome of entheogen use may depend on the client's personality structure (Cohen et al, 1960).

Mechanisms of Action

The mechanisms of action of entheogens are not fully understood. One of the major debates in this area is whether the psychological effects of entheogens, such as vivid perceptual changes or spiritual experiences, are necessary for their therapeutic effect. Writers who deny the necessity for a powerful psychological experience (Olson, 2021) believed that the association between dramatic subjective effects and positive outcomes does not imply causation. Rather, these subjective effects may only be a biological marker for 5-HT_{2a} receptor activation and increased neural plasticity (Ly et al., 2018), which means that - psychedelic analogues that do not have major psychological or spiritual effects may have the same potential (Cameron et al., 2021). If this line of research proves to be fruitful it would greatly undermine the spiritual and psychological claims of this treatment, which claims to allow access to levels of reality not available to our ordinary perceptual mechanisms. However, other research suggests that the underlying neurobiological mechanisms are necessary but not sufficient to confer the full, enduring benefits of these agents (Yaden and Griffiths, 2021.)

Brain imaging studies show that psilocybin decouples the default-mode network (DMN)[1] and the medial temporal lobes (Carhart-Harris et al., 2014). Psilocybin also decreases the activity of the DMN, which is regarded as a central orchestrator of global brain activity, having to do with "higher-level, metacognitive operations such as self-reflection" (Carhart-Harris et al., 2014, p. 5), and seen as "physical counterpart of the narrative self or ego" (p. 6). Carhart-Harris et al see the effects of these agents as "relinquishing the ego's usual hold on reality" (2014, p. 8). That is, psilocybin opens the brain to other levels of consciousness. MDMA increases the release of serotonin, which account for the feelings of elation, energy, and autonomic effects the drug produces (Davison et al., 1997). MDMA also inhibits the reuptake of serotonin, norepinephrine, and dopamine (Rudnick et al., 1992), as well as releasing oxytocin, a hormone that facilitates feelings of empathy, trust, and relatedness (Kirkpatrick et al., 2014).

In *The Doors of Perception*, Aldous Huxley described his experience with mescaline as "sacramental vision of reality" (1954, p. 15). He felt that mescaline enhanced his consciousness and removed filters to greater awareness, to the "divine source of all existence." Huxley suggests that mescaline diminishes the brain's "reducing valve," so that "Mind at large" can flood the subject's consciousness (1954, p, 6). Here, Huxley uses Henri Bergson's notion that the brain is a gate or reducing valve that selects from a wide range of sensations only what is useable at the moment. In this model, entheogens open a gate to allow transpersonal levels of the psyche to enter the egoic level and the ego loses its normal boundaries and its hegemony. The notion that psychedelics open a filter was confirmed by Carhart-Harris and Nutt (2012), who used fMRI to show that these compounds suppress neuronal activity in parts of the brain that act as "connector hubs" or filters. Many entheogenic experiences are suggestive of the tenets of the Perennial Philosophy described by Huxley (1945) and conform to mystical states described by all the spiritual traditions. No wonder the use of these agents to explore the unconscious has been described as analogous to the microscope and telescope in the exploration of the outer universe.

Do Entheogens Produce Genuine Mystical Experience?

Not only do subjects using psychedelic doses of entheogens experience psychological insights and emotional breakthroughs (Peill et al, 2022) they also have mystical experiences (Davis et al., 2021), and experiences of death transcendence (Schmidt and Liechti, 2018). There seem to be correlations between the type of subjective experience and the type of entheogen used. Dimethyltryptamine (DMT) is associated with experiences of cosmic unity, while psilocybin tends to produce ego-death and intense introspection (Zamberlan et al., 2018).

Religious scholars such as Zaehner (1954), have dismissed entheogen-induced experiences as nothing more than forms of inebriation. Zaehner suggested that mescaline experiences have nothing to do with the beatific vision of Christianity. In contrast, religious scholars such as Huston Smith and Walter Stace (1987) believe that entheogenic experiences are indistinguishable from genuine mystical experiences. The following is an experience produced by psilocybin that supports this idea:

Suddenly I became aware of a presence that was enormously powerful and nurturing. It/She reassured me that I could surrender to the experience. I had an odd sensation of separating from my body, and suddenly felt myself floating, exquisitely light and free. I seemed to exist as pure consciousness within brilliant light and felt blissful peace and joy. I became aware of two beings composed almost entirely of light. We discussed my path in life, significant events and their relevance to my life's purpose. The deep wisdom and compassion of these beings helped me understand and accept several painful life events and feel forgiveness towards people who had hurt me. I felt relief and emotional healing. Next, they led me to a golden platform that ascended seven levels, like a stepped pyramid. At the top was a blaze of brilliant, diamond light, radiantly clear, sparkling with flashes of color. I was awed and sensed that this was a divine presence. The light coalesced into the form of a goddess with an Asian face. No words were exchanged, just unspeakable reverence and devotion on my part, and unfathomable love on hers. I knew her to be Guanyin. She smiled at me, then turned her gaze at what appeared to be the earth far below, surrounded by the darkness of space. As I looked at the planet, I saw countless drops of light, which I knew represented every living being on the earth. My heart opened as I experienced an incomparable love for all life, and the deepest compassion I have ever known. I felt unconditional love for all, including rapists and murderers, whom I loved with the sadness of one who sees their suffering. I knew them as lost souls who had forgotten their true nature, and I felt a deep desire to help guide each one towards their birthright. Looking at Guanyin. I realized that my experience was simply a reflection of her divine nature, shared with me at this moment.

Needless to say, this experience was relevant to the subject's developmental history. She had been beaten, shamed, and ridiculed by her mother. Guanyin is the archetype of a loving, compassionate, divine mother, of the kind that she did not have as a child. The vision was therefore extremely helpful. The high level of spirituality revealed in this experience, together with its coherence, are evidence that it was an authentic spiritual experience.

In this context, James Cooke (2020) has outlined a range of ways in which psychedelics may have influenced religious traditions. For example, the ethnomycologist R. Gordon Wasson, who first brought psilocybin mushrooms to the West, believed that the ancient Hindus used the mushroom *Amanita muscaria* as a sacramental food, an idea that is widely accepted. Much more controversially, John Allegro (1970) suggested that the roots of Christianity included cult practices in which psychedelic mushrooms were ingested. He believed that Jesus himself was actually a mythological creation of early Christians under the influence of psychoactive mushrooms. Allegro's evidence was largely linguistic, based on his interpretation of the meaning of ancient words, and his idea was discounted and ridiculed by most scholars. His book was notorious at the time but the idea that mind-altering substances played a role in Judaism and Christianity has since been taken more seriously (Irvin, 2009). The religious historian Dan Merkur (2000) noted the repeated association of eating the biblical manna (bread from heaven) with episodes of religious ecstasy and visionary mysticism. He believes that manna was psychoactive because it contained ergot, a psychoactive fungus. The Bible story tells us (Exodus 16:8, 16:12, RSV) that after eating manna the Israelites saw the glory of God, which appeared in a cloud (16:10). Merkur believes that this knowledge was kept secret for fear of persecution, although it was well known to both Jewish and Christian religious authorities. He supplies evidence that manna was used sacramentally in ancient Israel and was responsible for the visionary experiences of Ezekiel and other prophets. Other speculations include the possibility that psilocybin mushrooms grew in the desert, or that the Israelites brewed a psychedelic compound from the bark of the acacia tree.

Safety

There is broad consensus about the physiological safety of serotonergic entheogens such as LSD, psilocybin, and mesacline (Nichols, 2016; Johnson et al., 2008) and about their non-addictive nature (Johnson et al., 2018). It is currently not clear whether chronic use of psychedelic agents may produce valvular heart disease, but this possibility has been reported. These agents should not be used by people taking serotonergic antidepressants or anti-migraine medications because of the danger of serotonin toxicity (Schifano et al., 2021). Other medications, such as antipsychotic agents and lithium, may interact pharmacologically with psychedelics.

In cases of extreme anxiety during a psychedelic session, anxiolytic medication may be necessary. Accordingly, these agents are only safe in the hands of trained facilitators, and their use requires informed consent on the part of the participant, when the risk/benefit ratio has been explained. Under the appropriate conditions, risks are minimal (Johnson et al., 2008), but episodes of psychosis may be triggered in vulnerable people (Sami, et al., 2015), so the presence of a borderline personality disorder, an anxiety state, or pre-existing psychosis are contraindications for their use. The risk that psychedelics might trigger a psychosis is small, except in the case of people with a personal or family history of psychotic illness, who should not use these agents.

Residual adverse effects may occur, including unpleasant flashbacks and depression, probably the result of experiences that were not contained, understood, and integrated (Aday et al., 2020). A recent study (Anderson et al., 2020) found that psychedelics can have lingering effects that include increased suggestibility and affective instability and may induce a vulnerable state both during and after the session. In a recent double blind study of single-dose psilocybin for treatment resistant depression (Goodwin et al, 2022), after three weeks, greater improvement was seen in patients receiving 25mgs than those receiving 10 mgs. or 1mg. This possibility needs further study. Small doses of these agents, such as 25 mgs. of pure psilocybin, are psychedelic and may produce psychodynamic insights, but they are not entheogenic, that is, they do not produce significant spiritual experiences. MDMA seems to have no major long-term adverse effects in clinical trials (Sessa et al., 2019a &b), although temporary anxiety, confusion, headaches, fatigue, nausea, and self-destructive impulses may occur acutely (Thomas et al., 2021). Recent studies have reported that long-term use of "classic psychedelics," meaning tryptamines, lysergamides, and phenylethylamines, actually improve mental and physical health (Simonsson, et al., 2021), perhaps because this practice is associated with personality factors such as being particularly open to experience. The other possibility is that the immunomodulatory effects and anti-inflammatory effects of these agents may be responsible for their effects on physical health.

The Importance of Set and Setting

The effects of entheogens may be affected by the environment (setting) in which they are used, and by the pre-existing mental set of the individual, including expectations about the experience, motivation, and the subject's relationship with the therapist or guide (Sloshower et al, 2020). Ideally, the environment is esthetically pleasant, comfortable, and calm, without potential disruptions such as phone calls. Some people prefer to be in a natural setting such as a garden. The subject is not left unsupervised. Sometimes music is helpful, and so are eyeshades. The home environment to which the subject will return, and social support after the experience, are also important in the integration of the material. Because entheogen sessions are long, often at least six to eight hours, it may be necessary for the therapist to work with a co-therapist to prevent exhaustion. It is important not to use entheogens as a substitute for ordinary therapy or to idealize entheogen assisted therapy.

There may be a danger in the decoupling of entheogens from their cultural and spiritual context, when they are brought into a Western therapeutic model (Labate et al., 2013). Agents such as peyote, psilocybin mushrooms, and ayahuasca have important historical and cultural roots, and in indigenous cultures their use is supervised by experienced individuals who underwent a long apprenticeship. Their use outside of traditional contexts raises the issue of colonization or cultural appropriation (George et al., 2020). Indigenous Nations who regard these agents as openings to the sacred are concerned about the lack of recognition of this dimension among Western researchers, the commercialization of psychedelic use, and even the possibility of patenting traditional medicines. Indigenous voices are notably absent from Western psychedelic research. The relationship of entheogens to cultural competence needs further study and the development of ethical guidelines that take this issue into account. Meanwhile, the study of entheogens requires their use with due respect, even reverence.

References

Aday, J.S., Mitzkovitz, C.M., Bloesch, E.K., Davoli, C.C., & Davis, A.K. (2020). Long-term effects of psychedelic drugs: A systematic review. *Neuroscience and Biobehavioral Reviews, 113*, 179-189.

Allegro, J.M. (1970). *The sacred mushroom and the cross*. Doubleday.

Bogenschutz, M.P., Forcehimes, A.A., Pommy, J.A., et al. (2015). Psilocybin assisted treatment for alcohol dependence: A proof-of-concept study. *Journal of Psychopharmacology, 29*, 289-299.

Cameron, L.P., Tombari, R.J., Lu, J., et al. (2021). A non-hallucinogenic psychedelic analogue with therapeutic potential. *Nature, 589(7842)*, 474-479.

Cohen, S, & Eisner, B.G. (1959). Use of lysergic acid diethylamide in a psychotherapeutic setting. *A.M.A. Archives of Neurology and Psychiatry, 81*, 615-619.

Carhart-Harris, R.L., Erritzoe, D., Williams, T., Stone, J.M., Reed, L.J., Colasanti, A., & Nutt, D.J. (2012). Neural correlates of the psychedelic state as determined by fMRI studies with psilocybin. *Proceedings of the National Academy of Sciences, 109(6)*, 2138-2143.

Carhart-Harris, R.L., Leech, R., Hellyer, P.J., Shanahan, M., Feilding, A., Tagliazucchi, E., Chialvo, D.R., & Nutt, D. (2014). The entropic brain: A theory of conscious states informed by neuroimaging research with psychedelic drugs. *Frontiers in Human Neuro-science, 8*, Article e20.

Carhart-Harris, R.L., Bolstridge, M., Day, C.M.J., et al. (2018a). Psilocybin with psychological support for treatment-resistant depression: Six-month follow-up. *Psychopharmacology, 235*, 399-408.

Carhart-Harris, R.L., Roseman, L., Haijen, E., et al. (2018b). Psychedelics and the essential importance of context. *Journal of Psychopharmacology 32*, 725-731.

Carhart-Harris, R.L., Bolstridge, M., Rucker, J., et al. (2016). Psilocybin with psychological support for treatment-resistant depression: An open label feasibility study. *Lancet Psychiatry, 3*, 619-627.

Cooke, J. (2020) https://realitysandwich.com/guide-to-psychedelics-and-religion/retrieved (Last Accessed Jan. 17, 2023).

Cosimano, M.P. (2021). The role of the guide in psychedelic-assisted treatment. In: Grob, C.S. & Grigsby, J. (Eds.), *Handbook of Medical Hallucinogens* (pp. 377-394). Guilford Press.

Cutner, M. (1959). Analytic work with LSD-25. *Psychiatric Quarterly, 33*(4), 715-757.

Davis, A.K., Barrett, F.S., May, D.G., et al. (2021). Effects of psilocybin assisted therapy on major depressive disorder: A randomized clinical trial. *J.A.M.A. Psychiatry, 78,* 481-489.

Davison, D., & Parrott, A.C. (1997). Ecstasy (MDMA) in Recreational Users: Self-Reported Psychological and Physiological Effects. *Human Psychopharmacology: Clinical & Experimental, 12*(3), 221-226.

Fadiman, J. (2011). *The Psychedelic Explorer's Guide: Safe, Therapeutic, and Sacred Journeys*. Park Street Press.

Fordham, M. (1963). Analytic observations on patients using hallucinogenic drugs. In R. Crocket, R. Sandison, & A. Walk (Eds.), *Hallucinogenic drugs and their therapeutic use* (pp. 125-130). C.C. Thomas.

Garcia-Romeu, A. & Richards, W.A. (2018). Current perspectives on psychedelic therapy: use of serotonergic hallucinogens in clinical interventions. *International Review of Psychiatry, 30*, 291-316.

George, J.R., Michaels, T.I., Sevelius, J., & Williams, M.T. (2020). The psychedelic renaissance and the limitations of a White-dominant medical framework: A call for indigenous and ethnic minority inclusion. *Journal of Psychedelic Studies, 4*(1), 4-15.

Goodwin, G.M., Aaronson, S.T., Alvarez, O., et al. Single-dose psilocybin for a treatment-resistant episode of major depression. *New England Journal of Medicine, 18* (1637-1648).

Griffiths, R.R., Johnson, M.W., Carducci, M.A., et al. (2016). Psilocybin produces substantial and sustained decreases in depression and anxiety in patients with life-threatening cancer: A randomized double-blind trial. *Journal of Psychopharmacology, 30*, 1181-1197.

Grof, S. (1976). *Realms of the human unconscious: Observations from LSD research.* E.P. Dutton.

Hartogsohn, I. (2017). Constructing drug effects: A history of set and setting. *Drug Science, Policy and Law, 3*(1).

Huxley, A. (1945). *The Perennial Philosophy.* Harper and Brothers.

Huxley, A. (1954). *The doors of perception.* Harper & Brothers.

Irvin, J.R. (2009). *The holy mushroom: Evidence of mushrooms in Judeo-Christianity.* Gnostic Media Research & Publishing.

Johnson, M., Richards, W. & Griffiths, R. (2008). Human hallucinogen research: Guidelines for safety. *Journal of Psychopharmacology, 22*, 603-620.

Johnson, M.W., Garcia-Romeu, A., & Griffiths, R.R. (2017). Long-term follow-up of psilocybin-facilitated smoking cessation. *American Journal of Drug and Alcohol Abuse, 43*, 55-60.

Johnson, M.W., Griffiths, R.R., Hendricks, P.S., et al. (2018). The abuse potential of medical psilocybin according to the 8 factors of the Controlled Substances Act. *Neuropharmacology, 142*, 143-166.

Kirkpatrick, M.G., Francis, S.M., Lee, R., de Wit, H., & Jacob, S. (2014). Plasma oxytocin concentrations following MDMA or intranasal oxytocin in humans. *Psychoneuroendocrinology, 46*, 23-31.

Labate, B.C., & Cavnar, C. (2013). *The therapeutic use of ayahuasca.* Springer.

Lafrance, A., Loizaga-Velder, A., Fletcher, J., Renelli, M., Files, N., & Tupper, K.W. (2017). Nourishing the spirit: Exploratory research on ayahuasca experiences along the continuum of recovery from eating disorders. *Journal of Psychoactive Drugs, 49*(5), 427-435.

Ly, C., Greb, A.C., Cameron, L.P., et al. (2018). Psychedelics promote structural and functional neural plasticity. *Cell Reports, 23*, 3170-3182.

Mahr, G. & Sweigart, J. (2020). Psychedelic drugs and Jungian therapy. *Journal of Jungian Scholarly Studies, 15*(1), 86-98.

Merkur, D. (2000). *The mystery of manna: The psychedelic sacrament of the Bible*. Park Street Press.

Metzner, R. (1998). *The unfolding self: Varieties of transformative experience*. Origin Press.

Metzner, R. (2015). *Allies for Awakening: Guidelines for Productive and Safe Experiences With Entheogens*. Berkeley, CA: Regent Press.

Mithoefer, M.C., Feduccia, A.A., Jerome, L., et al. (2019). MDMA-assisted psychotherapy for treatment of PTSD: Study design and rationale for phase 3 trials based on pooled analysis of six phase 2 randomized controlled trials. *Psychopharmacology, 236,* 2735-2745.

Nagra, J. (2022). Psychedelic Agents as Potential Therapeutics for Obsessive-Compulsive Disorder. *Impulse (19343361), 19*(1), 1-9.

Nielson, E., & Guss, J. (2018). The influence of therapists' first-hand experience with psychedelics on psychedelic-assisted psychotherapy research and therapist training. *Journal of Psychedelic Studies, 2*(2), 64-73.

Nichols, D.E. (2016). Psychedelics. *Pharmacology Review, 68,* 264–355.

Olson, D.E. (2021). The subjective effects of psychedelics may not be necessary for their enduring therapeutic effects. *ACS Pharmacology & Translational Science, 4*(2), 563-567.

Peill, J.M., Trinci, K.E., Kettner H., et al. (2022). Validation of the Psychological Insight Scale: A new scale to assess psychological insight following a psychedelic experience. *Journal of Psychopharmacology, 36,* 31-45.

Peluso, D., Sinclair, E., Labate, B., & Cavnar, C. (2020). Reflections on crafting an ayahuasca community guide for the awareness of sexual abuse. *Journal of Psychedelic Studies, 4*(1), 24-33.

Phelps, J. (2017). Developing guidelines and competencies for the training of psychedelic therapists. *Journal of Humanistic Psychology, 57,* 450-487.

Phelps, J. (2019). Training psychedelic therapists. In: Sessa B and Winkelman M (Eds.), *Advances in Psychedelic Medicine: State of the Art Therapeutic Application (pp. 274-294)*. Praeger Publishers.

Ross, S., Bossis, A., Guss, J., et al. (2016). Rapid and sustained symptom reduction following psilocybin treatment for anxiety and depression in patients with life-threatening cancer: A randomized controlled trial. *Journal of Psychopharmacology, 30*, 1165-1180.

Ruck, C.A.P., Bigwood, J., Staples, D., Ott, J., & Wasson, R.G. (1979). Entheogens. *Journal of Psychedelic Drugs, 11*(1–2), 145-146.

Rudnick, G., & Wall, S.C. (1992). The molecular mechanism of "ecstasy" [3,4-methylenedioxy-methamphetamine (MDMA)]: serotonin transporters are targets for MDMA-induced serotonin release. *Proceedings of the National Academy of Sciences of the United States of America, 89*(5), 1817-1821.

Sami, M., Piggott, K., Coysh, C., & Fialho, A. (2015). Psychosis, psychedelic substance misuse and head injury: A case report and 23-year follow up. *Brain Injury, 29*(11), 1383-1386.

Sandison, R. (1954). Psychological aspects of the LSD treatment of the neuroses. *Journal of Mental Science, 100*, 508-515.

Sandison, R. (1959). The role of psychotropic drugs in individual therapy. *Bulletin of the World Health Organization, 21*, 495-503.

Sandison, R. (1963). Certainty and uncertainty in the LSD treatment of psychoneurosis. In R. Crocket, R. Sandison, & A. Walk (Eds.), *Hallucinogenic drugs and their psychotherapeutic use.* (pp. 33-36). C.C. Thomas.

Sandison, R. (1997). LSD therapy: A retrospective. In A. Melechi, (Ed.)., *Hallucinogenic drugs in Britain* (pp. 53-86).

Schifano, F. et al., (2021). New psychoactive substances (NPS) and serotonin syndrome onset: a systematic review. *Experimental Neurology, 339*(1), p. 113638.

Schmid, Y. & Liechti, M.E., (2018). Long-lasting subjective effects of LSD in normal subjects. *Psychopharmacology, 235*, 535-545.

Schultes, R.E., Hofmann, A., & Ratsch, C. (2010). *Plants of the gods: Their sacred, healing, and hallucinogenic powers.* Healing Arts Press.

Sessa, B., Higbed, L. & Nutt, D. (2019a). A review of 3,4-methyl-enedioxymethamphetamine (MDMA)-assisted psychotherapy. *Frontiers in Psychiatry, 10*, 1-7.

Sessa, B., Sakal, M.C., O'Brien S., et al. (2019b). First study of safety and tolerability of 3,4-methylenedioxymethamphetamine (MDMA)-assisted psychotherapy in patients with alcohol use disorder. *Journal of Psychopharmacology, 35*(4), 375-383.

Simonsson, O., Sexton, J.D., & Hendricks, P.S. (2021). Associations between lifetime classic psychedelic use and markers of physical health. *Journal of Psychopharmacology, 35*(4), 447-542.

Sloshower, J., Guss, J., Krause, R., et al. (2020b). Psilocybin-assisted therapy of major depressive disorder using Acceptance and Commitment Therapy as a therapeutic frame. *Journal of Contextual Behavioral Science, 15*, 12-19.

Stace, W.T., & Smith, H. (1987). *Mysticism and Philosophy.* J. P. Tarcher.

Tai, S.J., Nielson, E.M., Lennard-Jones, M., et al. (2021). Development and evaluation of a therapist training program for psilocybin therapy for treatment-resistant depression in clinical research. *Frontiers in Psychiatry, 12*: 27.

Tennant, R., Hiller, L., Fishwick, R., et al. (2007). The Warwick-Edinburgh Mental Well-being Scale (WEMWBS): Development and UK validation. *Health and Quality of Life Outcomes, 5*, 63-75.

Thal, S.B., Bright, S.J., Sharbanee, J.M., et al. (2021). Current perspective on the therapeutic preset for substance-assisted psychotherapy. *Frontiers in Psychology, 12*, 2501.

Thal, S., Engel, L.B., Liam, B., & Bright, S.J. (2022a). Presence, trust, and empathy: Preferred characteristics of psychedelic carers. *Journal of Humanistic Psychology*, 1-24.

Thiessen, M.S., Walsh, Z., Bird, B.M., & Lafrance, A. (2018). Psychedelic use and intimate partner violence: The role of emotion regulation. *Journal of Psychopharmacology, 32*(7), 749-755.

Thomas, K. & Malcolm, B. (2021). Adverse effects. In: Grob, C.S. & Grigsby, J. (Eds.), *Handbook of Medical Hallucinogens,* (p. 414-440). Guilford Press.

Vizeli, P. & Liechti, M.E. (2017). Safety pharmacology of acute MDMA administration in healthy subjects. *Journal of Psychopharmacology, 31*, 576-588.

Von Franz, M-L. (1975). *C.G. Jung: His myth in our time.* G.P. Putnam's Sons.

Walsh, Z., & Thiessen, M.S. (2018). Psychedelics and the new behaviorism: Considering the integration of third-wave behaviour therapies with psychedelic-assisted therapy. *International Review of Psychiatry, 30*(4), 343-349.

Yaden, D.B., & Griffiths, R.R. (2021). The subjective effects of psychedelics are necessary for their enduring therapeutic effects. *ACS Pharmacology and Translational Science, 4,* 568-572.

Zamberlan, F., Sanz, C., Vivot, R.M., Pallavicini, C., Erowid, F., Erowid, E., & Tagliazucchi, E. (2018). The varieties of the psychedelic experience: A preliminary study of the association between the reported subjective effects and the binding affinity profiles of substituted phenethylamines and tryptamines. *Frontiers in Integrative Neuroscience, 12*(8), 1-22.

Zaehner, R.C. (1954). The Menace of Mescalin. *Blackfriars, 35*, 412-413, 310.

Endnotes

[1] The Default Mode Network is a subsystem in the brain that is active when the rest of the brain is relatively inactive, not performing a task, or when we are simply daydreaming. It is responsible for autobiographical memories and hence part of one's sense of identity.

The Importance
of Breakthroughs

Beyond The Masks of
Automated Experience

Romano Màdera

We believe we perceive reality, or at least a representation of reality. However, the enduring wisdom of all cultures, some modern and contemporary philosophies, as well as depth psychology and other soft sciences, warn us that this perception taken for granted might be understood instead as the enigmatic result of hidden processes, as a made up habit, in both a historical and cultural sense.

We live in a world of masks without knowing that they are masks. The world of relationships is often, for the most part, a world of social masks and roles played without knowing that they are roles. Nevertheless, even objects have a history—a history made up of human relationships, jobs, and exchanges that remain opaque to us. Even nature is a part of history: even uncontaminated nature is presented to us as a set of ideas and concepts, which prevailing opinions and trends of the time, not to mention the current deluge of images, have presented to us.

Our uncritical preconceptions mar almost everything. The techniques of de-automatization of perceptions in every culture have paved the way for a different perception and understanding, which we might call *spiritual*, precisely because it escapes prevailing habits of contact with the world and ourselves. Our present age of disenchantment with the world and refusal to deal with the *sacred* can make us over-perceive nature scientifically and technically. The area uncovered through de-automatization has much to do with the sacred.

The history of the use of psychedelic substances can be placed within this picture of the processes of de-automatization of experience.

Since perception is taken for granted as something automatic, what customarily comes about is a disguised darkening of the possibilities of the spectrum of consciousness, and an unconscious numbing effect over every inner conflict; when it fails to take over the subject, it can turn into a mere symptom. It behooves us to find ways to breach this wall. Every journey into these hidden depths implies an upheaval, an earthquake of the dominant inner plate tectonics, and for this reason, the techniques of depth psychology are free association, the analysis of dreams, slips, and misses, spontaneous drawing and sand play, active imagination, or any other way to express our imaginative capacity.

As for myself, what I can say about the possible use of psilocybin and LSD for cognitive and curative purposes: knowledge—not abstract but experiential—remains for me the basis of any cure; this is, however, conditioned by my encounter with psychedelic substances, my work as a philosopher and psychoanalyst and, above all, my commitment to try to think and feel even where thought ceases and becomes a mystery. For these reasons, I want to begin from lived thoughts and my own experience to talk about breaking the barrier of perception put in shape by customs and pre-judgments received and accepted in everyday life, and by prevailing ways of thinking.

Like so many in my generation—those born in the early years after World War II—from eighteen onwards I had "tripped" with marijuana, hashish, then psilocybin and LSD. The hellish stages were far more numerous than the comforting ones.

In hindsight, half a century of it, I have the impression of an assortment of conflicting instances: for a few years, the very intense political engagement in the extreme left had compressed individual conflicts, including my eluding confrontation with admittedly moralistic Catholic sensibilities. Uncomfortable with the guidelines implicit in sexual revolution-liberation, the result was years of malaise, which I felt I had to deny in the open couple experiments that seemed the only outcome of the search for a new and antipatriarchal relationship between the sexes. The rationalism implicit in Marxist reading and revolutionary commitment prevented any sentimental weakness, resulting in us being forced to wear an impassive mask to defend against any so-called sentimentality. Mourning for my father's death, to whom I was bound by being the younger and favorite son, found no place and, inevitably, made its way into the neurosis that followed.

Mourning, seen as what I thought was the narcissistic swill of bourgeois sentimentality was only to be repressed. I was sinking into a welter of emotion without being able to confess it even to myself. Only the diaries used to contain everything in them; only they could hold this kind of inner quartering and embody it because they were secret. They were not to be published, they were not to act, and I was to play nothing but my painfully mixed parts. Paper is more durable than life; it can carry it, gather its acid and sulfuric moods without making a crease, and hold up its dead weights without collapsing underneath. I was only inhabiting those papers. However, the play was getting more and more dangerous.

Different crisis factors were piling up: The death of my father. Then, after the end of the moderate far-left political Gramsci Group, the adventure of Autonomia Operaia, a movement of worker and student collectives without joint coordination and with tangents where the boundaries between political violence and armed struggle could easily be crossed. A thwarted relationship: a marriage for pretense, which soon transcended into a surreal experiment because of a broken couple turning into a non-couple (the aggravating factor was that part of me seriously believed in the necessary sacrifice of all sentimentality to build the new man, while another part was falling hopelessly and briefly in love with flings over in the span of a few months), because of the weight of that marriage that I could not end, crushed inwardly by guilt over our son, who immediately became the center and victim of a guerrilla war of recriminations, different but mutual. And finally, the lucid madness of wanting, in a Rimbaudian reminiscence, to unregulate all the senses, experimenting with psychedelics.

Nevertheless, in each of these eddies, I was saved by what I cursed at the time and to which I wished to be immune: a malaise of body and soul that crushed every further step. For one who defies his superego, transgression is paid for by panting to the point of near delirium in the jumble of symptoms. Yet it was precisely an experiment with LSD that gave me, unexpectedly at once, the exhilaration of touching the ecstatic dimension—at a time as far removed as ever from any attraction to mysticism—and the proof, in retrospect, that I had passed through a stretch of psychotic experience.

Many years later, I recognized, in Tart's research (1969), and in Hulin's (1993) magnificent book on wild mysticism, the description of the effects of that journey and the explanation of that mixture of anguish and bliss that had marked my experiences with hashish, LSD, and psilocybin.

On a few rare instances, and especially with the aid of an acid trip in Cesena in December 1973, the war of the psychic worlds between the anguish of resistances to the reality principle and identification with egoic masks, when threatened and surmounted by the flood of erasures: the bodily schema subjected to brutal dissimilarities, dilation and contraction to the infinitesimal of space and time, interpenetration of causes and ends in the chaos of luminescent points of ephemeral revelations, and the blissful delighted loss of the silly carnival of the world and life centered on the nothingness that we are, subsided.

The advent of the Non-Thing, of a Macbethian "non-thing," had transmuted itself into the cosmic-sized paradise of becoming everything: the appearance of the thin consistency of our ridiculous works disappeared as if it had been the effect of an illusionist's game. It was a dive and flyover into Joy, into an *excessus mentis* (beyond the mind's eye) that had disarmed all distressing defenses. On that day in 1973, I overcame, I don't know how or why, the barriers of fear of losing all control of the self, and the habits we call consciousness and will, which are indispensable to survive, work, and even to create enduringly, but at the same time barricade of the doors of perception.

We were a group of five in a nineteenth-century house in Cesena, where in every corner, the echo of Italian history from the Risorgimento onward could be perceived. But the center of the experience, on the surface of a pair of red-brick rhomboidal tiles, was the dialogue of shared insights with Federico De Luca Comandini, close friend of all the sorts of political events and expeditions of discovery of the seabed in which we hoped to find the transformative formula that had remained alien to surface revolutionaries. Impossible to say, of course. The shared impression was of a kind of immediate telepathy of mind-blowing consonance with visions of the same red-green structure that resembled the figurative tables of the carbon molecule, which we found out in retrospect. Federico remained lucid and understood at once the incommunicable that belonged to the event. Slowly, I, too, came to divest myself of the purpose—albeit after a few hours of actual, apparently controlled delirium—of going out on the street and beginning to announce the revelation. Even Liberiana Pavone was fortunately against this involuntary self-certification of madness.

In what did the revelation consist? Too easily it could be attributed, once the possession of the mania vanished, to the rare but not very rare possibility of the effects of LSD being capable of inducing temporary and artificial psychosis.[1] But neither is it reducible to the neurotic factors and psychotic angle latent in everyone. I still say this fifty years later, after constant analysis and philosophical exercises on myself and with others, patients and practitioners—and I have no sympathy for magic and irrationalism of any kind.

Personal determinants had a great deal of weight in my experience. First and foremost, the shelter and transfiguration of a looming personal failure on all planes of life: of an unprocessed loss; of a love that was ending, or rather that had already ended after having just begun, in the words of a jingle that sounded, at the time, pathetic and, at the same time, condemned me to ridicule. Yet, the vision accompanied me always: I think it had the splendor of truth. Nothing less.

In everything, beyond the fetish of obvious things, behind the crust that surrounds with utility the necessities of daily and everyday living, lives a world of nexuses that sediment relationships, actions and times that express lives, a human history that is viaticum for the other dimensions of nature. And in this immense beam of transcoloring light, and thus of chiaroscuro shadows of all forms, the self overcomes itself and becomes a subatomic reflection of the communion of worlds that reality turns out to be. Nothing particularly original, and for that very reason, all the more serious: the same experience as millions of mystical experiences. My way there was to pierce the shield of fetishistic perception—yes, precisely in Karl Marx's sense—beyond the falsifying, but perfectly real, dialectic of the reification of human relations and the personalization of the values of things.

In the light of today's understanding it was an individuative experience, according to the Jungian lexicon. Or an experience of ecstatic perception, in a philosophical sense: that is, "according to the whole." Or in a spiritual sense, which would be the ultimate goal of the path I call *biographical analysis*, tending precisely to the search for a meaning capable of blessing and supporting life, which makes us feel and recompose ourselves as the pulsating organ of the whole. [2]

From this experience came the fundamental insight that holds up my first book, *Identità e feticismo. Forma di valore e critica del soggetto, Marx e Nietzsche* (*Identity and Fetishism: Value Form and Critique of the Subject*). And even today, its second part, "History and Biography," is the basis of all my theoretical work, with some corrections. I add that it is not a self-referential delusion, like so many wastes of paper, but is attested by studies done thirty years later on the nexus between philosophical autobiography and the philosophy of autobiography in Nietzsche. And I'm saying this not because they quote that essay of mine, but even better, because they confirm its insights without knowing it.

After all, even my latest book, *Lo splendore trascurato del mondo. Una mistica quotidiana (The Neglected Splendor of the World: An Everyday Mystique)* is a consequence, a further ramification of that root and experience. If committed to truth, Enlightenment is seen over time and must stand the test of years; it must be remastered and redigested countless times. It has to pass the sharp and scratchy sieve of opposing experiences and black enlightenments—when pain, the kind that crushes you by crumpling up your body, leaves no escape in good thoughts, candy-colored intentions, and feelings.

That particular mystical feeling is by no means foreign to Jung's experience, and his autobiographical recollections also reference it. After recalling the "crucial experiences" of his life, Jung writes:

> It was then that it dawned on me: I must take the responsibility ... I knew that I had to find the answer out of my deepest self, that I was alone before God, and that God alone asked me these terrible things ... Often I had the feeling that in all decisive matters I was no longer among men, but was alone with God. And when I was "there," where I was no longer alone, I was outside time; I belonged to the centuries; and He who then gave answer was He who had always been, who had been before my

birth. He who always is, was there. These talks with the
"Other" were my profoundest experiences: on the one
hand a bloody struggle, on the other supreme ecstasy.
(1989, pp. 54-55)

Here Jung speaks, inevitably and like everyone else, within his
cultural framework, so he speaks of a God who is a kind of person, as in
the Judeo-Christian tradition. However, the two movements of struggle
and ecstasy seem to belong to mysticism of all latitudes. Moreover, a
page of Jung's from the 1912 book that would mark his break with Freud,
Symbols of Transformation, a book that had no less than four editions
over forty years—opens the first chapter of Hulin's (1993) *The Wild
Mysticism*, although very little is said about Jung in the text thereafter. It
is such a characteristic page for our subject that one cannot fail to quote
it in full. Here is what Joël, quoted by Jung (and taken up by Hulin from
Jung's book) writes about the primordial experience:

I am lying on the seashore, the sparkling blue of the
waves shines in my eyes lost behind a dream; from afar
light breezes are blowing—the sound of the undertow
reaches the shore—or the ear? I cannot tell—with a
rush that shatters it, changing it into an exciting and
soothing foam. Distance and proximity, outward aspect
and inward aspect of things, insensibly pierce one into
the other. The sound of the undertow resounds more and
more from near, more familiar, more intimate: now it
resounds in my head like the rumbling of a magnified
pulse; now it passes over my soul, filling it with echoes,
enveloping it, swallowing it, while at the same moment,
it pours outward, like a blue wave. Yes, outer and inner
are one. Sparkle and froth, roar and breath of wind,
rumbling—the whole symphony of sensations felt dilutes
into one sound, all senses become one sense merging
with feeling; the world exhales into the soul, and the soul
dissolves into the world. Our little life is surrounded, like
a sea, by a great sleep. Sleep our cradle, sleep our grave,

and home that we leave in the morning to return to in the evening, while our life is the short journey, the tense stretch between emerging from the original unity and returning to and sinking into it! Blue waves, the infinite sea in which bosom the jellyfish dreams of that primeval life toward which our confused intuitions still descend, filtering through the eons of memory since every experience holds both a change and the preservation of the unity of life. In the instant when they are no longer fused, in the instant when the one who goes through that experience, still blind and dripping, lifts his head from sinking into the river of experience, still all imbued with what he has experienced, in the instant when the unity of life amazed, bewildered, detaches from itself the change, holds it before itself as something foreign, in this instant of estrangement the aspects of the experience have taken shape in a subject and an object, and in that instant consciousness is born. (CW 5, § 500)

Just before this long and very dense quotation, Jung tries to place it in his psychological perspective:

The subsequent blending, whether pantheistic or aesthetic, of the sensitive, civilized man with nature is, looked at retrospectively, a reblending with the mother, who was our first object, with whom we were truly and wholly one. She was our first experience of an outside and at the same time of an inside: from that interior world there emerged an image, apparently a reflection of the external mother-image, yet older, more original and more imperishable than this—a mother who changed back into a Kore, into an eternally youthful figure. This is the anima, the personification of the collective unconscious. (CW 5, §500)

48

Thus Jung, on the one hand, remains on Freudian ground, genetically tracing the fusional (but it would perhaps be better to say: expansive-intensive) experience of oceanic feeling back to the relationship with the mother, and on the other hand, seeks an alternative to reductionism in bringing the origin back to his assumptions about the collective unconscious. But in his note, Jung takes up a consideration of Joël, who points the way to an overcoming of psychophysiological origins in a unity woven of differences:

> Life is not lessened in artists and prophets, but is enhanced. They are our guides into the Lost Paradise, which only becomes Paradise through being found again. It is not the old, mindless unity that the artist strives for, but a felt reunion; not empty unity, but a full unity; not the oneness attained through differentiation ... All life is a loss of balance and a struggling back into balance. We find this return home in religion and art. (CW 5, n. 31)

Karl Joël, therefore, thinks like Romain Rolland about the oceanic feeling that Freud could not understand except as a phantasmatic return to the mother's womb: their approach to mystical experience indicates that one cannot genetically reduce this communion with and in the whole without losing its most proper characteristics. The going beyond and beyond the boundaries of the ordinary experience of space-time, and the separation of subject from object, as the palpitating truth of a co-belonging that does not fade but transforms and transcends differences, enhancing them as lights of a co-starry sky.

But let us turn to Elvio Fachinelli. Fachinelli, while not the only Freudian-trained psychoanalyst among Italians to go far beyond Freud, Freudism, and Lacanism to the ecstatic dimensions of the mind, [3] is the most original. These, in his view, contain mysticism as one of the manifestations of the ecstatic, not the only one. According to Fachinelli (1969, p. 22), the *apex mentis,* apex of the mind, according to the medieval definition, is also the basis of the mind. Fachinelli continues the work of psychoanalysis but reverses its perspectives: from the defenses from the chaotic and seething ocean of the Id, to be replaced by other

49

and more mature containment strategies, to the acceptance of the oceanic feeling through a feminine supplement, "Non-inhibition, removal, denial, etc.: the different stratagems, the partial defenses of a general defensive setting. From the pointed forest of defenses, there is no getting out. But instead, welcome, accept, and trust intrepidly in what is on the horizon."

And again,

> Insistence on defenses is always, implicitly, insistence on offense, on the ability to offend. The connection of the vigilance-defense system with the more established masculine approach. Then welcome: feminine? The feminine would then be at the heart of many different experiences. And also of this experience of mine... Upon becoming a shaman, it is said men change sex. The depth of the necessary change is thus emphasized. However, the feminine as a receptive attitude does not do away with the masculine; it proposes a parallel change to it. The masculine is then delineated as a patient, a laborious, sometimes almost blind operation that precedes and follows the creative act. (Fachinelli, 1969, p. 22)

We read here the transcript of one of his experiences with "the pilot friend," the psychotropic substance that is isolated from teonanacatl, a sacred Mexican mushroom:

> San Lorenzo at the seaside. Windy September afternoon and rapid clouds frayed. From the edge of the beach where I stand, with my back to the town, the sea is a purple ribbon that rolls and unrolls without end. I have been standing still for more than an hour, perhaps. At the spot where I put my deck chair, sheltered, there is no wind, only an occasional gust ... I keep looking fascinated at the ribbon of the sea ... In certain places, something, anything stands timeless, and I watch it stand. But I am only looking at the thing that stands, its way of being

in the light. That tree is a living being, a living being trembling, swinging in the wind, a ball of yarn playing with the air in myriads of wads. The vibration of my every rib. Joy in being this ... The small, the limited, turns out to be inexhaustible, infinitely rich. It becomes total. (Fachinelli, 1969, pp. 75-76)

I don't think Fachinelli remembered that passage from Joël quoted by Jung; he probably hadn't even read it. Many passages in his book are close, quite akin, to the oceanic feeling experiences that, from Hulin onward, we can call "wild mysticism." Time slows:

Constant surprise at the clock. Doubt that it has stopped, how is it possible that so little time has passed. Living thickly, in thin sheets superimposed ... joy and dismay and certainty of having reached the essential ... splendor of life, pulsing of life - in its centerless, all-center bottom ... What is generated in emptiness, in extreme rarefaction, is what has been sought. One finds what in us, someone beyond the self, sought: God, art, science, or even, immediately, the suspension of the time of transience. In general: a new figure of the world. The finding is always singular and refers back to the seeker's singularity. But this arises from the 'common ground' of the body if it is true that the passage from emptiness to fullness presupposes the body as an indispensable mediator. (Fachinelli, 1969, p.23)

Fachinelli has great admiration and respect for Freud's genius. Still, precisely his research into the ecstatic dimensions of experience leads him to write that what prohibits Freud's step toward the ecstatic is the "poverty of theory." He says of Freudian psychoanalysis, it is as an "infantile project" of "incurable misery of the theory of sublimation," which claims to explain the genesis of the ecstatic and the mystical as sublimations of the desire to return to infant perceptions or the mother's womb: it is a demonstration of the utter inadequacy of the Freudian model of the mind. As Fachinelli says, if you want to explain what is sublime by something else, you are already off the mark: what is sublime is sublime from the beginning, if it is sublime at all! The Italian psychoanalyst shows how Freud "feared excessive joy." Perhaps this fear leads him to combine the death drive that tends toward wiping out all tension with an oceanic feeling. Too much evidence, not only of ecstatic moments but of entire lives, should make us doubt the wisdom of Freud's hypothesis.

Ecstatic perception can distance us from the habit of agreeing on a plane neutralized by the overwhelming flow of the echo of wholeness, just as it can reunite us with the whole as typical, as another witness recounts the unexpected opening of the doors of perception:

> I think it happened on the boat on the lake, or arriving at the port of Laveno; a specific moment not sought, unexpected, sudden in which I clearly felt the profound significance of this belonging to a community not restricted, but enlarged to such an extent as to embrace everything and everyone. To be part of it: this awareness instantly translated into a feeling of peace and harmony. These words come to mind: communion, undifferentiated union, love generalized and not aimed at anyone or anything specific, zeroing or reducing needs and expectations; there was no room for the superfluous because it was superfluous at that moment. (Fachinelli, 1969, pp. 75-76)

Whether it arises from a need to escape monotony or its opposite, whether it is an implicit demand to detach oneself from the meaninglessness of life (made up of work far from any possible expression of people's abilities and aspirations, and the disappointment of desire for recognition in love relationships, family and friendships), in any case, the ubiquitous, keenly searched for, and frequently celebrated value of the experience of ecstatic-mystical perception are certainly symptoms of the desire for intensity and a poignancy of life and meaning. And this remains stifled or devalued in the more common ways of life.

The connection between this overflow into different streams of ecstatic aspiration and the fading, often to the point of disappearance, of religious feeling, belonging, and practices is intuitive. As if the rituality of religious ceremonies and symbolism sounds faint and outdated to contemporary sensibilities. Since even that which goes against the grain is inevitably affected by the spirit and customs prevailing in our societies, the desire to transcend the well-armed frontiers of the economic-consumerist finalization of our lives also takes its forms of manifestation from the dominant traits of our cultural epoch.

Thus, the tension to an ecstatic perception of necessity is embodied in the prevailing current that wants every effective response offered as a thing, as a means, as the immediacy of effect, and as a commodity available on the market. Hence the drive to exceed the limits of perceptual standards through drugs capable of altering the state of consciousness, of artificially induced mystical experiences. We all think of drugs, especially psychotropic drugs, from LSD and lysergic acid to the varied procession of psychedelic substances—that is, "manifesting the psyche"—such as psilocybin, mescaline, peyote, ayahuasca, etc., both natural and chemically created. But artifice could also describe all the innumerable ascetic techniques that, in the history of different cultures, have been experimented with to achieve ecstatic perception by altering the normal state of consciousness. These are the so-called Altered State of Consciousness (ASC): from silent meditation to maintaining specific postures, from fasting to night vigils to the continuous repetition of a mantra or prayer to music and dance.

This is also a way of looking differently at all ascetic techniques, often debunked and taken for obtuse moralism, accused by critics of religion, for more than two centuries now, of denying the world, the earth, the senses, and so on. Flipping these into their paradoxical opposite, we might say that the intent of the fiercest ascetics is, at times, to arrive at corporeality, the state of being corporeal, so that they become the sentient host of the spirit. What we are looking for, Hulin (1993) says, when we speak of "wild mysticism" and its core of universal meaning is, above all, "the existential, and primarily affective, dimension of the phenomenon" (Hulin, 2012, p. 22), beyond the techniques and disciplines that can facilitate it. Indeed, being wild indicates that experience can give itself in infinite ways, far beyond particular rules of behavior and any possible technique. It is certainly typical of the world of global capitalism to be driven to find technical-mercantile solutions, available as objects that can be bought and consumed quickly, rather than to engage in a discipline of a whole life consecrated to the transformation of one's way of being, acting and perceiving. Hence the rarity of monastic vocations in contemplative orders and the mass prevalence of psychotropic substances. A pill is well worth a lifetime of abstinence. We could also say we seek ecstatic-mystical dimensions at discounted prices and immediate effect. But still, without moralizing blind to historical change, we can, and must, try to understand the underlying need-desire that animates this dissatisfaction with the kind of life prescribed for living productively and care-free. I will therefore take an example of my experience with LSD from a message sent to me for conversations on the wild mystique of radio show *Uomini e Profeti* by a great cartoonist, Tullio Pericoli. It is a message that surprised me because it tells of an experience conducted with Elvio Fachinelli and gives us back, in a few penetrating strokes, the understanding of psychedelic substance-induced experiences. Pericoli's story is taken from *Crossroads*, one of his books published by Adelphi (2019): "A long friendship linked Fachinelli and me, and in his book, he tells of his personal experience with mescaline - psilocybin in pills."

> Elvio remembers that before he did it on himself, he did it on me, using me, with my consent, him being present as a guinea pig. He curled up on a small chair to my right, like a cat waiting for food, and I stood at the easel in front of a painting that had already begun. It depicted a small group of people, four or five, facing a balcony, with the wall of the house behind them made of falling pieces ... First pill. Caught up in work, I almost forgot about Elvio nearby; the painting was coming along nicely, and I went on quietly. Quiet, however, he was not; every now and then, I sensed signs of impatience emanating from the side of the chair where he was squatting. He was waiting for the pill's effect, which could not be seen. Second pill. Elvio sat back down, and I went back to work. I took a

small tube of red and covered a figure with large brush strokes. 'Here it is! The red! The red! Here is the effect!,' 'Look, Elvio, that this red was already decided upon; I had already thought of it before I started the painting.' I was beginning to feel guilty; the tablets were like water. Elvio was disappointed, and I was for him. 'Give me another one,' I asked him. Third pill. The painting was still in front of me, the same, waiting for me to proceed with the work, when another smaller one, hanging on the opposite wall, began to light up. The green became true green, the red was taking on more dimensions, and what my hands touched were no longer objects but souls.

Everything began to be part of me, and I of the whole: I touched everything with love as if it had become a fragment of my body and skin. Elvio disappeared. Faint, sweet sounds of him remained. He now had a fetching smile, and everything approached me, embracing me with magnetic attraction: even the sky, the clouds, the street with parked cars, and the wide-open window. Elvio grabbed me. I was about to jump or go down and fly into the street from the fifth floor. He ended up at his house in the evening with Herma, his wife, and some friends. I think.

I have chosen to take up this short story not only because it broadens our knowledge of Elvio Fachinelli, of his provocative curiosity (for those times and the psychoanalytic milieu), but because in a few lines, as in Pericoli's style, it tells us of the disorienting ambivalence of induced experiences, without preparation exercised in a spiritual discipline, of alterations of consciousness that can convey both the bliss of feeling enveloped by the All and the erasure of the limits of our possibilities. Aldous Huxley summarized this kind of experience in a dazzling title: *The Gates of Perception*. The title, no accident at all, comes from William Blake's 1793 book *The Marriage of Heaven and Hell*;[4] debatable as it may be, Huxley claims Martin Buber and his Vedanta teacher, Swami Prabhavananda, both attacked. Huxley hints at the continent that can be opened when one crosses the boundaries of everyday consciousness. He writes, "All one can do is go to the mental equivalent of Australia and look around." Here *Australia* is the metaphor precisely for the antipodes of our perceptual habits. Travels excellent and terrible, beautiful and horrible together; everything is random. Said my analyst, Paul Aite, when I, young and back from a fairly reckless life, once proposed to him to take LSD in session, "It's like going fishing with bombs! Better to go fishing with dreams and sand play!" That's right, you catch a lot of fish, perhaps, with psychedelic substances, but the carnage is sometimes disproportionate: you and the boat on which you sail may blow up along with them. A certain amount of caution is, therefore, in order. However, one must guard against excessive fear, undoubtedly influenced by the political-cultural campaign that, for LSD, struck at a widespread tendency in the 1970s youth counterculture movement to question a one-dimensional view of life and the world. The term deliberately echoes Herbert Marcuse's *One-Dimensional Man* (1964). The result was in 1971 outlawing the use of lysergic acid diethylamide 25, which had been discovered (in one of many cases of serendipity) by Swiss chemist Albert Hoffmann in 1938.

It all depends on the use, motivations, and environment, relational first and foremost, that shape the field of experience in a situation. All the more so since research nowadays on psilocybin has landed on fascinating results for possible pharmacological use. Psilocybin mushrooms have been used ritually for centuries by South American natives. In the 1960s and 1970s, Stanislav Grof, to name but one, experimented with psychedelic substances with the terminally ill; today, these experiments are being taken up by leading scientific institutions. From 2012 to 2016, Robin Carhart-Harris demonstrated, using functional magnetic resonance imaging (fMRI), that psilocybin and LSD decrease the functionality of certain brain control functions by letting various stimuli be perceived in a more vivid, less usual way. But the so-called psychedelic renaissance is now mainly concerned with the use of psilocybin, which has milder effects than lysergic acid in cases of severe depression and appears to act on circulating serotonin by affecting mood and behavior.

Meanwhile, this process has already been initiated in several U.S. states (Oregon and California first), and Australia. Oregon and California governments have decriminalized psilocybin possession and they and

Australia granted permits for possible drug treatment. MDMA, or ecstasy, is also being tested for efficacy in cases of post-traumatic stress disorder (PTSD), just as other synthetic derivatives of psychedelic substances are being tested for efficacy treating various forms of addiction. Their possible effectiveness against dementia, depression of the terminally ill, and cluster headaches are also being studied. Of course, the old use of these substances for creative and recreational purposes—essentially to feel more perceptually and mentally stimulated, remains the most popular. The difference is that today we try to justify it by hypothesizing that increased nerve cell contacts produce the effects of a more incredible feeling of perceptiveness due to taking these substances. The result is an increase in microdosing, the daily use of tiny amounts of LSD or psilocybin. This rehabilitation of psychedelics is of marginal interest concerning the nexus with the search for experiences of ecstatic states of perception that border on, or even identify with, the states of consciousness that we can call common mysticism.

It is in this nexus and the openness of this possibility that those who desire it and are capable of contact with the deep layers of the psyche—after a sufficiently long period of analysis—can be accompanied by an experienced analyst on a journey of exploration facilitated by the measured use of psychotropic substances. That this practice is still banned in many countries worldwide, including Italy, is another matter entirely related to politico-cultural factors and legal prohibitions that we must observe for the time being but with which we are not expected to agree.

References

Fachinelli, E. (1969). *La mente estatica,* Adelphi.

Hulin, M. (1993). *La mystique sauvage.* Presses Universitaire de France.

Hulin, M. (2012). *La mistica selvaggia,* Ipoc.

Jung, C.G. (1989). *Memories, Dreams, Reflections.* A. Yaffé, Ed., R. & C. Winston, Trans. Vintage Books.

Podvoll, E. (1990). *Recovering sanity.* Shambala Publications.

Tart, C., Ed. (1969). *Altered states of consciousness.* J. Wiley and Sons Inc.

Endnotes

[1] On the links and differences between the effects of psychotropic substances, see Podvall, 1990, in particular pp. 195-203.

[2] L'Analisi Biografica a Orientamento Filosofico (Biographical Analysis philosophically oriented) is the practice of the Società di Analisi Biografica a Orientamento Filosofico (SABOF) part of Associazione Philo-pratiche filosofiche.

[3] In his last book, *La mente estatica,* published by Adelphi on the same year of his passing, in 1969.

[4] See also Huxley's 1954 *The Doors of Perception*, and Pollan's 2018 *How to Change Your Mind.*

The Path to the Transcendent Function: Dreams, Visions, and Psychedelics

Nancy Swift Furlotti

As I was thinking about how I was going to begin this paper, I had a dream:

> *I was with a large crowd of men standing at the edge of a low cliff next to the ocean. Our attention was drawn out across the water to the sky, first with loud noise then the sight of three very large vessels, a submarine, a large bus, and a large passenger jet coming together in the sky/water in front of us swirling around in a large dance, twisting around each other in a matrix that was not just air but was water-earth-air that had a translucency and transparency that seemed to move in and out of one dimension into another. I couldn't believe what I was seeing. It was awesome—in non-slang meaning— numinous, fascinating, and terrifying at the same time.*

I woke up and wondered what this meant. It was beyond personal, coming from the archetypal realm, something huge, potentially dangerous, destructive, unusual. Large ships like these three don't behave this way. They were like huge blue whales flipping and rolling around each other, yet not in the ocean but in some unknown matrix that included three levels of our recognizable and symbolic life, ocean/underworld, earth/reality, and the sky/spirit realm. They were all made of metal, and all were vessels that carried humans. They were creations of our cultural, rational scientific development. They were strong, protective, technological, useful and each one was a part of our everyday life—well, maybe not the submarines, although they could be. In the dream they did not destroy each other or crash and fall, hurting the humans on the ground. They were playful. It was an archetypal vision of three powerful and unlikely creations outside of my reality pointing to a different reality, a much more fluid reality where unimaginable things can happen. These vessels of transportation represent libido—the life energy that propels us forward and carries us on our life's journey. Here, in this dream it is not a ship on a river moving towards the ocean, or a ship on an ocean journey which would indicate how the unconscious waters of life carry us along. This was a mix of water, earth, and air and three different vessels, each equipped for its own journey in its own dimension. It is significant to add two other dimensions to the task.

I didn't know anyone standing in the crowd with me, surrounded by the male crowd Jung referred to as the animus. This was my dream so it must have to do with my rational extraverted thinking function, being scientifically minded and being shown a vision of the impossible, except that here it is not impossible. It is a challenge to my rational thinking. My introverted intuitive function is having fun with my second function! There was no feeling, just fascination, and the hope that they do not destruct.

It was an experience of crossing the veil from one dimension into another and seeing what is possible in that other dimension. And maybe it is a view of how the technological, rational masculine attitude has gotten out of hand, is let loose in all levels of life as we see with ChatBots and augmented reality. Are we heading to the singularity where God is tech, where Nature recedes and the inanimate take over? Is it a warning that this can get out of control and destruct? With the absence of the feminine, and how she is under attack culturally, I do admit this is one of my biggest worries.

This is the type of dream one cannot forget. It is gripping and I will remember this for the rest of my life. Here I have actually had an experience out of time, out of the dimension of my reality. My small world view has enlarged. There is something out there that animates inanimate objects, metals, and minerals that we think of as static and unchangeable. It is beyond AI, it is inherent in the nature of the matrix of the universe— the ability to move in and out of dimensions, through elements, and time.

In the past if I had not had psychedelic experiences, I would think the end of times were upon us or some huge catastrophe was about to befall me, forcing a massive change of life or viewpoint. This dream is an example of the similarities of visions in dreams and psychedelic experiences. Thankfully, I have had experiences where reality was torn away from me while I observed and entered the process, both willingly and unwillingly.

My first such experience was with mescaline at age 16. I was in Hawaii for my older brother's wedding when I joined an outing with my other older brother and a couple of his friends. He had gotten mescaline capsules from a friend who happened to be the son of the Chancellor of UCLA at the time—it was 1968. We were on Maui and spent the day at the Seven Sacred Pools of Hana on the far side of the island, away from tourists and towns. It was a joyous day in nature with all sensations coming alive and I became aware of all of them. I was a different animal transforming from an intuitive to a sensate being. It was an experience of pure joyous play and exploration in pools of water, waterfalls, volcanic rock, tropical forest with all the animals and sounds that inhabit that land. I was safe with my favorite older brother and his two kind and funny friends. This was the best possible initiation I could have had to psychedelics. It was then I learned of more than one reality, with a multitude of realities coming at me at once. What was so important in this first experience was that it took place in a beautiful, safe setting and I was surrounded by caring, kind people.

Bipolar disorder runs in my family and my father had a severe case with mixed mania, or what we now call mixed affective state, committing suicide when I was seven. I grew up in a world where reality was always changing; there was a very thin veil between where I stood and the other side, the darker side. My father frequently crossed over and returned. These experiences of a shifting reality left me knowing both sides and spending my childhood into adulthood building a more solid barrier between the two for my own protection. My early experience in Hana showed me the other side could be harmless, actually comforting and interesting. Later during a number of LSD experiences in college, I was reminded that there was a lot to be afraid of behind that veil. One had to tread carefully. I watched as a friend slipped into schizophrenia as the result of a bad trip. LSD was more of a head trip and I didn't like its effects. At first it was interesting with wildly changing hallucinations like bees the size of eagles dive-bombing over our heads, swirls of colors, but as time wore on my jaw clenched and I became more fearful and paranoid. It was not a good experience and I stopped accepting the free offers of blotters or window pane LSD. It brought out the worst in me, opened up my shadow side, and let it all flow out. I had no way of integrating what my experience was at the time. Thankfully, I had a bit more of a barrier between reality and the unconscious shadow as I experienced what my father must have lived with in his depressions and manias. It was totally frightening. This is where psychedelics are dangerous for those not prepared for the experience, not contained and safe. I felt lucky to be able to endure the unpleasant trips. Others were not so lucky.

All these experiences growing up gave me an intuition of different dimensions of the psyche, some frightening and dangerous, others interesting and creative. It was a natural that I resonated with Jung from the moment I began reading his writings. He spoke my language with his understanding of the three layers of the cosmos and striving for a balance between them all. Hence, I pursued psychology rather than physical sciences or mysticism, and allowed my dreams to lead the way. They became my entrance into that other realm, taking the place of hallucinations as a softer, much kinder ticket to the other side, although sometimes fierce and terrifying too, as the one described above.

Much later in life, I tried psilocybin with a Jungian friend who knew what she was doing by preparing a mixture of psilocybin mushroom with San Pedro Cactus (Schultes et al., 1998, p. 62) and THC. We laid blankets and pillows on her deck overlooking a river and settled in for an evening of intense, unknown experience. The trip lasted about six hours, coming on quietly at first, then with its full force. The visual images and lessening of consciousness were greater with my eyes closed. If I needed to remember where I was, I would open my eyes, but then return to the other world where a deep and profound universal wisdom was showing me the reality of existence. I visualized a huge dragon shaped creature or energy pattern arching across the cosmos, pulsating with light and life. It seemed to be wide open, as if the body of the dragon was sliced and pulled apart to act as a huge container for all the souls of the worlds. They were the flashes of light and energy that would come and go from this belly-vessel. The dragon moved with the rhythms of the cosmos and was just as large, containing its energy. It was stunning, gripping, and transformative to witness the vision of all souls/soul energy functioning together, for a higher purpose. We were all the same substance, transporters of light, coming and going to and from earth and other unknown realms. I will never forget that powerful vision.

In the Chinese zodiac, I am a water dragon and find comfort in its image. The soul-carriers of light remind me of the beliefs in Gnosticism and Kabballah having to do with recovering the broken shards of glass and light that have fallen to earth after God's creation and returning them to God to form his wholeness. Each of us is responsible for contributing to the wholeness of God by making conscious what is lost and forgotten within our dark unconscious. So many philosophical ideas and religious beliefs swirl around this concept, which has a fundamental archetypal basis. Jung came to this in his *Answer to Job,* and so did Erich Neumann in his many writings, especially in his *Depth Psychology and a New Ethic.*

We are familiar with Jung's dreams and visions, while not so with Erich Neumann's. In his letters to Jung during WWII, while struggling with the concept of evil and God's relation to it, Neumann described a profound vision he had after which the world forever looked different:

> I seemed to be commissioned to kill the apeman in the profound primal hole. As I approached him, he was hanging, by night, sleeping on the cross above the abyss, but his—crooked—single eye was staring into the depths of this abyss. While it at first seemed that I was supposed to blind him, I all of a sudden grasped his "innocence," his dependence on the single eye of the godhead, which was experiencing the depths through him, which was a human eye. Then, very abridged, I sank down opposite this single eye, jumped into the abyss, but was caught by the Godhead, which carried me on the "wings of his heart." After that, this single eye opposite the apeman closed and it opened on my forehead. (Bit difficult to write this, but what should one do). (Jung & Neumann, 2015, p. 331)

Neumann discussed evil in relation to his psyche's clarification in the dream as being something he had to experience; it was not sin but a necessary action. In his vision, he jumps into the abyss, rather than falling. He is held by something greater in all his actions, both good and bad. Sin becomes irrelevant in relation to this new divine. A new morality compels one to integrate as much of the unconscious or the opposites that are God as one is able. This includes evil.

Jung remained concerned because of what he recognized as the limited consciousness forming ability of humans, and therefore believed the actual transformation of evil takes place in the unconscious, through the changing symbols in relation to the God-image and the Self. Yet it remains up to each one of us to recognize this. This recognition comes through our dreams, visions, and even psychedelics if we understand the wisdom offered.

Neumann was forever changed by his powerful vision, as I was from the vision induced by psilocybin. It is the change in one's view of the world and of one's sense of self that is precious. The vision itself is an activation of the greater Self, the wisdom of the unconscious that bridges opposites to release the transcendent function, revealing the 3rd element, the new viewpoint or sense of being. This is the apex of Jungian analysis. We strive for the experience of wholeness and a return to the unitary reality that was fundamental to our early life in the uroboros, but now with a newfound consciousness of this wholeness, light and dark, and all opposites. My cosmic dragon vision was such an experience. I can't say that I wasn't going to achieve this profound knowledge without psychedelics. I most likely would have, and was well on my way, but the intensity and quality of the vision sped up the process and left me with a sense of knowing, not speculating with my shadow intruding to discount the vision. It was too powerful to discount or minimize. It was absolute and was deeply incorporated into my life.

Writers on the topic of psychedelics talk about the experience leaving one with greater understanding of the cycle of life, the meaning of death, love, and compassion. All those elements are part of the change that takes place. While Jung spoke of the limited consciousness forming ability of humans, he was accurately accessing humans from his personal experience as a psychiatrist and analyst, and from observing the changes both positive and negative in cultural and human development.

According to a private conversation I had with Sonu Shamdasani shortly after the publication of *The Red Book*, he revealed that there was strong evidence that Jung tried mescaline, yet in later writings he warned of its use, perhaps because it has the potential to trigger a psychosis and might be too potent for many unprepared people. During Jung's life, many people were contained within a religious organization. This is not true today. The world is a different place and people have many experiences that were not available during his lifetime. There is greater interest in and discussion around different methods of treating mental health, psychedelics being one.

What We have Learned from Neuroscience

Psychedelics are being studied for use with people with cancer and end of life issues. These people are running out of time. In my experience, when one is approaching the end of life, time speeds up as does the inner work on preparing oneself for death. Dream and vision images can be stronger and more abstract. Psychedelics help go to the heart of what is needed to find peace at the border of this transition from life to death—as long as it is determined the person has the resilience to handle this powerful experience and is in a safe, contained vessel before and during the process. It is recommended by many researchers that no one who has a psychosis in the family should be eligible to participate in psychedelic therapy. I am glad I snuck past that rule! The experience was just what I needed to grasp the depth of my family illness and further my individuation.

Scientists throughout the years have studied the effects of psychedelics on the brain as a way to understand how we perceive ourselves, and our relationship to the world. They dramatically alter our perception and our brain chemistry, dropping us into a state similar to dreaming. One pioneer, Aldous Huxley, in his book, *Doors of Perception* (1970, p. 16), described his experience after taking a single dose of mescaline:

Half an hour after swallowing the drug I became aware of a slow dance of golden lights. A little later there were sumptuous red surfaces swelling and expanding from bright nodes of energy that vibrated with a continuously changing, patterned light.

Neuroscientist Solomon Snyder described the phenomenon of synesthesia where the senses overlap with each other so that touch can be experienced as sound, or sound can be experienced as vision (1996, p. 180). As ego boundaries are broken down, one feels connected to others and the universe. Huxley commented,

> To others again is revealed the glory, the infinite value and meaningfulness of naked existence, of the given, unconceptualized event. In the final stage of egolessness there is an obscure knowledge that All is in awe—that Awe is actually each. This is as near, I take it, as a finite mind can ever come to perceiving everything that is happening everywhere in the universe. (1970, p. 16)

Heinrich Kluver in his book, *Mescal and Mechanisms of Hallucinations* (1971), described a psychedelic experience of mescaline use in 1927 by the physicians, Knauer and Malony at Emil Kraepelin's clinic at the University of Heidelberg. Kraepelin coined the term dementia praecox, the precursor to schizophrenia:

> Beautiful crimsons, purples, violets, blues and greens quickly succeeding one another. The background of this gorgeous color panorama was first like faintly illuminated ground glass; it is now a silvery tint, and is deepening into a yellow like pure gold ... On pressing upon my eyes, the whole picture seemed to materialize. The wires became more solid, more real and quite distinct from the background. The wires are now flattening into bands or ribbons, with a suggestion of transverse striation, and colors of a gorgeous ultramarine blue, which passes

in places into an intense sea green. These bands move rhythmically, in a wavy upward direction, suggesting a slow endless procession of small mosaics, ascending the wall in single files. (Kluver, 1971, p. 14)

From the early research, it seems there are visions common to psychedelic experiences: geometric figures and kaleidoscopically changing forms of grating or lattice, tunnels, funnels, vessels, or spirals; familiar objects like faces and landscapes that change from one to the other; or unusual and monstrous forms and landscapes. Colors are brilliantly vivid and changing as if alive with energy. Objects change size. These descriptions are similar to both my psychedelic experiences and my dreams. Both, including visions, emanate from the same place in the brain.

Jung wrote in *The Red Book*:

The gifts of darkness are full of riddles. The way is open to whoever can continue in spite of the riddles. Submit to the riddles and the thoroughly incomprehensible. There are dizzying bridges over the eternally deep abyss. But follow the riddles. (2009, p. 308)

It is no surprise that Jung may have ingested mescaline since psychedelics were the object of experimentation for many scientists during their early careers, including William James. Sigmund Freud experimented with cocaine and became addicted. Jung, however, developed a way to initiate visions without the use of drugs, through concentration, perhaps much like lucid dreaming, and many of his visions came upon him spontaneously. He had studied Eastern philosophies and yoga in great depth before embarking on his personal journey of experimentation, laid out so beautifully in *The Red Book* (Jung, 2009, p. 273), in which he shared eight waking visions he had during 1913-1914, one of which is as follows:

I wandered to the northern land and found myself under a gray sky in misty-hazy cool-moist air. I strive to those lowlands where the weak currents, flashing in broad mirrors, stream toward the sea, where all haste of flowing becomes more and more dampened, and where all power and all striving unites with the immeasurable extent of the sea. The trees become sparse, wide swamp meadows accompany the still, murky water, the horizon is unending and lonely, draped by gray clouds. Slowly, with restrained breath, and with the great and anxious expectation of one gliding downward wildly on the foam and pouring himself into endlessness, I follow my brother, the sea. It flows softly and almost imperceptibly, and yet we continually approach the supreme embrace, entering the womb of the source, the boundless expansion and immeasurable depths. Lower yellow hills rise there. A broad dead lake widens at their feet. We wander along the hills quietly and they open up to a dusky, unspeakably remote horizon, where the sky and the sea are fused into infinity.

This vision has the feeling of a psychedelic experience and contains content consistent with Kluver's descriptions of mescaline visions: a landscape changing before one's eyes; changes in the apparent size of things; distortion of time and space; an altered sense of self; the unification of self with the unending source of creation; cosmic emotions of ecstatic states (Kluver, 1971, p. 13-55). "The experiences in the mescal state are not easily forgotten. One looks beyond the horizon of the normal world, and this beyond is often so impressive or even shocking that its after-effects linger for years in one's memory" (Kluver, 1971, p. 19).

The psychedelic experience can be profoundly positive or destructively horrible. It can start out well and then become a nightmare. But in either case, it allows one to step outside the frame of consciousness or, as psychoanalysts would say, to fall into the unconscious. As the dream research shows, it is questionable whether one is completely unaware while unconscious. The NREM dream state may most closely resemble a lack of awareness and unconsciousness. There are, nevertheless, so-called unconscious states that co-exist with awareness. Awareness and consciousness are not the same things. To take the Jungian concept of complex, for example, when one falls into a complex one is unconscious of the motivating factors creating an emotional disturbance, meaning that the ego is not in charge. I would say the executive function, among others, has shut down while the limbic system has taken over and is running the show with irrational emotion. It is the ego that gives one a sense of self-ness and corresponds to consciousness. The ego coordinates thoughts and emotions, much like the executive function of the brain. Without a sense of self or ego, one can still be aware in a physical way, although not psychologically. Consciousness from a psychological point of view can be defined as one's ability to control, influence, or evaluate. To the extent the ego is partially present while in a complex, one can be modestly conscious of oneself, while one also remains aware physically in time and space. Jung referred to these small nodes of consciousness and potential awareness in the unconscious as *scintilla*. They are the sparks of light that reside in the unconscious. It is clear from this comparison that when one is in a complex, one is in an altered state of consciousness. Jung explained the experience using his own words, and while he did not have the advantage of our understanding of contemporary neuroscience, he nevertheless, intuited the relationships and structures quite well. There are, also, similarities between dreaming and complexes. It is in this same way that dreaming is also considered an altered state of consciousness:

> Although Eugene Aserinsky and Nathaniel Kleitman's discovery that brain activation in (REM) sleep was associated with hallucinoid dreaming shook the dream theory tree quite strongly, it did not evoke the wider interest it deserved as the harbinger of integration between experimental psychedelism, psychology, psychiatry, and traditional neurobiology… Both Freud and James believed that dreams, psychotic hallucinations and quasi-religious visions all depended somehow, on alterations in brain function. (Hobson, 2001, p. 19)

We know that during sleep we move through various stages including NREM and REM, cycling up and down from deep sleep to near waking sleep over the course of the night. At each stage, the brain is activated differently and influenced by different brain chemistry. The limbic system and the visual associative cortex are activated in dreaming while the executive cortex, among other areas, is inhibited. The aminergic demodulation noted for its support of flight or flight response, results in letting go of logical narrative sequencing, while memory, attention, and volition are diminished. Emotion is enhanced. In REM sleep, the motor areas are inhibited while the visual and emotional areas are in high gear. This is not the case in psychedelic usage where the motor areas are not shut down. It is also true in lucid dreaming where the blood flow to the dorsolateral prefrontal cortices increases so that they are as active as in the waking state:

> First, we can alter consciousness voluntarily and without the use of drugs to achieve many of the formal desirata of the drug-induced psychedelic states. These include the simulation of psychosis, with exotic visual imagery; the simulation of magical behaviors… the cultivation of ecstatic elation; and the experience of highly erotic sexual adventures… as did Emmanuel Swedenborg, whose induction procedure included intentional sleep deprivation to potentiate the REM process on which lucid dreaming rides. (Hobson, 2001, p. 95)

This may explain C.G. Jung's ability to induce visions. It seems that the dorsolateral prefrontal cortex, deactivated in REM sleep, is active during lucid dreaming, thus opening the pathways for memory, self-reflective awareness, and volition while also allowing the bizarreness and imagery of REM sleep. It is also activated during the use of psychedelic drugs.

> Any drug that produces dreamlike visual imagery during waking will simulate the visual activation pattern of dreaming while still permitting wake state visual processing to proceed. The result will be a

72

phenomenological and physiological hybridization of conscious state and brain state. (Hobson, 2001, p. 56)

Psilocybin and LSD resemble in structure the neuromodulator, serotonin, while mescaline is closer to that of norepinephrine or dopamine with some similarities to serotonin. But it has proved difficult to determine exactly how they work (Snyder, 1996, p. 196).

People can go from sleep into hypnagogic or hypnopompic hallucinations, sleep walking, or lucid dreaming and experience a continuation of REM sleep dreaming while moving into a waking state. The boundaries between states are not clearly delineated. It shows the great difficulty in containing dreaming to sleep. During REM sleep, the norepinephrine and serotonin neuromodulatory systems are inactivated while, "LSD... causes instantaneously dreamlike waking as it blocks serotonergic neuromodulation" (Hobson, 2001, p. 125). For both, there is a shift from aminergic to cholinergic dominance. The similarity between the dream bizarreness, vivid colors and emotionality of REM sleep is similar to the descriptions of psychedelics, and it seems the activation on the brain is the same. As Snyder says, "All of the major psychedelic drugs have a close chemical resemblance to the neurotransmitters norepinephrine, serotonin, and dopamine" (1996, p. 195).

Albert Hoffman discovered the hallucinogenic effects of LSD-25 by accident and realized by ingesting a small but very potent amount that it, "acted directly on the brain, altering its chemistry in the direction of psychosis and dreaming" (Hobson, 2001, p. 253). During his trip, Hoffman was able to observe what was going on, so he clearly was not asleep in the sense that he was not unconscious. He suspected that the stimulating effects on the visual parts of his brain were the result of a depletion of serotonin. The visual changes were not just visual but visuomotor, creating a sense of continuous motion, much like in dreaming. Serotonin can be impaired naturally in dreaming, or pathologically in depression, or chemically with the use of LSD. When this is the case, the limbic areas are activated creating strong and negative emotions. This has to do with LSD's enhancement of the serotonin, 5-HT system. With LSD, the imagery is not narrative as in dreams, but geometric and kaleidoscopic. One can have auditory hallucinations that interact with the visual. Of course, one large difference between dreaming and LSD is that during dreaming the outside world is shut out (assuming the unconscious is not aware of anything in this state, which is questionable). Under the influence of LSD both inside and outside stimulus affect the individual's experience:

> Single cell recordings in the raphé nuclei of the brain stem show that the serotonin-containing cells are actively suppressed during REM, the stage of sleep most strongly correlated with dreaming. The serotonin system exerts a restraining effect on the acetylcholine neurons that actively and directly mediate the REM sleep events responsible for visual system activation and dream hallucinations. Thus when the serotonin system is suppressed, either naturally in REM or pharmacologically by LSD, the cholinergic system is released and visual hallucinations become more probable.
> (Hobson, 2001, p. 257)

Many of the phenomenology are the same between dreaming and drug induced psychosis, which is what Hobson calls an LSD trip. Cognition, emotion, perception, attention, are similar but what is different is the intensity of sensation. It is greater with LSD than dreaming because reception of external stimuli is shut down in dreaming, except for the falling into sleep stage when the door to the outer world is still ajar. LSD makes the waking state more dream-like while at the same time suppressing REM sleep and dreaming. Since LSD interferes with the inhibitory role of serotonin, which promotes waking, it allows a dream-like state while awake. LSD as well as psilocybin work in the same way on the brain, causing serotonin to stop firing. Mescaline, however, does not cause an abrupt cessation like LSD does. It affects the dopamine system. Perhaps this is why my experience of mescaline was smoother than that of LSD, which I would describe as sharp.

The psychedelic state corresponds to Jung's description of psychosis—when one has fallen into the unconscious. One moves from consciousness with a sense of self and ego control to a loss of ego. The difference between falling into a complex and psychosis is a matter of degree. This means the ego is no longer able to withstand the internal forces pressing upon it and voices and visions are unleashed. Although, some have thought that Jung was psychotic because of his active imaginations in *The Red Book*, he maintained control over his ego the entire time he was in the unconscious. He was the objective observer of his own inner drama. The drama did not supersede him. He was able to dialogue with these inner figures, maintaining his integrity. He was aware of what it meant to be psychotic from his early work at the Burghölzli Hospital in Zurich and may have sought out the experience himself just as many around him and after him had done through the use of psychedelics or other techniques to open the doors of perception to the many dimensions of the psyche:

> George Ajhajanian's research may also illuminate how LSD influences the user's sense of self. The greatly accelerated firing of the locus coeruleus presumably provokes a powerful, patterned release of norepinephrine from nerve terminals throughout the brain... This extremely enhanced level of alertness might possibly account for the "transcendent" mental state produced by psychedelic drugs. In other words, in a state of such heightened awareness, the drug user may become conscious of an "inner self" to which he or she is normally oblivious. (Snyder, 1996, p. 203)

The Importance of Rituals

This may be this mechanism that allows the individual to experience the transcendent, the "inner Self" that opens the door to the greater cosmos and unitary reality. From the neuroscience research, it seems clear that dreams, visions caused by substances, or activities such as holotropic breathing, isolation, dancing, drumming, and torture of the body induce changes in the brain that allow a heightened level of awareness, a mystical transformative experience. Many cultures use these techniques to arrive at this experience. For example, the classic period Maya used bloodletting as a way to induce extreme pain causing, unbeknownst to them, a shift in the brain's neurotransmitters resulting in the longed-for presence of the *vision serpent*. In this way, the individual was able to contact powerful ancestral spirits and give the most precious life-substance, blood, as tribute to their Gods. A thorn-lined rope or stingray spine was drawn through the tongue, the skin of the arm, or the penis, and the resulting blood fell into a basket and was captured on strips of paper cloth. The paper was then burned as an offering of ash and smoke as it floated up to the spiritual world, to the ancestors. The following three lintels from Yaxchilan[1], structures 21 and 23, AD 725, depict this ritual bloodletting process to invoke supernatural visions.

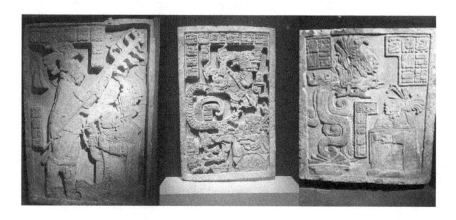

The Maya not only used bloodletting as a means to induce visions, but hallucinogenic drugs such as cactus, plants, and mushrooms were also common there and throughout all of the Americas for healing rituals and religious ceremonies. These included peyote or mescaline, psilocybin, Turbina corymbosa, the skin of the toad Bufo marinus, Jimson weed, wild tobacco, water lily, Salvia, and San Pedro Cactus. Some are still used in ritual ceremonies to induce altered states of consciousness to communicate with divine powers, and to offer tribute with the goal of maintaining a heathy balance in the cosmos. These rituals have been practiced for well over 3000 years, and perhaps far longer. We have a lot to learn from this long history of experience. They can show us how to think about and prepare for the life changing experience, how to process it afterward, how to see it as a vital part of the health of the culture and every individual who makes up the whole of that culture. One could say they are religious experiences, but today many people have lost the connection to the essence of what this means, and our collective mental health has suffered. Revisiting these experiences and rituals opens the door to the forgotten world that includes many dimensions. Erich Neumann wrote in his book, *The Roots of Jewish Consciousness, Volume Two*:

> The ecstatic situation is where all existence is reborn. Its continuous realization corresponds to the highest level of being ... But just as ego stability was one of the genuine preconditions for prophecy in antiquity, now one of the preconditions for genuine ecstasy is a focus of the world. It is as if the dissolution of consciousness into nothingness had to be seen essentially as the apex of a parabola, where the soul hurls itself into nothingness, in order to pass through this point and return to the world in the other direction. In one step, in a process of progressive extraversion, it comes back through the stages of creation, returning newborn to the world. (2019, p. 32)

Conclusion

It seems clear from the research on psychedelics over 70 years that, when used carefully and therapeutically, the experience results in "a realignment of ego-defenses and boundaries" (Pahnke & Richards, 1966, p. 94). This leads to a rapid resolution of symptoms: depressive and anxious, alcoholism, addictions of all kinds, post-trauma, and fear of dying. This is due to a changed and enlarged attitude toward life involving one's goodness and intrinsic worth as a member of the human race, resulting in feeling the full harmony of emotion and intellect (Pahnke & Richards, 1966, p. 90). The individual is left with greater sensitivity, increased tolerance, and compassion:

> It would seem better for a person to have a drug-facilitated experience of the mystical consciousness, enjoy the enriched life that may follow, and serve other

persons during the greater part of his life than to live a life that may be inauthentic and withdrawn until old age, when such an experience may occur by means of ascetic practices. (Pahnke & Richards, 1966, p. 89)

This experience is not an absolute. It requires a combination of the right set-up, allowing the drug to be the effective trigger. Careful preparation and execution include making sure the patient is open and ready to participate. Psychological problems may have to be explored before a breakthrough into mystical consciousness is possible. Screening procedures and timing are crucial, ensuring a sense of trust and safety with the analyst who will accompany the individual through the process (Pahnke & Richards, 1966, pp. 84-89). Just as a beautiful, safe setting in nature was crucial for me, a comfortable room, music, soft light capturing a ritual setting prepares one for the anticipated experience—caring for the physical environment as well as the emotional atmosphere.

Afterwards, it is crucial that the insights be integrated. "Unless such an experience is integrated into the on-going life of the person, only a memory remains rather than the growth of an unfolding process of renewal that may be awakened by the mystical experience" (Pahnke & Richards, 1966, p. 89). This is where Jungian analysts are uniquely trained, not only to build trust and safety, but to understand the symbolic/ archetypal meaning of the elements that appear in the visions and how to work with them as part of the patient's individuation process. This part of the work may take a long time to help the patient integrate all the feelings and insights. It may not always be a wonderful experience, it can also be full of feelings of guilt, grief, or hostility. We Jungian analysts are used to dealing with everything that emerges from the psyche, to be able to tolerate strong affects and incomprehensible images. It is what we are trained to do—to help integrate the opposites as we follow the path to the transcendent.

References

Furlotti, N. (2023). *Eternal echoes: Erich Neumann's timeless relevance to consciousness, creativity, and evil.* Chiron Publications.

Huxley, A. (1970). *Doors of perception.* Harper & Row.

Hobson, J.A. (2001). *The dream drugstore: Chemically altered states of consciousness.* MIT Press.

Jung, C.G. & Neumann, E. (2015). *Analytical psychology in exile: The correspondence of C. G. Jung & Erich Neumann.* Princeton University Press.

Kluver, H. (1971). *Mescal and mechanisms of hallucination.* Chicago: University of Chicago Press.

Neumann, E. (2019). *The roots of Jewish consciousness, volume two: Hasidism.* A. C. Lammers, (Ed.). London: Routledge.

Pahnke, W.N., & Richards, W.A. (1966). Implications of LSD and experimental mysticism. *Journal of Religion & Health, 5,* 175-208.

Schultes, R.E., Hoffmann, A., & Ratsch, C. (1998). *Plants of the gods: Their sacred, healing, and hallucinogenic powers.* Healing Arts Press.

Snyder, S.H. (1996). *Drugs and the brain.* Scientific American Library.

Endnotes

[1] "Yaxchilan," the Place of the Split Sky, lies on the banks of the Usumacinto river in what is now Guatemala. The city was constructed in phases between 400- 800 AD by successive Maya rulers, among them Lord Shield Jaguar and his son Lord Bird Jaguar, who reigned during the seventh and eights centuries AD. Among the buildings in Yaxchilan are two structures (23 and 21) which contain a series of limestone panels commemorating the accession rituals of these two rulers.

Each panel formed the upper lintel of a doorway, so that participants in the ritual passed beneath them. Two sets of these lintels are on display in the gallery at the British Museum, while one set remains in Mexico at the Museum of Anthropology.

Maya rulers summoned deities to oversee events such as their enthronement, the dedication of temples and monuments, and their military campaigns. The gods sanctioned the monarch's actions and conveyed their divine power to human affairs. The first carving, Lintel 24, depicts Lord Shield Jaguar and his principal wife Lady Xoc engaged in a bloodletting rite that took place on October 28, 709 AD. The king stands on the left brandishing a flaming torch to illuminate the drama that is about to unfold. Kneeling in front of him wearing an exquisitely woven huipil, Land Xoc pulls a thorn-lined rope through her tongue. The rope falls onto a woven basket holding blood-soaked strips of paper cloth.

On the second lintel from Structure 23 at Yaxchalin, the sacrificial offering of blood conjures up a visionary manifestation of Yat-Balam, founding ancestor of the dynasty of Yaxchilan. In the guise of a warrior grasping a spear and shield, this ancestral spirit emerges from the gaping front jaws of a huge double-headed serpent rearing above Lady-Xoc. She gazes upward at the aspiration she has brought forth. In her left hand she bears a blood-letting bowl containing instruments of sacrifice, a sting-ray spine and an obsidian lancet.

The third lentil 15 repeats the bloodletting in lintel 25. The serpent coils up through a beaded blood scroll and from its mouth emerges the ancestor whom the Lady has contacted in the rite. British Museum, Mexico about 2000 BC-1500s, Room 27.

Psychedelics and Jungian Principles

Can You Bear It?

Murray Stein

> "You are aware of only one unrest;
> Oh, never learn to know the other!
> Two souls, alas, are dwelling in my breast,
> And one is striving to forsake its brother."

(Goethe, *Faust*, Pt. 1: 1110-14)

Can psychedelics advance individuation? If so, how? And can they be used in conjunction with analysis? In these questions, there are many issues to consider. Two important ones are:

1. The patient's history and present ego-functioning. Do they support the judgment that ego strength is sufficient is to bear the influx of powerful unconscious material that can potentially be unleashed by psychedelic substances? Normally in analysis the unconscious appears in the form of dreams, waking visions or fantasies, and in projected contents that can be processed and made conscious. This work is done gradually and carried out over extended periods of time. There is time to process the unconscious material as it emerges naturally and spontaneously in these forms. There are of course exceptions such as psychotic breaks, panic attacks, and other borderline episodes. In working with these unconscious materials, the psyche's defenses are respected because they exist for a good reason, namely to protect a fragile ego structure. The process of making unconscious material conscious is gradual

and attuned to the natural flow of material as it becomes available. The analyst has the opportunity to observe the patient's capacities to integrate unconscious material gradually over an extended period of time. At some point, the analyst is able to form an opinion of the patient's ego capacities for receiving archetypal material and being able to use it for constructive integrative purposes. The decision could then be made to advance the process of individuation through use of psychedelic substances of one kind or another if there seemed to be a good reason for this. What these reasons might be can be discussed, and there will be differing opinions based on clinical considerations.

2. The second large issue to consider is what is latent in the unconscious of the patient. This content could be positive or negative, benign or malignant, relatively mild or extremely powerful. Answering this question is more difficult than answering the first. How is the analyst to know "what rough beast is slouching to Bethlehem to be born?" We recall Jung's story of a physician who came to him for analysis because he wanted to train and become a psychoanalyst himself. The initial dream warned Jung that he should not pursue this path, and he consequently advised him to stay away from delving further into the unconscious. Jung spotted a latent psychosis in his personality. This man's ego would not be fit to bear the onslaught of the unconscious even though his conscious functioning looked quite normal on the surface. "I had caught him in the nick of time," Jung writes, "for the latent psychosis was within a hair's breadth of breaking out and becoming manifest. This had to be prevented" (Jung, 1961, p. 136). This was Jung's clinical judgment. This man would not have been a suitable candidate for a psychedelic experience.

In what follows I will use some myths and literary references to discuss the possible outcomes of opening the conscious mind to the depths of the unconscious through the use of psychedelics, assuming this is what psychedelics do. My comments revolve around the two questions asked above: How much can the patient bear? And what might the patient have to bear as a result of a "breakthrough" of archetypal content into the world of ego-consciousness due to psychedelics? In considering these questions, I take my lead from Jung's description of Mercurius as the "spirit of the unconscious."

The first story is both cautionary and promising, and it is certainly familiar to students of Jung (CW 13, §§ 239-249). It is the famous Brothers Grimm Fairy Tale, "The Spirit in the Glass Bottle." A young woodcutter hears a voice calling out deep in the forest, begging to be released from captivity. Looking around, he discovers that the voice comes from a sealed bottle in the roots of an oak tree, whereupon he excavates it and takes out the stopper. Immediately, a spirit springs forth, grows into a giant monster, and threatens to break his neck. In this moment of crisis and loss of control of the situation, the young man is able to keep his wits about him and address the threatening spirit. The spirit announces himself to be Mercurius, and a dialogue ensues. Had the young man panicked, he would have been lost. He had a strong enough ego to face the threat of annihilation rationally, and instead of freaking out he was able to trick the spirit back into the bottle. We do not know why he had this ego capacity except that he had some education thanks to his poor father's sacrifice. This must have given him the confidence to confront Mercurius so effectively. (The story reminds me of Jung arguing and debating with the figures he conjures up in his active imagination as recorded in *The Red Book*.) Mercurius improbably shows himself in this story to be quite stupid and easily tricked. After being imprisoned now for the second time, Mercurius offers his magical powers to the woodcutter and promises not to injure him if he will release him again. Astonishingly, the young man trusts him and again releases him. Is this an example of "second naiveté?" With the gift of Mercurius, the woodcutter is enabled to complete his university studies, and after a time he becomes "the most famous doctor in the world" (Zipes, p. 367).

The brilliantly successful outcome of this story depends on two factors: the ego strength of the protagonist and the cooperation of the spirit of the unconscious (Mercurius). Within the context of our discussion, this would be the case of an individual with a well-enough developed ego who is thereby able to extract maximum benefit from a psychedelic experience even if the experience was frightening and threatening at first. Being able to put Mercurius back in the bottle and then carrying on further negotiations with him is an essential move to be able to make in order to achieve this success. There is a release, loss of control, recovery, and further dialogue out of which the transcendent function, i.e., an ongoing relationship, is established. I have known of such cases, and the testimony they offer is quite convincing. The psychedelic drug opened a bottled-up unconscious spirit that gave them a new direction in life, which in the long run was a blessing to themselves and others. They became physicians of the soul and indeed some became quite famous and successful within their professional contexts. The cases of successful outcome that I know of personally did not take the psychedelic drug as part of an analysis, however, but rather as part of a social scene they were in at the time. Later they worked on the experience within the context of analysis and deepened the relationship between ego and the unconscious through the use of dream work and active imagination.

A more complex example is the case of Goethe's poetic character, Faust. While this story also ends well for the protagonist, the routes it takes are much more convoluted and ambiguous. The spirit of the unconscious here is, like Mercurius, a potentially destructive force named Mephistopheles, who brings a whole new direction into the stale life of the scholar Faust, but at a high price. This is to say that the psychedelic experience may have a life-changing effect on a person, but even at its best and most productive the outcome may turn out to be ambiguous morally and psychologically. It leads to a sharp departure from the conventional life, but to what extent does this instigate greater individuation in the sense of integration of the opposites and achievement of psychological wholeness?

The poem opens with Faust in his study, utterly bored with books and academic learning. He is burned out. He has reached the limit of knowledge as offered in his extensive library, and he longs for direct knowledge and experience of the mysteries. About such matters, Jung would agree with Faust, "the intellectuals know nothing… for intellectuals know neither themselves nor people as they really are" (Jung, 1979, p. vi). So Faust, like Jung, looks to esoteric traditions and opens a book by Nostradamus, where he comes upon some mystical symbols. These will offer him a psychedelic-like experience by opening the windows to the spirits of the unconscious.

First, he conjures the spirit of the air, a high spiritual agency, but this figure is beyond his reach. He cannot do anything with it. This is sometimes the case with psychedelic experience: it is too distant from consciousness to dialogue or engage with consciously. Next, he conjures the spirit of the earth, who appears to him vividly and shows him the wonders of the invisible world. To this spirit Faust responds enthusiastically, and in a kind of feverish attitude he attempts to claim identity with this spirit. He wants to live in the world of this vision, one with the spirit, but the spirit rejects him abruptly telling him he is projecting: "Du gleichst dem Geist, den du begreifst,/ Nicht mir!" ("You resemble the spirit you understand, not me!") (Goethe, 512-513, my translation). Whereupon the spirit exits and leaves Faust abandoned and devastated: "I am not like the gods! That was a painful thrust;/ I'm like the worm that burrows in the dust" (Goethe, 652-653). Faust feels bitter and humiliated, and in this mood he is tempted to commit suicide. "Why is that bottle as a magnet to my eyes?" (Goethe, 687), he cries out as he is drawn to the poisonous liquid. This is the outcome of his encounter with the spirit of the unconscious, Mercurius. The return to ego reality is too painful for Faust to bear.

This is similar to the condition of a young man who came to me for analysis after having had a devastating experience after taking a dose of LSD. His story was that under the influence of the drug he had heard the voice of God judging him to be sinful and unworthy. This harsh and final judgment was repeated several times. He could not defend himself or speak up. He was left in Hell. This was a depression similar to Faust's, and he also contemplated suicide. Although he was no longer suicidal when I saw him, he had not recovered his former agency even after several years. He was living at home with his mother, isolated, dejected, and unable to face the world. Unlike the clever woodcutter, he had not been able to benefit from his encounter with the spirit of the unconscious. With Faust, he could cry out: "I'm like a worm that burrows in the dust,/ Who, as he makes of dust his meager meal,/ Is crushed and buried by a wanderer's heel" (Goethe, 653-655). He was left bereft, abandoned on the shores of an inhospitable and meaningless world. The ego was not able to handle the accusation of a powerful archetypal figure unleashed by the drug. No doubt, this judgmental God resident in his unconscious was present and ready to pounce on him because of his earlier personal history. Had he been in analysis, perhaps precautions would have been put in place and work done in the usual analytic fashion to bring this complex to consciousness in a more gradual way that would have allowed the fragile ego to deal with it in a less traumatizing way.

Following the story of Faust further, we find him somewhat recovered from his suicidal depression after hearing the church bells ringing during Easter celebrations. The atmosphere of traditional religious ritual has rescued him from the abyss of despair, temporarily at least, and once again he can tolerate life in the temporal world. This represents a kind of therapeutic intervention. It makes life in the temporal world tolerable. But the previous breach in the fragile membrane between this world and the archetypal unconscious has left an opening, and now the spirit of the unconscious in the form of a playful poodle enters and follows him home. This is Mephistopheles in disguise. This time the spirit stays around, and indeed offers Faust an experience of a kind he has not known before:

> Right in this hour you will obtain
> More for your senses than you gain
> In a whole year's monotony
> What tender spirits now will sing,
> The lovely pictures that they bring
> Are not mere magic for the eye:
> They will delight your sense of smell,
> Be pleasing to your taste as well,
> Excite your touch, and give you joy. (Goethe, 1436-1444)

This sounds like the drug, Ecstasy! But again, this experience leaves Faust depressed when it's over and Mephistopheles departs:

> Betrayed again? Fooled by a scheme?
> Should spirits' wealth so suddenly decay
> That I behold the Devil in a dream,
> And that a poodle jumps away? (Goethe, 1526-1529)

Mephistopheles resembles what Jung describes as Mercurius, the "archetype of the unconscious" (Jung, CW 13, § 299). He is the shadow personality of the Christian-dominated consciousness of Dr. Faust, and as such he "tempts us out into the world of sense: he is the *benedicta viriditas* and the *multi flores* of early spring, a god of illusion and delusion of whom it is right said: 'Invenitur in vena / Sanguine plena' (He is found in the vein swollen with blood)" (Jung, CW 13, § 299). Mephistopheles will eventually draw Faust out of his scholar's library into a new life filled with all manner of activity and pleasure in exchange for his soul upon his death. Faust accepts the offer because he does not believe in the afterlife so he has nothing to lose, he thinks. From this point in the story forward, Mephistopheles takes the lead in Faust's furiously paced individuation journey.

Does psychedelic exposure have this effect of unleashing individuation in a stuck and moribund personality trapped in personal and cultural complexes? Individuation as we understand it requires making contact with the spirit of the unconscious and cooperating with it in a joint venture. We speak of forging a transcendent function, a link between the higher functions of the psyche—rational thinking, reflection, ethics, ideals—and the irrational shadow personality with its emotional depths, intuitions and psychological complexities.

This relationship that Faust finds himself in with Mephistopheles is a kind of transcendent function. The linkage that is established does not break during Faust's lifetime. The unconscious spirit, in the form of Mephistopheles, takes him into experiences of life that had been unknown previously. A whole new world opens to him as he is led from one adventure to another. Mephistopheles is both his guide and protector. It is clear that Faust's life experience is greatly expanded and enriched through the guidance of this devilish companion. Mephistopheles incites Eros and releases his sexuality; he introduces him to other physical pleasures and opens the way to the pursuit of power and fame; he even makes possible the numinous encounter with the archetypal anima figure, Helen, the most beautiful woman in history, and a mystical *coniunctio* with her produces a charming divine child. However, tragedy and guilt follow on the heels of his conquests: the child he gives to Gretchen, his first conquest, is murdered, and she is imprisoned and dies by suicide; his child with Helen, the bold Euphorion, flies too high, crashes and dies at their feet, whereupon Helen leaves him and returns to her home in the Underworld.

Faust's life finally ends at the age of 100 in a burst of creativity, an idealistic land reclamation project that is meant to set up a new garden of Eden for the people. But this turns out to cost the lives of the innocent couple, Philemon and Baucis. Faust has become a deluded visionary, all the while enabled by the spirit Mephistopheles who is biding his time in anticipation of taking Faust's soul with him to Hell. Is this the endpoint of living under the guidance of the spirit of the unconscious? Does the psychedelic road lead to this result?

We know from the Prologue in Heaven at the beginning of Goethe's poem, which he called his life's work, that the Lord God is present throughout, invisible but in ultimate control of Faust's fate. The Self has empowered the archetypal shadow personality manifested in Mephistopheles to have access to the ego (Faust), to give the ego what it unconsciously wishes for—pleasure, power, recognition. Mephistopheles opens the door to experience. Faust had been trapped in words and texts and had no access to the spirits he studied and wrote about. In the end and with the help of Mephistopheles, Faust's was not a particularly happy life, but it was a rich one and full of experience of all kinds. We could say that his opening initially to the unconscious when he consulted the book of symbols etched by Nostradamus and conjured the spirit of the unconscious—his first psychedelic experience—led ultimately to a connection with the spirit of the unconscious (Mercurius), which made possible a rich and multifaceted individuation process that would not been possible had he remained true to his one-sided scholarly vocation. In the end, the pact with Mephistopheles to have Faust's soul upon his death was annulled by the Lord God who sent his angels to escort his soul to Heaven. Despite being burdened by sin, guilt, and tragedy, Faust was lifted up to the realms of Divinity and achieved wholeness, perhaps because he felt remorse for the pain he had caused others in his furious quest for life and continuous action.

The question I am asking is: Can you bear it? The two instances I have referenced—the woodcutter in the Grimm's fairytale and Faust in Goethe's poem—have been able, due either to good enough ego structure (the woodcutter) or to the help of the Self (Faust). The onslaughts of the unconscious spirit (Mercurius, Mephistopheles) were strong but not too much for them, and in the end they benefited from the connection to the spirit.

Another example of a mythical figure who could bear it is the Virgin Mary. She experiences a visitation by an angel who announces her future. This is a visitation from the spirit, not Mercurius this time but the spirit of the Lord, another dimension but no less dangerous for the unprepared. She will bear a son who will totally determine her destiny. She can bear it. She is a figure who can give birth to the spirit and endure the consequences of this visitation to the end, when she is, like Faust, transported to the Heavens by an angelic company. This would be an instance of a breakthrough from the unconscious that changes one's life course, installs an individuation process, and results in both suffering and exaltation. Sometimes a psychedelic experience can open the way to such a development. It depends on the nature of the content breaking through (in Mary's case, the divine Logos, an archetypal animus) and on the stability of the ego that receives the annunciation. Mary also had the helpful assistance of a good husband, Joseph, who supported her individuation process despite its unfavorable appearance to collective gossip.

A counterexample to the Virgin Mary is the story of Coronis who attracts Apollo and is impregnated by him. This is a numinous psychedelic-like breakthrough experience for the young woman, but she is not faithful to her divine lover and sleeps with a human partner. In other words, she does not take her encounter with Apollo seriously enough and becomes distracted by other interests. When Apollo discovers this, he asks his sister, Artemis, to kill Coronis, which the faithful sister does in due course. Apollo then intervenes and rescues the fetus, who later becomes the great healer, Asclepius, who learns the arts of healer from his father, Apollo, and the centaur, Chiron. The ego could not bear the child of her Olympian lover and was destroyed because of her infidelity. Nevertheless, the child born of this union of conscious and unconscious archetypal spirit did survive thanks to his heavenly father. And something new and humanly helpful came out of this encounter between conscious and unconscious. One thinks of great authors and artists like Nietzsche who have created masterworks but died at an early age because they could not bear the burden of their grandiose visions.

Individuation requires linking up the ego with the unconscious personality, an inner daimon. Jung speaks often of his two personalities, number one and number two. The relationship between them was worked out of the course of the *Red Book* experience and continued in a fashion throughout the rest of Jung's life. There was an astonishing moment at Jung's spontaneous lecture at Eranos in 1939 on the topic of Rebirth. Suddenly he paused and, referencing Castor and Pollux, declared: "We are that pair of Dioscuri, one of whom is mortal and the other immortal, and who, though always together, can never be made completely one" (Jung, CW 9i, § 235). We all have an inner divine other, and "we are comforted with that inner friend or foe, and whether he is our friend or our foe depends on ourselves" (Jung, CW 9i, § 235).

Castor and Pollux (the first mortal, the second immortal) were born to Leda as twins but had different fathers (Tyndareus and Zeus), a case of heteropaternal superfecundation. These brothers get along very well, work and play together, and in the end Castor is also immortalized and they become the Gemini in the astrological skies. I believe Jung's relationship with Philemon was of this order, largely cooperative and playful. This relationship with his inner immortal other gave Jung the presence of a great individual, which was attested by so many who knew him. However, Jung also often spoke of his personality number two as a daimon, one who bequeathed on him a strong obligation to carry out projects that seemed beyond his capacities. He suffered from the relationship with his transcendent Other, but he also created his greatest works because of this relationship. In Jung's case, this relationship came about through the practice of active imagination, not psychedelic drugs. About the latter, Jung was cautious and warned people that the breakthroughs elicited by these substances would bring heavy obligations in their train. To bear these obligations and fulfill their requirements would be the task of a lifelong journey, of individuation.

So the question is: Can you bear it?

References

Goethe, J.W. von. (1963). *Faust*. Translated and with an introduction by Walter Kaufman. Anchor Books.

Jung, C.G. (1961). *Memories, dreams, reflections*. Aniela Jaffé (Ed.). R. & C. Winston (Trans.). Vintage Books.

Jung, C.G. (1979). 'Foreword', in J. Jaffé, *Apparitions*. (pp. v-vii). Spring Publications.

Zipes, J. (Trans.) (1987). *The complete fairy tales of the Brothers Grimm*. Bantam Books.

Psychedelics: Another Tool in Analytical Work?

Aurea Afonso Caetano

"Our way of looking at things is conditioned by what we are... All psychology has the character of a subjective confession, mine included..." (Jung, 1961, pp. 134-138)

In our increasingly rationalistic and pragmatic culture, where market demands impose themselves, the question of the effectiveness of psychotherapy has become more important every day. The financial equation, expressed through the cost-benefit binomial, has been prevalent; it is evident that issues regarding the various costs associated with "mental illnesses" are so significant that they have been widely discussed in various global economic forums.

I consider it relevant to present some data that justify the importance and necessity of discussing the inclusion of a new tool in our already extensive therapeutic arsenal. Despite being a Jungian analyst and therefore more inclined to work with dreams, images, amplifications, and numinous experiences in the therapeutic relationship, I believe that objective data can facilitate and expand our clinical practice.

The costs associated with mental illnesses have been increasing worldwide, and even more intensely in recent years. In 2013, the U.S. government estimated that forty-four million Americans, out of a population of approximately 325 million, suffered from some form of mental illness, with anxiety and depression being the most common.

The World Health Organization (WHO) is an agency within the United Nations system that aims to direct and coordinate international health efforts. In May 2013, 194 health ministers adopted the World Health Organization's "Mental Health Action Plan," recognizing mental health as a priority for global health and committing to taking action to mitigate this problem. The issue of mental health was also extensively discussed at the World Innovation Summit for Health (WISH) in Qatar in 2013. It is estimated that in 2010, approximately 10% of the global population suffered from some form of mental illness, making it a matter of general importance (Patel & Saxena, 2014).

According to a study published by the Lancet Commission (neurocaregroup.com, 2023), the direct and indirect costs associated with this type of illness have been increasing considerably, with projected expenses of over sixteen trillion dollars between 2011 and 2030, related both to treatment and the impact of individuals with mental illnesses leaving the workforce. This cost already exceeds the amount spent on individuals with cancer, diabetes, or heart disease. This subject is so important that it has been a topic of discussion in recent World Economic Forums held annually in Davos, Switzerland. In 2020, mental health care was recognized as a social and economic imperative.

'The call for investment received attention for a very good reason: current mental health funding levels are woefully inadequate. In 2015, global funding for development assistance for health was estimated at $36 billion. Of that, only $110 million went toward mental health." (WHO, 2023)

Mental health is a lot more than the absence of illness: "it is an intrinsic part of our individual and collective health and well-being." As this "World Mental Health Report" shows, to achieve the global objectives set out in the WHO's "Comprehensive mental health action plan 2013–2030" and the Sustainable Development Goals, "we need to transform our attitudes, actions and approaches to promote and protect mental health, and to provide and care for those in need" (WHO, 2023).

In the 2022 report, presented and analyzed the most recent data on global mental health. The numbers figures show that there are 970 million people living with mental disorders worldwide, of whom 52.4% are women and 47.6% men. Among this population, 31% experience anxiety disorders, 28% suffer from depression, 11.1% have developmental disorders, 8.8% have ADHD spectrum disorders, while the remaining portion is divided among bipolar and conduct disorders (4.1% each), autism spectrum disorders (2.9%), schizophrenia (2.5%), and eating disorders (1.4%).

> As the world comes to live with, and learn from, the far-reaching effects of the COVID-19 pandemic, we must all reflect on one of its most striking aspects – the huge toll it has taken on people's mental health. "Rates of already-common conditions such as depression and anxiety went up by more than 25% in the first year of the pandemic, adding to the nearly one billion people who were already living with a mental disorder." (WHO, 2023)

In health economics, there are two types of assessment. The first refers to the costs associated with the disease, which can be direct (related directly to the treatment of the disease) and indirect (all other costs related to the impact of the disease, such as loss of income, absenteeism from work, early retirement, violence, and premature mortality). The second concerns the economic or cost-benefit assessment, which involves comparing two or more treatment options and the benefits they can bring; there is a triad that always involves the choice between available alternatives (comparability), the benefits obtained (greater than the costs), and user preference (Razzouk, 2013).

The collection of such data raises important questions. The first is: what is considered a mental illness? Criteria such as those described in the DSMs help us define this issue in objective terms, but they are not without controversy. Furthermore, what is the most cost-effective (or cost-benefit optimal) way to help individuals who are experiencing psychological distress, have received a diagnosis, or are facing difficulties in their integration into the world and job market to, as soon as possible, return to their so-called normal and productive functioning?

> Therapeutic effectiveness has become a fundamental criterion in a biotechnical and pragmatic culture. The effectiveness of a treatment is measured by its ability to make the individual return to normality as quickly as possible in order to perform their social functions. (Bastos, 2002; my translation)

This is a part of the discussion; the other equally important part relates to how we Jungian analysts define an individual experiencing psychological distress and what a trajectory toward normal, productive functioning means to us. Or yet, what is normal and what is pathological? Are these boundaries clear to all of us? How evident are these limits?

Advancements in genetic studies, particularly in the field of epigenetics, show us that the old distinction between nature and culture should be disregarded—among many other traditional polarities, this one also seems to have fallen to the ground (or rather, it seems to have been transcended, to use Jungian terminology). We know that the development of an organism occurs through constant interaction between the genotype it carries and the experiences it has with the sociocultural milieu in which it lives. Genetic influences and the environment are interrelated and determine development; environmental influences can determine, restrain, or enhance the expression of developmental processes, but they do not unilaterally determine them (Konner, 2013). How can we talk about mental illness?

Personal Equation or How We Work

Jung's great openness and curiosity for everything related to nature and human nature is clearly reflected in his own words: "I am a man; I consider nothing human to be alien to me" (Jung, CW 18, § 91, n. 10). This understanding of human nature pervades Jung's life and work. We call this the *Jungian Attitude* and it is the attitude that reflects our experience in our work as analysts. This attitude postulates totality and diversity, the existence of a relationship between the psyche and a world that is alive and indissoluble. In the words of Brazilian analyst Roberto Gambini, "Jung is attitude" (Casement, 2007, p. 363).

> The Jungian attitude explores the object, thought or image in a movement known as *'circumambulation.'* This circular exploration favours the knowledge or acknowledgement of multifarious aspects of the same reality, providing a deeper and more comprehensive understanding that opens us to a world of multiplicity, complexity and nonlinearity. Based on the concept of psychic energy, Jung talks about the importance of movement and thus proposes that pathology is an expression of lack of fluidity, a rigidity. (Caetano, 2018)

Psychotherapy, as we know it today, originated within the context of medicine as an activity with scientific aspirations. Sigmund Freud, a trained neurologist, initially worked in the laboratories of brain physiology and anatomy and later took up a position at the general hospital, where he encountered cases of hysteria, which were commonly diagnosed at that time.

Carl Jung, who had a degree in psychiatry, began his work as a physician treating patients at the Burghölzli psychiatric hospital in Zurich. It was at this institution that he started using the word association test for diagnosing psychiatric disorders.

From the early stages of his work, Jung proposed what would become a significant paradigm shift: both the patient and the therapist are equally affected in the analytical process. The working duo consists of two human beings engaged in constant conscious and unconscious interaction. The person or personality of the therapist is just as important as that of the patient in this work. According to him: "For two personalities to meet is like mixing two different chemical substances: if there is any combination at all, both are transformed" (CW 16, § 163).

We know how important the concept of personal equation was to Jung. In his view, the personality of the therapist was more important than the technique. His commentary on the Chinese text of *The Secret of the Golden Flower* reads:

> In reality, everything depends on the man and little or nothing on the method. The method is merely the path, the direction taken by a man: the way he acts is the true expression of his nature. If it ceases to be this, the method is nothing more than an affectation.... (CW 13, § 4)

Throughout his work, Jung emphasized and reaffirmed the impossibility of developing a singular method of work; the way he constructed his theory over time is clear evidence of the profound exercise of his personal equation.

Latterly adopted by Jung, the term personal equation "became the leitmotif of the pretension of complex psychology to be a superordinate science, the only discipline capable of encompassing the subjective factor held to underlie all the sciences" (Shamdasani, 2003, pp. 30-31).

Each of us has a different viewpoint shaped by the relationship between our individual reality and the collective, the conscious and the unconscious, our subjectivity, and the objective level of reality. Through his study of psychological types, Jung concluded: "the insight that every judgment made by an individual is conditioned by his personality type and that every point of view is necessarily relative" (Jung, 1961, p. 183).

According to Jung, there is a living and indissociable relationship between the psyche and the world; there is totality as well as diversity. "For Jung, the idea of totality is intrinsically associated with a dynamic and systemic view of the being and the world, in which the parts interrelate in a compensatory and complementary manner within a single whole" (Penna, 2013, p. 138; my translation).

This viewpoint of the human being that gives meaning to the world is also the viewpoint of the analyst, who, in the relationship with their patient, seeks the meaning of that experience. According to Jung, "Our psychology is therefore an eminently practical science. It does not investigate for investigation's sake but for the immediate purpose of giving help" (CW 17, § 172). And also, "I have set up neither a system nor a general theory, but have merely formulated auxiliary concepts to serve me as tools as is customary in every branch of science" (CW 18, § 1507).

Papadopoulos, when discussing the issue of the personal myth, states:

> As Jung believed that each person should strive to discover their own personal myth, Jungian analysts should do the same, and the foundation of their theoretical and clinical approach should be their own unique and individual personal myth. Therefore... paradoxically, anyone who calls themselves "Jungian" is essentially not following Jung's message and therefore cannot be called Jungian. (1998, p. 165)

Each of us therapists with a Jungian orientation use specific techniques in our work. Each of us, in our own way, according to our personal equation, not only chooses but also creates techniques or tools that facilitate our clinical work. The objective of each technique is to facilitate access to and relationship with unconscious material in order to achieve greater integration of all aspects of the psyche. To bring the unconscious into consciousness, to establish a healthy dialogic relationship that allows for transformation, and the healing of the symptoms afflicting our patients.

A survey conducted in Brazil in 2015 with therapists of Jungian orientation obtained a total of 282 valid responses. One of the questions raised in this study, among others, pertains to the techniques employed by each therapist. Working with dreams is one of the oldest and most commonly used techniques in our practice: 98.23% of the participants in the survey stated that they use this technique in their clinical work. Dreams, as Jung and Freud stated, are "the royal road to the unconscious" (Freud, 1900/1973). For Jung, dreams are symbolic in that they arise from the relationship between the conscious and the unconscious. The interpretation of dreams and of all symbolic material is one way to approach the contents of the unconscious. Another way is through amplification, which aims to both make explicit and amplify what is revealed by the dreamer's unconscious. While dream interpretation allows individuals to engage with their personal context, amplification provides the opportunity to shed light on and amplify the content of symbolic material, not only dreams. It involves the association with universal images, thereby elucidating what could be a collective or common content for all of humankind.

Another way of establishing this dialogue is through the technique of active imagination, a kind of dreaming with open eyes, where a conversation between consciousness and the unconscious takes place. 50% of the participants in this survey reported using this tool. Through this technique, consciousness or the conscious ego actively connects to an image or images that emerge and allows the inner images to flow by merely following them. The active nature of active imagination refers to the way the ego intervenes in the imagination and its capacity to interact in a controlling, modifying and transformative manner in the imaginative event. In this way, aspects of the unconscious can be integrated into consciousness. Jung's most fundamental ideas emerged from his experiences with active imagination.

> ... [T]he model of symbolic formation described by Jung can be experienced in Active Imagination: the unconscious emerges, is perceived and assimilated, and when in dialogue with consciousness, with the awakened ego, both the conscious and the unconscious undergo changes; this can be observed in symbols in transformation as well as in new symbolic formations. (Kast, 1991, p. 190)

Painting, sculpting, expressive techniques in general can be possible tools to facilitate the conversation between the conscious ego and the contents that arise from the unconscious. The objective is always and once again to facilitate the exchange and to increase the possibility of transit between unconscious contents and consciousness, thus promoting psychic transformation. Once the conscious-unconscious flow is improved and dialogue is established, the creative relationship between the various aspects of the psyche can occur. This technique is used by 63.83% of the therapists who responded to the survey.

Sandplay therapy, used by 24.47% of the participants in this survey, has also been increasingly employed by Jungian analysts. It involves the possibility of non-verbal processing that takes place through the creation of scenes in a sand tray. Several studies demonstrating its effectiveness have been published, and analysts often work exclusively with this technique without the need to verbalize or put into words what is being placed and experienced there.

A meta-analysis conducted by the American Psychoanalytic Association (2014) describes some active ingredients for the success of psychotherapy. Clinicians, researchers, and theorists have concluded that the therapist-patient relationship is one of the most important factors for the success of psychotherapy. This meta-analysis of 79 studies shows a significant correlation between therapeutic alliance and favorable psychotherapeutic outcomes. It also emphasizes the importance of using specific techniques as active ingredients in psychotherapy to help patients make changes within themselves and in their lives (Smith-Hansen, 2014).

Jung Now?

As he was more concerned with the expansion of his knowledge than with the reaffirmation of his discoveries, Jung continued until the end of his life to be an avid researcher, willing to broaden his field of interest, revise his theory whenever confronted with new data, and explore new possibilities of understanding. This open-minded attitude led him to consider the existence of a Jungian school to be inadequate. He once stated: "I want people to be, above all else, themselves. 'Isms' are the viruses of our time, responsible for disasters greater than those caused by any medieval plague or pestilence" (Post, 1992, p. 12).

One cannot help but think of the relevance of this statement in today's world. Jung already perceived the fundamentalist and rigid quality of all schools, religions and groups organized around a central idea. In them, the individual human being becomes enmeshed and confused with the group and their freedom of functioning is deeply compromised. The emphasis placed on the importance of recognizing one's personal myth corresponds to the need for integral and authentic expression. Only that which holds true meaning for the individual in question can be real, and only an individual aligned with their deepest expression can be authentic.

For Jung, his own theories and formulations were always "suggestions and attempts to formulate a new scientific psychology based, in the first place, on immediate experience with human beings" (Jung, 1961, p. 143). He elucidated two of his most fundamental concerns in this account: the attempt to conceive of a psychology rooted in scientific principles, and the understanding of direct experience—contact with one's inner reality—as a form of knowledge. In other words, there is no possible knowledge without considering the whole personality. So-called scientific knowledge must account for the individual viewpoint or introspection that underlies every and any scientific viewpoint.

Therefore, it is impossible to consider Jungian theory, and even more so any current Jungian practice, outside the personal context of the psychotherapist in question. Furthermore, it is not possible to conceive of a theory detached from the cultural context of its time.

Samuels states that we are still developing Jung's radical proposal regarding the need to create a culturally sensitive psychology. According to him: "... Jung was perhaps the first to anticipate the ethical and political disaster of a one-size-fits-all, colonial psychology. Hence, he is one of the founding fathers of transcultural and intercultural psychotherapy" (2014, p. 625).

Jungian analysis explores the processes that occur in the encounter between two individuals, and each encounter is unique. We are simultaneously unique as therapists and equal to the clients we see; various aspects of our personality can be constellated as each process is unique.

Therefore, we can say along with Jung that each new case requires pioneering work, and routine proves to be a blind alley. The tasks of psychotherapy challenge not only our understanding and sympathy but the whole human being (Hopcke, 1995). "The doctor is inclined to demand this total effort from his patient, yet he must realize that this same demand only works if he is aware that it applies also to himself" (CW 16, § 367).

In our daily work, we evoke memories; in our interaction with others, we assign new meaning to our experiences, we reshape mental configurations, and in doing so we reconstruct not only the mental landscape but also our neural landscape. It seems that psychodynamic therapists often struggle to recognize the materiality of our work, the constant labor in the relationship with our patients that transforms our experiences, regardless of the level at which they occur. In our everyday lives, we seek to expand consciousness and reshape patterns, and we do so through the affective exchanges that we now understand to be the foundation of the architecture that structures the functioning of every human being.

We do not know, however, what the best path to follow is, what is right or wrong, good or bad for the patient with whom we engage. We are always in search of exchange; psychic development, at whatever level it happens, takes place in the wholeness of being.

One of the questions we seek to answer in our research is related to the individual's relationship with theory. In other words, how we therapists with a Jungian orientation construct and solidify our theoretical framework, and how we apply it in our daily work. Reflecting on this also involves figuring out what our personal myths are and what pathways we choose to follow toward our individuality as therapists with a Jungian orientation.

The discussion regarding the use of psychedelics in Jungian analysis fits into this paradigm. To find and express one's personal myth is also to give meaning to Jung's theory and to continue the exploration to reach a place that is both an end and a new beginning in the process of being a therapist—a whole and unique professional with each of their patients, thinking and employing the best possible tool for each case.

What about Psychedelics?

"If the doors of perception were cleansed everything would appear to man as it is, infinite." (William Blake, *The Marriage Between Heaven and Hell*, 1793)

From an etymological perspective, the term *psychedelic* is a composition of two other words of Greek origin: *psykhe* (ψυχή), which means *mind* or *soul*; and *deloun* (δηλοῦν), which means *to make visible* or *to manifest*. It is important to note that the Greek word *psykhe* carries a similar connotation to the German word *geist*, which is usually translated as *spirit* and can be understood in the Platonic sense of *essence,* or as an invisible principle that supports and gives meaning to life (Guia do Psiconauta, 2016). The term mainly indicates the potential for experiences of self-knowledge.

The origin of the term traces back to the letters exchanged between Humphry Osmond, a British psychiatrist and one of the pioneers in studying the use of LSD as an adjunct in the treatment of various pathologies, and Aldous Huxley, who, as we know, had already experimented with mescaline and later with LSD. In one of these letters, while discussing what the best term would be, Huxley sends a rhyme along with his suggestion: "To make this trivial world sublime, take half a gram of phanerothyme. To fathom Hell or soar angelic, just take a pinch of psychedelic" (Bisbee et al., 2018).

Almost a year after this letter, Osmond published in the *Annals of the New York Academy of Sciences* the name he had chosen for that class of substances and the reasons that led him to that term.

> I have tried to find an appropriate name for the agents under discussion: a name that will include the concepts of enriching the mind and enlarging the vision... My choice, because it is clear, euphonious, and uncontaminated by other associations, is psychedelic, mind manifesting. (Osmond, 1957)

Despite the term's initial association with LSD experiments, it was mescaline, not LSD, that served as the prototype hallucinogen capable of triggering ecstatic and visionary experiences, at least until the early 1940s. The pharmacological properties of mescaline, which alter the state of consciousness, had been known since the early days of the Spanish conquest and colonization of Mexico. Furthermore, mescaline not only appealed to scientists, artists, and intellectuals, but also fostered an increasingly close, intimate, and extensive contact between them (Ribeiro, 2020).

Close to the turn of the 20th century, Louis Lewin, a brilliant German pharmacologist, came into contact with the peyote cactus during a trip to the United States and began studying its psychoactive properties. Later, Lewin expanded upon the botanical-psychoactive classification devised by Linnaeus (considered the father of taxonomy) and proposed a new nomenclature: *euphorica*, for opioid substances; *inebriantia*, for alcoholic beverages; *excitantia*, for stimulants in general; *hypnotica*, for sedatives that emerged during that time, like chloral hydrate; and *phantastica*, for hallucinogenic substances.

By creating the term *phantastica*, to which mescaline served as a kind of prototype, Lewin sought to emphasize the pharmacological properties capable of sharpening the senses to the point of distorting them into dream-like illusions, without compromising the level of consciousness or critical awareness of the ongoing psychic alteration. It is quite different from the term *hallucinogenic*, which refers to the appearance of images devoid of a real object with a complete absence of critical awareness of such distortions—a situation rarely (if ever) observed with this class of substances.

Each person with their own personality, through their individual work, confessing their subjectivity. One of the earliest accounts of LSD being used as a supplementary tool in psychotherapy among us Jungians comes from Dr. Ronald Arthur Sandison. He was born in 1916, started his pre-clinical studies in 1934 and qualified with a MBBS in London in 1940. In 1945, he became a trainee psychiatrist at Warlingham Park Hospital, Surrey. There, fascinated by the dreams patients experienced during insulin coma therapy, he developed an interest in Jungian psychology (Sassa, 2010).

In 1952, Dr. Sandison joined a tour of mental hospitals in Switzerland. Besides visiting Burghölzli Hospital in Zurich, he had the opportunity to visit Sandoz Pharmaceutical Laboratories, where he learned of the work being done there with LSD (Hill, 2010). He returned to London with a supply of 100 vials of the drug and, impressed by the altering effects of LSD on human consciousness, "Dr. Sandison began using it in low doses with patients who were deemed stuck at different stages in their processes. He soon noticed positive results, even in cases of severe illnesses " (Sassa, 2010).

In 1954, Sandison published a paper with his colleagues Spencer and Whitelaw describing LSD-assisted psychotherapy on 36 patients in which the treatment was overwhelmingly positive and without adverse effects (Sandison, 1954). In 1955, he developed the world's first purpose-built LSD unit in the grounds of Powick, where up to five patients could receive LSD simultaneously in rooms equipped with a couch, a chair, and a blackboard for drawing emerging images. The Powick model became the blueprint used throughout Britain and the world for LSD treatment. In 1955, Sandison addressed the American Psychiatric Association about his work. Then, in 1961, he chaired the Royal Medico-Psychological Association meeting, which was devoted entirely to LSD therapy (Sassa, 2010).

Dr. Sandison identified three distinct types of psychedelic experience: dream-like hallucinations, reliving of forgotten personal memories, and imagery from the collective unconscious. Some accounts suggest that Dr. Sandison attempted to seek out Jung in Zurich to share the results of his experiments with him. However, he was reportedly advised against it since Jung was strongly opposed to the use of LSD. Despite Jung's limited knowledge of the responsible therapeutic use of psychedelic substances, Dr. Sandison understood that Jung's psychology paradoxically provides penetrating insights into the nature of psychedelic experiences and the practice of psychedelic psychotherapy.

Jung did not do any research on the use of psychedelics, but he made comments about it in letters to the Dominican priest Victor White and to Betty Eisner, a psychologist who was one of the early pioneers of psychedelic-assisted psychotherapy in the 1950s and 1960s. "While he was appreciative of the potential of psychedelics in helping researchers explore the unconscious, he was critical of some of the ways it was being done during the 1950s and 60s" (Clark, 2022).

After nearly half a century of prohibition due to the war on drugs waged by the powerful U.S. Food and Drug Administration (FDA), we are currently experiencing what has been called the Psychedelic Renaissance. Many articles and books have been published in recent years describing scientific research studies. In the early 2000s, physician Rick Strassman performed a research study with dimethyltryptamine (DMT) in the United States, which is considered one of the milestones of this Renaissance.

Since then, there has been a substantial body of literature, for instance, on psilocybin (the active ingredient in so-called magic mushrooms) used in the context of psychotherapy, particularly in the treatment of depression and anxiety in patients with terminal illnesses (Beserra, 2021).

In 2015, the Associação Psicodélica do Brasil (Brazilian Psychedelic Association) was founded. However, there is still no legislation in place in Brazil to regulate the use of psychoactive substances in clinical settings. Even though some psychedelics such as ayahuasca are not prohibited, we are not prepared for the introduction of this experience into our clinical practice.

Beyond the issue of legal use, our therapy sessions typically last 50 minutes, which is not enough time for the complete psychedelic experience, from ingestion to the termination of the effects and the processing of the content raised by the interaction with the substance used (Guia do Psiconauta, 2016).

We have been working, albeit timidly, on listening, exploring, and contributing to the elaboration of the accounts of our patients' autonomous experiences outside sessions. The therapeutic use of some substances has been facilitated by a 2011 regulation issued by the ANVISA (Brazilian Health Regulatory Agency), which authorizes individual use of unregistered medications. According to the regulation, the agency may authorize access to medication that: presents scientific evidence of its indication, or is in any phase of clinical development, provided that the initial data are promising, and the severity of the disease and absence of available treatments are proven (Leite, 2021).

We are experiencing a revolution in the field of mental health, a paradigm shift, as the model of separation between biological, biochemical, and psychological aspects is increasingly questioned. What is being referred to here is the interdisciplinary field that has linked psychopharmacology with anthropology. Today, there is a growing acceptance of this discussion, but it is still heavily influenced by a medicalizing and biologizing bias; therefore, I see an increasing need for the field of psychology to fully engage in the discussion about the use of psychedelics in healthcare, and in psychotherapy (Beserra, 2021).

Brazil is marked by traditional uses of ayahuasca among Indigenous Peoples and by its religious use in urban centers, which was introduced in the 1930s by Raimundo Irineu Serra and has since expanded extensively throughout the country and abroad (Labate, 2004). The religious use of ayahuasca is practiced by various groups in Brazil, such as Santo Daime, União do Vegetal, and Barquinha, among others, and it has its own regulations.

Osorio and colleagues conducted a preliminary study on the antidepressant effects of a single dose of ayahuasca in patients with treatment-resistant depression (Osorio, 2015). And the first randomized, double-blind clinical study with ayahuasca in the treatment of treatment-resistant depression was conducted by Palhano-Fontes (2019) with 29 participants, of whom 14 received ayahuasca and 15 received a placebo. Each psychedelic experience is unique, and clinical work can take various forms: it can involve sharing experiences or making sense of challenging experiences, colloquially described as bad trips (Salerno, 2020).

> We observed significant antidepressant effects of ayahuasca when compared with placebo at all-time points. MADRS scores were significantly lower in the ayahuasca group compared with placebo at D1 and D2 (p = 0.04), and at D7 (p < 0.0001). Between-group effect sizes increased from D1 to D7 (D1: Cohen's d = 0.84; D2: Cohen's d = 0.84; D7: Cohen's d = 1.49). Response rates were high for both groups at D1 and D2, and significantly higher in the ayahuasca group at D7 (64% v. 27%; p = 0.04). Remission rate showed a trend toward significance at D7 (36% v. 7%, p = 0.054).
> (Rapid antidepressant effects of the psychedelic ayahuasca in treatment-resistant depression: a randomized placebo-controlled trial)

The SBrPA (Brazilian Society for Analytical Psychology) annually holds an event called Moitará. The name is of indigenous origin and means a meeting for exchanges between tribes. Each year, a theme from Brazilian culture is chosen, and experts from various fields are invited to discuss and broaden perspectives on the chosen theme. The 31st Moitará took place virtually as we were still emerging from the Covid-19 pandemic. The chosen theme was *Power Plants and other Psychoactive Substances - Science and Spirituality*. The event attracted over 300 participants and featured many renowned speakers, as Brazil has a long history of using psychedelics in health protocols.

Among the various panels, some addressed, albeit still timidly, the analytical work of exploration, elaboration, and guidance of experiences with psychoactive substances that occurred outside clinical settings. It was concluded that Jung's Analytical Psychology, with its emphasis on the deepening and development of personality, profound experiences and spirituality, greatly facilitates the integration of these experiences. We recognize from accounts of recreational experiences that the that analytical work can be done with the material that arises and could be used as clinical material.

Final Considerations

As I finalize this text, *Psychedelic Science 23*, the fourth conference hosted by the Multidisciplinary Association for Psychedelic Studies (MAPS), is taking place in Denver, Colorado. The current event has around 12,000 registered attendees and 500 speakers, showcasing the latest research using psychoactive substances as supplementary tools in the treatment of conditions such as PTSD and depression. The previous conference was held in 2017 and had approximately 3,000 participants.

On the last day of the event, some indigenous leaders took the stage and questioned the limited space given to indigenous peoples. "Why are we not invited (to the studies), we who are the true holders of such knowledge?" There is an important discussion occurring between the pharmaceutical industry and the "anthropological and community-oriented psychedelic field, which condemns patents on substances that have been inherited through ancestral use by indigenous people" (Leite, 2023).

It is expected that the results from a phase 3 trial for treating PTSD with MDMA may lead to the approval of the protocol by the FDA in 2024. Psilocybin, as an adjunct for depression, is next on the path toward regulation (Leite, 2023). One of the honorees at the event, Dr.

Roland Griffins, spoke about how psychedelics can be a way to bringing spirituality into the realm of science (Krepp, 2023).

Data initially presented highlighted a significant increase in the global incidence of mental illnesses. Thinking about new tools is a way to contribute to the restoration of health. Thinking along with Jung entails embracing his radical proposal of an eminently practical work rooted in the personal myth and the full exercise of the individuality of each therapist, and, more precisely, that of each patient-therapist duo.

As suggested by Samuels, we are still developing Jung's radical intuition of the need to create a culturally sensitive psychology. It is impossible to consider Jungian theory, and even more so any current Jungian practice, outside the personal context of the psychotherapist in question. Furthermore, it is not possible to conceive of a theory detached from the cultural context of its time.

References

Bastos, L.A. (2002). Psicanálise Baseada em Evidências. *PHYSIS: Revista SaúdeColetiva* (pp. 391-408).

Beserra, F. (2021). Da ayahusca ao MDMA, spicodélicos podem ser aliados na terapia. *Revistq Contato, 135* (22-26).

Bisbee, C.C., Bisbee, P., Dick, E. (2018). *Psychedelic prophets: the letters of Aldoux Huxley and Humphrey Osmond.* Mc Gill- Queen's University Press.

Caetano, A.A. (2018). Complex in memory, mind in matter: walking hand in hand. *Journal of Analytical Psychology* (510-528).

Casement, A. (2007). *Who Owns Jung.* Karnack Books.

Clark, G. (2022). Carl Jung and the Psychedelic Brain. *International Journal of Jungian Studies, 14* (97-126).

Forbes. https://www.forbes.com/sites/onemind/2020/02/03/at-davos-2020-mental-health-seen-as-a-social-and-economic-imperative/?sh=5ebd480"97d57 (Last Accessed 10 June 2023).

*GuiadoPsiconauta.*https://guiadopsiconauta.wordpress.com/2016/06/28/origem-do-termo/ (Last Accessed 28 June 2023).

Hill, S.J. (2010). In appreciation for Dr. Ronald Sandison and his pioneering practice. *MAPS bulletin, XX-2* (p. 31).

Hopcke, R.H. (1995). *Persona.* Shambala.

Jung, C.G. (1961). *Memórias, Sonhos e Reflexões.* Rio de Janeiro: Nova Fronteira.

Kast, V. (1997). *A imaginação como espaço de liberdade.* São Paulo: Edições Loyola.

Konner, M. (2013). Play, Plasticity and the Perils of the Conflict-Problematizing Sociobiology. In: D. Narvaez, (Ed.) *Evolution, Early Experience and Human Development.* Oxford University Press.

Krepp, A. https://www.poder360.com.br/opiniao/por-dentro-do-maior-evento-psicodelico-do-mundo/ (Last Accessed 4 July 2023).

Labate, B. (2004). *A reinvenção do uso da ayahuasca nos centros urbanos.* Campinas: Mercado de Letras.

Leite, M. (2021). *Psiconautas.* Fósforo.

Leite, M. A volta triunfal dos psicodélicos. *Folha de São Paulo.* (19 June 2023).

neurocaregroup.com. https://www.neurocaregroup.com/news-insights/report-predicts-burden-of-mental-illness-will-cost-us16-trillion-by-2030 (Last Accessed 19 June 2023).

Osmond, H. (14 de march de 1957). A review of the Clinical Effects os Psychotomimetic Agents. *Annals New York Academy of Science,* 418-434.

Osorio, F.D. (2015). Antidepressant effects os a single dose of ayahuasca in patientes with recurrent depression: a preliminar report. *Revista Brasileira de Psiquiatria, 1,* pp. 13-20.

Palhano-Fontes, F.E. (2019). Rapid antidepressant effects of the psychedelic ayahusca in treatment-resistant depression. *Psychological Medicine, 39*(4) (655-653).

Papadopoulos, R. (1998). Jungian Perspectives in New Contexts. In: A. Casement, *Post Jungians Today.* Routledge.

Patel, V., & Saxena, S. (2014). Transforming Lives, Enhancing Communities-Inovations in Global Mental Health. *The New England Journal of Medicine, 370* (498-501).

Penna, E.D. (2013). *Epistemologia e Método na Obra de Jung.* São Paulo: EDUC.

Post, L. (1992). *Jung e a História de Nosso Tempo.* Civilização Brasileira.

Ribeiro, M. https://siterg.uol.com.br/cultura/2020/07/28/a-mescalina-e-o-nascimento-do-termo-psicodelico/ (Last Accessed 20 July 2023).

Salerno, C. (2020). *Psychedelic Integration: grounding the journey.* Fonte: Psychedelic.support: https://psychedelic.support/resources/psychedelic-journey-integration/

Samuels, A. (2014). Political and Clinical developments in Analytical Psychology. *Journal of Analytical Psychology, 59* (641-660).

Sandison, R.S. (1954). The Therapeutic Value of Lysergic Acid Diethylamide in Mental Illness. *Journal of Mental Science, 100* (419) (491-507).

Sassa, B. (November de 2010). Dr. Ronald Arthur Sandison. *The Psychiatrist.* Cambridge University Press.

Shamdasani, S. (2006). *Jung e a Construção da Psicologia Moderna.* Aparecida: Ideias e Letras.

Smith-Hansen, & P.R. (2014). The Active Ingredients of Succesful Psychological Treatment. *Journal of the American Psycho-analytical Association, 62* (493-499).

WHO (https://www.who.int/teams/mental-health-and-substance-use/ world-mental-health-report (Last Accessed 10 June 2023).

Integration of Jungian and Psychedelic Training and Practice: A Conversation

Miriam Stein
Anne Flynn

The involvement of Jungian Analysts in Psychedelic Assisted Therapy and Training is a vexed question. What, indeed, is the appropriate relationship for an analyst, with a unique orientation and training, to the new modality of psychedelic assisted therapy?

The upsurge in the use of psychedelic drugs as medicines to experience breakthrough states of awareness corresponds with the recent development of Psychedelic Assisted Therapy Training (PATT) programs for their guided use. Both are reflections of the collective *spirit of the times*, which Zygmunt Bauman (1996; 2000) has defined as "liquid modernity." Bauman describes the essential qualities as mobility, lightness, and great fluidity. He observed that, instead of construing ourselves as "pilgrims" in life committed to undertaking a deep, focused search for meaning, people in our time are more like "tourists," skimming the surface in their desire for many and varied experiences.

Jung, by contrast, was oriented to the *spirit of the depths*. He observed that many like him had become "weary of scientific specialization and rationalistic intellectualism" (CW 15, § 86), a central characteristic of modernity. He sought to redress what he regarded as an imbalance in the spirit of his times. In the context of this one-sidedness, Jung observed a longing that arises for "truths which broaden rather than restrict them, which do not obscure but enlighten, which do not run off them like water, but penetrate to the marrow" (CW 15, § 86). He cautioned, however, against simply appropriating new spiritual paths and experiences, using them to "veil from ourselves our real human nature with all its dangerous undercurrents and darkness" (CW 15, § 88), without the necessary psychological work.

The question arises whether techniques characterized by the spirit of "liquid modernity" may also enable or augment a connection with the spirit of the depths? Jungian theory is based on accessing, experiencing, and being impacted by the depths through opening to and experiencing states that are alien to the ego. It would follow that if it were possible that the guided use of psychedelics could pave the way for that opening and experiencing, the involvement of Jungian Analysts in PATT may offer a new, appropriate way to work within the spirit of the times to augment the realization of and union with the spirit of the depths.

Training Models

Jungian Analysts may encounter analysands who have taken psychedelics, and there are analysts who have had psychedelic experiences. However, in addressing the questions of whether and how an analyst may fruitfully incorporate psychedelic therapy, it is important to understand a fundamental difference in orientation between the two training models and the implications arising from this difference.

In the recent psychedelic research and literature concerning training in the use of psychedelic therapies, PATT is presented as a treatment model. The prevalent MAPS (Multidisciplinary Association for Psychedelic Studies) training, the basis of PATT for this chapter, has a primarily pathogenic focus on the treatment of participants' symptoms and diagnosable mental illness, such as depression, anxiety, PTSD, pain, and addictions. This may be due in part to their research goals: hoping to demonstrate the effectiveness of the drugs and thereby attract support for legalization, as well as funding to enable the expansion of psychedelic training and treatment, and to ensure ongoing access and availability. Nonetheless, this approach shapes the model such that the primary active agent in treatment and therapeutic change is the drug or medicine itself. The role of and relationship with the guide is considered secondary, followed by the few suggested integration sessions after the psychedelic experience.

Some exceptions to this pathogenic focus include Phelps' and Henry's ambitious integrative model, *Foundations for Training Psychedelic Therapists* (2022), and a New York University program developed by Guss (2021): *Psychoanalytic Perspectives on Psychedelic Experience*. These training models instead highlight the need for a guided psychedelic experience to be oriented to "the natural design and intelligence" of an individual's capacity for self-healing, thereby re-establishing "a fundamental trust in the unfolding of life," and letting "go of trying to control it" and "to help people remember who they are in their fullness" (Phelps & Henry, 2022, p. 95). Rather than an emphasis on symptomatology and its treatment, they address "remembering the disconnected parts of ourselves" (Phelps & Henry, 2022, p. 93). Their models may have more in common with a Jungian orientation.

Jungian training and practice, in contrast to the MAPS training, operates largely within a salutogenic model of inquiry, one that focuses on "unravelling the mystery of health" (Antonovsky, 1986), rather than concentrating on the pathogenic attention to illness and symptoms. A salutogenic orientation, therefore, asks different questions when gathering information about processes that may directly foster well-being, resilience, development, and creativity. The goal of a Jungian analysis in this respect is teleological and not primarily oriented to treating specific symptoms or promoting adaptation to normative functioning. Instead, given the omnipresence of suffering and conflict, Jung, like Antonovsky, concerned himself with understanding the fundamental human problem of fostering balance and order out of chaos. While Jung accepted the valuable role in appropriate instances of a pathogenic approach, he was more drawn to understanding the neglected area of the creative and prospective dynamics of how unconscious processes can unfold for the development of a wider consciousness.

Accordingly, within a Jungian milieu of meaning-making and progressions on the path of individuation, psychedelic use would not be the principle active agent. Instead, as with dreams, visions, active imagination and synchronistic experiences, the loosened experience of consciousness brought on by psychedelics would be a secondary means to approach the contents and dynamics of the unconscious, personal and collective. In so doing, an analysand begins to submit to holding the tension between manifest opposites and moral conflicts, between what is conscious and known, and the unconscious unknown, in a process of centroversion. In response, from the depths of psyche, potentially unifying symbols are produced, offering a new possibility to consciousness, as the centering process points to the coherent and encompassing sense of Self.

This attempt to work with and transcend psychological opposites through their personal meaning constitutes the process of individuation, and is the basis of an analytic modality that goes beyond specific pathology to be cured by a drug. It emphasizes, at its core, a process in which the Self is the active agent, confirmed by its realization (Stein, 2021, pp. 243-253). This is the basis of Jung's view that the ongoing longing for and commitment to the inner experience of transformation creates a new, coherent sense of wholeness, and, for some, a numinous sense of totality: the transpersonal experience of unity and interconnectedness with all beings and the cosmos. These theoretical and practical emphases on integration of these multiplicities necessitates a comparatively long period of training, including the ongoing experiential component of personal analysis. This too is an important difference between the two training models.

PATT of a Jungian Analyst

Regardless of these differences in orientation, the medicinal use of psychedelics has already made a major impact on the field of mental health and the creation of new training programs. To some, PATT and Jungian thought and training may appear to overlap on the basis that Jung was personally and theoretically interested in numinous experiences as providing the most direct connection with that which is unknown by and alien to the ego. However, the salience he attributed to being close to the numinous was in service of a particular and continuous process, as illustrated in Jung's formula for the Self in his work *Aion* (Stein, 2012) and the alchemical expositions throughout his work. This dedicated inner work and trust in the process of self-reflection does not arise from a single experience, as it is considered by most Jungian analysts to be a lifetime process.

The use of psychedelics or other medicines is clearly not at the heart of the Jungian psychoanalytic enterprise. Nonetheless, in our contemporary context of liquid modernity, it is timely to examine if and how it may be possible for the two training and practice models to interact. For Jungian analysts, this inquiry is especially pertinent given the movement in many countries toward legalizing the use of psychedelics and related substances.

Anne Flynn is one of few analysts who has completed an approved MAPS training in the use of Psychedelic Assisted Therapy (PAT) as part of the one-year Naropa training, including the experiential component. We had several engrossing conversations about this new field, and the potential for overlap between Jungian Analysis and Psychedelic Assisted Therapy through the lens of their differing training models and orientation. Although not intended to be an exhaustive analysis, we offer this as an initial exploration of what may be possible.

MS: Before we dive into some of the specifics of your training in Psychedelic Assisted Therapies at the Naropa Institute, I'm interested in what you were hoping to find?

> **AF:** It was actually my first psychedelic experience as a young adult which gave me a glimpse of the world behind the world, that drew me later into Jungian training—that it was vast and strange and somehow true in its fullness. I suppose it was my first awareness that there existed a non-ego unconscious aspect to mind. So my decision to do the training in Psychedelic Assisted Therapy came from wanting to reconnect with this inner truth, to come home to what I now understand as a desire to access the creative source—the unconscious, both personal and collective, with the hope of generating something new, previously undiscovered. These kinds of feelings of wonder and awe which had always motivated me towards creative pursuits had diminished over time. I had an inkling that the shift in perspective occasioned by the psychedelic experience would open up this connection to the creative source. Also,

at the time I made this decision to do the PATT, my father was dying. I saw how he resisted death. I felt his fear. I knew that psychedelic therapy was used very successfully in treating end-of-life existential issues. In a very broad sense I think we all face fear of our own mortality; it is at the root of much human anxiety and suffering, and I wanted to investigate that problem.

MS: Did you feel that there was something missing for you in the Jungian training and approach?

AF: Not as such. In the end, the guided psychedelic experience component of the training provided more of a deepening of the experience begun in my personal analysis and informed by Jungian theory. The powerful affective experience of psyche during my psychedelic journey truly coalesced with my intellectual understanding developed in my Jungian training. In some ways I guess my own personal equation figured in this, in that I had become overfocused on the intellectual—one of the reasons I was drawn to Jungian training, which in turn reinforced this for me. But the PATT upended this one-sidedness. The psychedelic experience generated greater fluidity between the different ways I perceive phenomena.

MS: Can you describe the format and scope of your PAT training?

AF: The Naropa University Certificate on Psychedelic Assisted Therapies training is a 10-month online and in-person program. It covered the history of the use of psychedelic substances in healing, including its use among Indigenous People; ethics; social justice; competencies in administration of MDMA, psilocybin, ketamine therapies, and plant-based medicine practices; as well as essential aspects of trauma-informed care and spiritual integration. They also addressed research outcomes for these substances on numerous symptoms, as well as the neurobiology of their impact. Many questions were raised and discussed concerning socio-cultural inequity issues as to availability of PAT, as well as the effect of the medicalization of psychedelics on the psychotherapy industry, and the impact of this rapid rise of interest in western cultures on indigenous practitioners and societies.

The MAPS training was in-person and was imbedded within the program. An experience with non-ordinary states was required for completion. The context and purpose of the MAPS training is that of a research study, hoping to show that psychedelics are effective medicines to treat PTSD and trauma related pathologies and symptoms. There was an emphasis on *first do no harm*. Essentially, the didactic program addressed the many concrete practical and ethical concerns particular to a guided psychedelic experience, given how susceptible and vulnerable people are while on psychedelics. These were aimed at helping participants develop their intentions (Set) and the non-intrusive but supportive role of the facilitator (Setting) in order to create the optimum conditions for a productive experience, with respect for ethical boundaries, potential transference and counter-transference concerns, and cultural sensitivities. They covered topics like screening, contra-indications, consent, safety, dosing, music, and aesthetics. The approach was mostly non-directed, based on empathic support and presence to assist the participant's unfolding experience and the body's own healing process. Interventions, theories of mind, etc., were not dealt with in detail. And the method of post dosing Integration was left to the individual therapist.

Impact on Professional Practice

MS: Having completed the PATT, and when the substances are legalized, do you plan to professionally accompany people through all 3 stages of their psychedelic process: Set, Setting and Integration?

AF: Probably not. I have been and will continue to work at the Integration phase for now—this is the piece I see as most consistent with Jungian analysis. I haven't worked through how the physical aspects of a psychedelic journey might impact a long-term analysis, especially in relation to issues of transference and counter transference, physical vulnerability, the extended length of time required by the journey, the need for reassurance, and for touch—not just for comfort, but for safety as well. This potentially tricky area regarding the frame and boundaries within the therapeutic relationship was touched on, but not explored in terms of the impact on an analytical relationship. Also, there are certain patients for whom I might question their unconscious (or conscious) intention in requesting psychedelic therapy to begin with. Psychedelics break down boundaries, and it is possible that such individuals (for example with borderline personality or borderline defenses) may be focused on that concrete aspect of the analytic relationship rather than on the actual deeper intrapsychic work. Individual psychological differences between kinds of patients seeking psychedelic therapy wasn't really looked at in detail either, with the exception of excluding individuals with a history of psychotic tendencies.

Deficits of MAPS Program

MS: Did you find any deficits in your MAPS training in terms of integrating the psychedelic experience?

> **AF:** Yes—my concerns with PATT lie mainly around the lack of time and attention given to the Integration therapy phase. This may be due to how new this field is, and how the information around the role of integration in PATT is still emerging. We know from research that neuroplasticity, an increased capacity for new connections in the brain, is enhanced following the

psychedelic session. This presents a critical opportunity for reset. So not addressing and reflecting with a skilled therapist on new salient meanings or insights derived from an experience seems like it could defeat the purpose of using the medicine for psychological expansion and growth. Even though I get that as a research study, it was more narrowly focused on testing the efficacy of the protocol in alleviating PTSD and trauma related symptoms. But it's the meaning making that comes from integration following the psychedelic experience that is the most interesting part of the whole process for me, especially in relation to difficult experiences.

MS: Something related also strikes me as problematic concerning the PAT training and orientation, which I welcome your views on. Despite the *overt* pathogenic orientation and goals of MAPS and similar PATT models, I notice a confusing lack of distinction in some of the language that is used. For example, words and phrases like 'journey,' 'transcendent,' 'holding opposites,' or 'self-directed healing' allude to a more salutogenic orientation toward a sense of wholeness that is potentially available to us all. However, this is done without clear reference to either a theoretical or practical framework that lays out what is meant by these terms and their inter-relationship, as well as what directly enables a salutogenic process and how that might occur. Notably, the use of such terms isn't connected theoretically or practically to a suggested therapy approach in the integration phase. Was this your experience in the MAPS program?

> **AF:** Yes, basically. Although the idea of an inner healing intelligence is very consistent with Jung's idea of the Self, the method of support for 'Integration' is not linked to any specific theoretical model but left to the individual therapist. Theories of mind, of consciousness and the link between conscious and unconscious states, for example, were not addressed in the training. The MAPS model is focused on the efficacy of the drug itself and trusts in the medicine to activate and connect to the

individual's 'inner healer,' in order to correct and redirect the psyche. But what the 'inner healer' is and how it may develop was not addressed in any detail. Similarly, I had hoped to learn more in the Naropa training about the nature of mystical experiences. This was only touched on very briefly and not within a process model. PATT was essentially presented as a self-directed, non-directive approach that encourages limited interventions, primarily to redirect the participant's energy if they begin to loop or get stuck in their processing. Trusting the capacity of the participant's personal process and agency in their own healing was emphasized.

Having said that, the training pointed to trauma informed therapies, such as Internal Family Systems Therapy, to guide the processing and integration of the experience. These therapeutic modalities were not comprehensively laid out. In the MAPS training, Integration work serves two main objectives: maximizing the benefits of a psychedelic experience and minimizing or dealing with adverse drug effects. Other suggested practices to achieve these two goals are: bodywork, creative pursuits, and spiritual practices, such as meditation. The PAT training did not address or endorse analyzing or interpreting the content of the experience.

MS: This is a little confusing isn't it, as these are potentially useful directive techniques. From what I understand, Internal Family Systems Therapy is primarily a reductive, concrete, and relational approach to therapy, emphasizing an historical, causal hypothesis in regard to the present symptoms experienced. Whilst this may be very helpful for ego resilience work, it would seem to miss out on the powerful creative impact of prospective symbolism, both personal and archetypal, manifest in symptoms, as well as in psychedelic images, personifications, and processes? Such methods also neglect the importance of synchronistic experiences through receptivity to such acausal meaning events.

AF: Absolutely. Of course, a lot of trauma work is concerned with injury based on personal experience, but as Jungians we are trained to look at factors beyond the personal. This raises a critical distinction between Jungian and Psychedelic training: the consideration of the collective unconscious. As Jungians we know that there are images in the unconscious that exist on a non-personal level and that as many of the contents of the unconscious are collective and mythological, they may not have come from personal lived experience. This was not acknowledged. There was no reference to symbolic thinking or to the archetypal imagery that is contained in symptoms and in their psychedelic experiences and process. Although studies were mentioned that found a correlation between mystical experiences and positive outcomes for healing, there was limited discussion as to the meaning of the mystical experiences, understanding their prospective value, or on how to work with them consciously in the Integration phase. As Jungians, we are trained in the mythopoetic language of the unconscious. This was not a part of MAPS training or the Naropa Psychedelic Assisted Psychotherapy program.

Benefits of a Jungian Training

MS: I want to reflect on your last answer expressing concerns about some deficits in the training model, as it raises the potential benefits that a Jungian training and approach brings to the conscious integration of psychedelic experiences. I'm thinking, in particular, of the pivotal role of archetypal symbols in bridging the divide between our conscious and unconscious nature as a "health giving counterweight to the inherent dissociability of the psyche" (Jacobi, 1974, p. 98). In Jung's later writings he referred to the luminosity of the collective unconscious: "In the unconscious are hidden those 'sparks of light' (*scintillae*), the archetypes, from which a higher meaning can be 'extracted'" (Jung, CW 14, § 700). This manifestation enables the first opportunity to consciously reflect on differences, on paradoxical and previously irreconcilable matters of self, on the question: what myth am I living? As well, Jung noted that the appropriate practice of active imagination eliminates the threat of internal chaos when faced with multiple unconscious contents. In this way, it becomes possible to meet and engage with a key dynamic archetypal property of a complex, without either being swallowed up by the unconscious instinct at play, or remaining on an intellectual level of understanding. Thus some of the dynamism of the archetype is experienced and embodied in new personal meanings (Jung, CW 8, § 414). The spontaneous coming together of pivotal unconscious and conscious elements of one's personality is what James referred to as a "bursting point" (Jung, CW 8, § 413). Much attention was given in our training to the issue of titrating the analysand's experience of unconscious material (e.g., through the use of methods like active imagination), and of being sensitive to the choice about when to raise and lower the heat in the analytic container, such that receptivity to its healing impact might be enabled. In this way, in the context of the particular analytic relationship, unconscious elements would no longer be felt as oppressive, but greeted as necessary strange partners within one's personality as a whole, creatively helping prepare the way forward.

I can't finish these observations without asking about the related issue of inflation, and ego's tendency to cannibalize and possess mysterious numinous experiences, resulting in the conviction of being special and even God-like. In our training, we were encouraged to examine such things through dialectics, such as the restoration of the persona that may occur following a period of deep analytic work and insight. Were these problems of inflation and deflation dealt with theoretically and practically in your Psychedelics training?

> **AF:** No, not really. And I agree it needs to be. A Jungian training by contrast, is at one level an initiatory experience into symbolic thinking. The sustained duration of both the theoretical instruction, and the accompanying experience of analysis and clinical supervision amount to a very full process and immersion, in which the candidate experiences all aspects of an initiation accompanying a change of state. The psychedelic experience may provide a

128

condensed version of an archetypal initiatory experience, which can be overwhelming and disorienting without scaffolding to help gradually draw personal meaning from the encounters. This can enhance the risk of falling into either inflation or deflation. Jungian training examines the aspects and stages of such a journey in great detail. In doing so it draws on historical studies of alchemy, fairy tales, and mythology for amplifications of the symbolic meaning and potential of the contents and processes experienced. These stories show all kinds of wrong turns and dangers as well as possible ways through by means of an increase in consciousness and embracing what is possible. I think this makes the psychedelic experience much more comprehensible to Jungians than therapists trained in non-depth, behaviorally or relational oriented therapies. For example, the unleashing of unconscious compensatory contents that results from the lowering of the threshold of consciousness can be terrifying if not understood as access to undifferentiated opposites in the landscape of the unconscious. It struck me, for example, that the archetypes of descent and initiation and the symbolism that attends those archetypes would provide an important perspective in understanding and navigating the non-ordinary experience of psychedelic journeys. In addition, the intensive study of dreams, and working analytically with dream series, seem directly relevant to making meaning of the psychedelic induced 'journey.'

MS: Jung believed in the helpful corrective role of the unconscious, initially from his personal experience and then reflected in his elaborated theoretical perspective. This same sentiment is expressed in much of the training and practice literature on psychedelic therapies. Nonetheless, I share your concerns about how helpful a therapist may be in the Integration phase of the process without having undergone a long-term personal analysis, supervision, and lengthy training themselves. Do you have further thoughts on this, especially having undergone a personal psychedelic experience?

> **AF:** My sense is that the psychedelic experience did allow access to primary process material, what Jung might have referred to as fantasy thinking in his essay on two types of thinking (Jung, CW 5, part II). In Jungian terms, the psychedelics move the ego away from its predominant position and temporarily open up the ego-self axis so that the mind has an opportunity to move along the continuum of ego and non-ego states. Since my rational mind was still operating in the background and it had the benefit of maturity, which I did not have at the time of some of my earlier affective experiences, this enabled an updating of some of the associations and thoughts which had become associated with those affects. I doubt whether this would have been the result if I had been less experienced, or if I had not undergone a full Jungian training and analysis over many years. I believe, for all the reasons you have suggested and from personal experience that Jungian training is the most effective choice for working with and integrating psychedelic and other non-ordinary experiences and states, especially difficult ones. As Jungian clinicians we know the value of holding the space for such experiences and have helpful methods for attending to the images symbolically that arise in such states.

MS: From many of your comments so far, I'm inferring that you would particularly endorse the value of Jung's Synthetic method: receiving the person's material symbolically to understand its creative potential, even 'foreknowledge' (Jung, CW 8, § 175) for the present, and even future. An analyst's capacity to hold the personal, historical level of meaning alongside the archetypal, and to use interpretation judiciously, requires lengthy training in tools and theoretical distinctions. These include, for example: working with transference and counter transference, amplification, understanding the difference and relationship between personal and archetypal images and personifications, synchronicity, and being able to distinguish different kinds of archetypal manifestations, for example, to recognize and highlight unifying symbols or symbols of totality, like particular geometric forms, mandalas, or personifications as Self-images. The fostering of receptivity in this way is important in the co-creation of analytic process, such that authentic new pathways and solutions to seemingly irreconcilable conflicts and suffering may emerge.

> **AF:** I do think psychedelic assisted therapy generally favors a synthetic approach. And I have personally experienced and have heard from others about that kind of 'foreknowledge' or realization of new ideas that arose as a result of the radical dissolution of old nonadaptive paradigms. These are not unlike the kinds of images that come up in artwork or dreams—images of emergent processes that have not yet been materialized. Also, there is no consensus as to what it is about the psychedelic experience that is healing. Some literature points to biological explanations; for example, we know that psychedelics activate serotonin receptors, but it is not clear what role this plays in healing. Studies also suggest that the use of psychedelic medicine is not a magic bullet but works in conjunction with therapy. Even among those who experienced immediate relief from their symptoms following a journey, it was never clear to me how much of that was attributable to the medicine as opposed to expectations of cure, and the attention and support provided during the preparatory phase of the treatment.

Benefits in Undertaking a PATT Program

MS: Let's turn now to benefits in undertaking a PATT program. Phelps and Henry (2021) report that research data from several studies suggest that therapists who have had personal experience with psychedelics show greater "empathy and effectiveness" (Richards 2015, p. 148) in their psychedelic psychotherapy work. Do you believe it is of benefit to have undergone some kind of guided psychedelic experience yourself in order to do this work with others?

> **AF:** I do. The common fears that accompany a psychedelic journey are that one will die or lose one's mind. This definitely enhances the setting for the experience, which we know is a critical factor in the experience. I felt reassured and comforted during my own personal psychedelic experience knowing that those facilitating my experience had been through something similar and had survived and learned from it. I think most Jungians would benefit from a well-curated psychedelic experience designed for inner exploration with the understanding that they are deepening their relationship to the unconscious. I don't think it is the only path to an understanding of this material, merely a reliable opportunity to deepen one's experience with it. Moreover, continuously searching to bring unconscious contents into consciousness is the goal and the focus of Jungian training, for ourselves and for most of our patients.

MS: I'm imagining that therapists who have had mystical experiences and other meaningful non-ordinary states may have similar advantages in this work. I'm also interested in any changes and benefits you experienced from your PATT professionally.

> **AF:** Up until this point I have only been involved in the Integration phase when working analytically with people who have had guided psychedelic experiences. I have found that the psychedelic experience really propelled their analytic process by facilitating access to previously unavailable unconscious imagery and symbols, and through an enhanced willingness to trust and to

open to vulnerability in the therapeutic relationship. Accompanying a patient in this journey is a profound honor and responsibility. I became more aware of how courageous they are being. When people bring in their experiences, it is not linear or coherent and hence very confusing to them. I am more relational in my frame now. I don't feel I am gratifying if, for example, I acknowledge their fear and invite them to hold it and to explore further together. By holding the experience lightly, amplifying certain images and offering symbolic interpretations as appropriate, I am enabling their capacity to relate more consciously to the archetypal elements of these psychedelic experiences and psyche.

Overall, the Psychedelic training sensitized me to the value of affective numinous experiences in moving the individuation process forward. The tool of psychedelics provides embodied evidence of larger non-ego powers in the psyche that need to be explored and brought into consciousness. I have seen patients accelerate their self-understanding as well. Fixed identities that were cemented through traumatic experiences and attachments become more fluid. The personality expands. After the Psychedelic training, and in working analytically with patients who use psychedelics, I am less concerned about the danger of unleashing unconscious contents, and more aware of the value of facilitating the capacity to be responsive to shadow parts. The analysis heats up!

It also re-sensitized me to the value of Setting in our analytic work in general. I give this more care and attention now. I am also more acutely aware of how to create a sense of safety and trust, not just in a psychedelic context, but through the relationship as a container. Through my personal psychedelic experience, I also became hyperaware of the importance of aesthetics in promoting emergent states and material. For example,

I found that the evocation of nature orients the psyche to the embodied cycles of being—of the need to shed something old in order to create something new. Music was also critical. It becomes a vehicle for psychological movement by mirroring the arc of the experience. I suppose I am generally more focused now on the importance of embodiment, and embodied forms of therapy, and how that might impact and interact with the symbolic.

MS: Can you share something of your personal guided psychedelic journey, in terms of its impact on your psychoanalytic views, practice and personally?

AF: I took this a year ago. Archetypally, it felt like a descent to the underworld through intentionally dropping myself into the stream of psychic images as Jung did in his personal research for *The Red Book*. According to Jung, the Western notion of a descent is characterized by a journey downwards, where the traveler meets the ground of experience through which they gain some knowledge or a gift that links them to the divine, and precipitates a reversal. This journey seeks a union of opposites and discovers union through fullness. It leads up to a moment of union between self and other which transcends ego limitations and forms the totality that is the transcendent creative. For me it was a mystical experience, culminating in a sense of awe and gratitude for all aspects of life.

My journey gave me a renewed respect for Jung's own experience and experimentation, and for the value of embodied experience, particularly of the numinous manifestation of unconscious contents, personal and archetypal. These are highly affective experiences and as such are difficult to work with intellectually. I have an increased appreciation for practices which engage the unconscious through creative, nonverbal means, and a renewed respect for the irrational. I also have a renewed trust in the way an individual's unique subjective experience creates their life. In fact, I cannot overestimate how much it enhanced my confidence in psyche's use of process to move life forward toward growth and health. The feeling I came away with was that everything that I have experienced, even if perceived as negative, is as it should be and that it directly contributed prospectively to my growth. Just as Jung said: "But the right way to wholeness is made up, unfortunately, of fateful detours and wrong turnings" (CW 12, § 6). And as Neumann articulated in his writing on the importance of numinous experience for individuation (1948, pp. 375-419), the maladies of my experience also contained the impetus for my quest toward individuation and were necessary to it. As a child, I'd had numinous experiences but the prescribed path toward them became associated with my strict catholic upbringing. As a result of a series of early experiences, affect associated with the numinous became associated with fear and was blocked. The psychedelics restored access for me and broke this fear association.

MS: Do you believe that a psychedelic journey offers something different or extra in terms of accessing unconscious material and opening to a new, more encompassing and enlivening center of being? Did it help you face your mortality squarely as you had initially hoped?

> **AF:** Absolutely. I think the psychedelic journey can take one to places in the internal landscape that may be beyond what one may encounter in analysis. It did that for me and rekindled my creative flow, which I feel more connected and committed to in my day-to-day life. And there were three marked behavioural changes immediately after my psychedelic journey, which although I hadn't specifically held as prior intentions, related overall to care of the

vessel—taking care of my whole self. After surfacing from my psychedelic experience, I felt as if I'd just done 20 years of analysis in one week. My immediate thought emerging from this intense journey was: Jung nailed it! As for mortality, I emerged with a sense of acceptance for all aspects of life, including death. I can understand why psychedelic therapy is being used successfully with end-of-life patients.

MS: As we draw this fertile conversation to a close, and by way of a thank you for sharing your personal experiences, Anne, I offer another story of re-enchantment following out of this world experiences of a somewhat literal kind. In a radio interview, Chris Hadfield, a retired Canadian astronaut shared his numinous experiences while journeying to the moon (ABC, 2023). He described the sense of "overwhelming beauty and magnificence," which flowed through him while seeing sunsets and sunrises every 45 minutes. These intense feelings were accompanied by a profound realization that he was "no longer looking up at the universe, but literally going through space together with the world." Returning to earth after 6 months in space, however, he felt he had "thumped back into the world." He was confronted by the question: "What do I do with this experience now, with the wonder of it all?" Hadfield felt a deep sense of gratitude alongside a duty "not to squander the richness of it all." By way of an answer, a desire emerged to share these precious gifts by finding a way to help others to create new choices and experiences for themselves. For Chris Hadfield, this took the form of working with others on projects that foster human well-being through the combination of science, comedy, and music. He noted that, for him, the non-verbal creative tool of music became especially important as a way to connect empathically with others and to "transmit ideas intuitively" (ABC, 2023).

The same essential question, "what do I do with this now?" demands a personal answer for all participants following their guided psychedelic journey. How do I honor the privilege of touching and experiencing the mystery of and connection between my individual and collective human existence? To do so, requires us to resist certain currents of liquid modernity—our spirit of the times, which favors the continuous seeking of novel, stimulating experiences, for quick fixes of intensity, pleasure and happiness. Jung felt a deep alignment with Chinese Daoist philosophers in this regard, and was greatly influenced by Wilhelm's translation of the alchemical treatise, *Secret of the Golden Flower.* He shared the warning given by Wilhelm about looking externally to the exotic for quick solutions. This applies equally today in regard to the rapid uptake of psychedelic medicines: "What has taken China thousands of years to build cannot be grasped by theft. We must instead earn it to have it" (Jung, 1962, p. 144). He notes that they understood that "redemption depends on the work the individual does upon himself. The Tao grows out of the individual" (Jung, CW 13, § 80). It is only in this way, piece by piece, that "the center of gravity of the total personality shifts its position. It ceases to be the ego ... and is located in a hypothetical point between the conscious and the unconscious which might be called the self" (Jung, CW 13, § 67).

It appears from your answers that examining this deeper question of "who am I?," or "who is who?" (Neumann, 1948, p. 384) can form the life changing basis of post-psychedelic Jungian integration work toward a more broadly encompassing and coherent sense of Self. For those like you, Anne, who have prepared fertile psychological ground prior to an assisted psychedelic journey, and afterward continued the honest self-reflective work of integration (gathering and centering), this new tool which enhances fluidity and connection between psychic states, may hasten as well as directly contribute something rich to the age old human process of individuation. As described by Jung: "a sort of release from compulsion and impossible responsibility," and a realization through which "the subjective 'I live' becomes the objective 'It lives me'" (CW 13, § 78). In a sense, this contemporary surge of interest in the role of the numinous through the new lens of psychedelics, raises its profile in contemporary Jungian training, asking for more attention.

References

Antonovsky, A. (1987). *Unravelling the mystery of health: How people manage stress and stay well*. Jossey-Bass.

Bauman, Z. (1996). From pilgrim to tourist: Or a short history of identity. In S. Hall & P. Du Guy (Eds.), *Questions of cultural identity*. (pp. 18-36). Sage Publications Inc.

Bauman, Z. (2000). *Liquid modernity*. Cambridge: Polity Press.

Guss, J. (2021). "Psychoanalytic perspectives on psychedelic experience: Clinical and theoretical implications of the integration of psychoanalysis and psychedelic therapy." In *NYU Postdoctoral program in psychotherapy and psychoanalysis* – Handout.

Hadfield, C. (2023, March 19). *The singing astronaut*. Australian Broadcasting Commission Radio Interview.

Jacobi, J. (1974). *Complex archetype symbol in the psychology of C.G. Jung*. Princeton University Press.

Jung, C.G. (1962). Appendix: In memory of Richard Wilhelm. In Wilhelm, R. *The secret of the Golden Flower: A Chinese book of life*. (pp. 138-149). Harcourt Brace & Company.

Neumann, E. (1948). Mystical man. In Campbell, J. (Ed.). *The mystic vision: Papers from the Eranos yearbooks*. (pp. 375-419). Routledge & Kegan Paul.

Phelps, J. & Henry, J. (2022). Foundations for training psychedelic therapists. In *Current Topics of Behavioral Neuroscience, 56*, 93-110.

Richards, W.A. (2015). *Sacred knowledge: Psychedelics and religious experience*. Columbia University Press.

Stein, L.A. (2012). *Becoming whole: Jung's equation for realizing God*. Helios Press.

Stein, L.A. (2021). *The Self in Jungian psychology: Theory and clinical practice*. Chiron Publications.

Indigenous Healing Perspectives

Therapist's Experience with Expanded States and Psychedelic Field: Perspectives Rooted in Jungian Psychology & Shipibo Indigenous Healing Traditions

Jerome Braun

In psychedelic assisted therapy, the depth, height, and breadth of a therapist's experience with expanded states can directly impact the client's potential healing. In other words, the therapist's mindset, therapeutic orientation, cultural complexes, skill set, and direct experience with psychedelic states can foster and sometimes hinder the client's therapeutic processes toward healing, integration, and individuation. Acknowledging as much does not diminish the autonomy and power of the client's individual psychological constitution, inner healer, and entelechy (inherent patterns directed toward individuation). Expanded states refer to states of mind that extend beyond the individual's quotidian psychological functioning and cultural paradigm. Expanded states occur spontaneously, can be cultivated, or induced through innumerable means, such as meditation, breathing techniques, trauma, or with psychedelics. In psychedelic assisted therapies, expanded states are warp and woof of the healing process, making available states of mind beyond those of a rational-empirical, individualistic, and predominantly Western paradigm. At times, in these expanded states, psychological and energetic portals open an individual's ego consciousness to connect with intelligences beyond the ego complex, unveiling glimpses of a bigger self and experiences of interconnectedness.

The therapist's experiences of expanded states enhance perceptibility of phenomena in a psychedelic field that constellates like a crucible, simultaneously containing both therapist and client during psychedelic therapy. This psychedelic crucible is not limited to empirical experiences but includes manifestations of the unconscious as well as beyond-human phenomena available through psychedelic treatments. This psychedelic field encompasses conscious, unconscious, and sometimes otherworldly realms.

The invisible-yet-real psychedelic field consists of empirical, psychological, energetic, and spiritual dynamics interacting simultaneously. The psychedelic field creates a veritable temenos (sacred healing space) that wholly connects the therapist, client, neuropsychological states induced by psychedelic medicines, and an interpenetrating energy exchange beyond everyday experiences. Sometimes the psychedelic field may access prenatal memories otherwise not consciously available to the individual, encounters with deceased beings, and sometimes appearances of other-than-human intelligences. At times, psychedelic experiences do not fit a Western cultural worldview, but psychedelic-assisted therapies rooted in a Jungian perspective can procure meaning of these enigmatic experiences. Additionally, mutual dialogue between Western psychedelic providers and Indigenous healers can benefit both groups. The mutual collaboration of cultural appreciation and exchange is important for the development of integrated psychedelic treatments. With reciprocal support to Indigenous peoples who know these enigmatic terrains, these integrations can surpass psychedelic treatments developed solely through the lens of a Western rational-empirical egocentric paradigm. This chapter explores perspectives based on my Jungian psychoanalytic practice, psychedelic-assisted therapy, and my ongoing, in-depth work with Indigenous Shipibo-Konibo healers in the Peruvian Amazon.

Importance of Jungian Psychology for Psychedelic Research & Therapy

The Psychedelic Renaissance—the current movement of psychedelic research and treatment—is like the mythical phoenix, a golden bird rising from the ashes, renewing itself, and symbolizing regeneration and hope for a better life. Psychedelic research in the U.S. was shut down by the Nixon administration in 1970 (Phelps, 2017), and

European countries also curtailed psychedelic research soon thereafter. In just a little more than two decades—research resumed in the U.S. in 1996—the Psychedelic Renaissance has risen from obscurity and expanded across North America and Europe (Phelps, 2017). This has changed mainstream cultural views about psychedelics with hopeful news of effective treatments for posttraumatic stress disorder, addiction, end-of-life anxiety, and clinically resistant depression. Buried in the collective unconscious for decades, the Psychedelic Renaissance is currently creating a new collective mythology on how to conduct psychedelic treatment and post-psychedelic integration therapy.

Jungian psychology is a likely choice for psychedelic treatments and integration with its breadth and depth of understanding of the dynamics of the personal and collective unconscious, ego-Self axis, and ancestral wisdom; however, psychedelic researchers are endorsing cognitive behavioral and egocentric therapies as predominant treatment models. When Jungian psychology is referenced in psychedelic treatments, the concepts of shadow and archetype are often the only Jungian concepts mentioned. Of course, these two Jungian concepts are highly valuable; however, Jungian and post-Jungian psychology provide many other applicable concepts for understanding and navigating perplexing and complicated psychedelic experiences, such as ego-Self axis (Edinger, 1972), typology theory (CW 6, §§ 556-671), cultural complexes theory (Singer et al., 2004), entelechy (CW 9i, § 278), psychoid unconscious (CW 8, § 368; CW 14, § 786), *unus mundus* (CW 10, § 780; CW 14, § 660), and dyadic communication with intelligences beyond the ego complex.

Although Jung (1975) warned of dubious benefits of psychedelic medicines, he admitted that his knowledge of psychedelic medicines was scant. In two letters he indicated the paucity of his knowledge about psychedelics. In his 1954 letter to Anglican priest, Fr. Victor White (Jung, 1975, pp. 172-174), and a second in 1957 written to psychologist Betty Eisner (Jung, 1975, pp. 382-383) who was conducting LSD research with patients in psychotherapy, Jung wrote disparagingly of psychedelics. He felt taking psychedelics allowed access to the unconscious with insufficient ego structure to handle material released from the unconscious and the burden of increasing one's moral responsibility (Jung, 1975, pp. 382-

383). To avoid presentism in judging Jung's stance, scientific psychedelic research was limited in his time. It is important to look afresh at what post-Jungian psychology brings to contemporary psychedelic treatments (Clark, 2021; Prakash, 2017; Swank, 2021; Mahr et al., 2020).

In my Jungian psychoanalytic practice, as a trained and certified psychedelic assisted therapist, I offer psychedelic treatment as an adjunct option to clients' therapy when it is appropriate and beneficial to their therapeutic process. Since 2017, I have also been incorporating into my therapy practice teachings from three Indigenous Shipibo-Konibo healers who live in the Peruvian Amazon. These healers use a psychedelic brew consisting of the ayahuasca vine (Banisteriopsis caapi) and leaves of the chacruna bush (Psychotria viridis). Additionally, they employ thirty-seven sacred plant medicines which are not psychedelic but heal through imaginal, medicinal, and energetic states. These three healers, Maestro Nelson Barbarán Gomez, Maestro Javier Vasquez Gomez, and Maestra Anita Perez Sinacay, offer me ongoing training and insights into their ancestral traditions beyond Western models of healing, and in exchange I offer them psychological guidance from a Jungian perspective. Currently I combine Jungian analysis with psychedelic assisted therapy and Indigenous healing traditions.

In 2016, individuals began calling my Jungian psychoanalytic practice, searching for therapy to help them understand and integrate psychedelic material that they experienced with recreational use, in underground psychedelic gatherings, or abroad in Indigenous ceremonies. At that time, in a similar vein to Jung's stance, I was not well informed about the benefits of psychedelic treatments, and I was skeptical of their therapeutic value. So, I began to research psychedelics and accepted these clients into my practice. Astonishingly, I witnessed rapid, deep, and sustained resolution of their psychological conditions by attending psychedelic gatherings. The shadow side of these gatherings, however, left some clients with another layer of trauma, not due so much to the medicines but to the unskillfulness, or worse, malfeasance, of some facilitators of these psychedelic gatherings. Through a series of synchronicities and prescient dreams, a year later, continuing intense research about psychedelic treatments, I found my way to the Peruvian

Amazon to experience ayahuasca-chacruna for myself, resulting in my ongoing close relationship with three Indigenous Shipibo-Konibo healers.

Whether viewed merely as neurochemical compounds, viable treatment for psychological disorders, or as mystical sacraments, Jungian psychology in conjunction with Indigenous healing traditions offer a veritable map for the process of individuation with psychedelic experiences. This map offers an orientation and understanding of experiences beyond the ego complex, personal and collective unconscious, ancestral wisdom, and the bigger Self. Psychedelic research, governmental regulations, patent restrictions, corporate influences, and social media buzz combine to influence the Psychedelic Renaissance as a new collective myth. With that in mind, it is imperative as a psychedelic assisted psychotherapist to differentiate one's own personal paradigm from the burgeoning collective mythology about psychedelic medicines.

Therapist's Experience with Expanded States

No matter how much one reads about psychedelics to develop a skill set to be a psychedelic assisted therapist (although this is an integral part of being proficient), the therapist's direct experience with expanded states is essential for learning how to navigate phenomena of the psychedelic field to assist clients through their psychedelic experiences and integration in post-psychedelic therapy. Reading about the neurochemical effects and psychological impacts of psychedelic medicines is necessary for harm reduction, determining dosages, and understanding the processes of these medicines; however, the therapist's direct experience with expanded states gives the therapist familiarity and know-how to more fully assist the client in psychedelic therapy.

Expanded states refer to modalities of perception that are outside the individual's conventional way of relating to the world and to others. Expanded states are portals beyond the limitations of the ego complex. Expanded states not only alter the senses of perception of the physical world but also expand perceptions beyond ego boundaries—beyond the sense of separation of self from others. These avail perceptions of energy, experiences beyond time and space, perceptions of deceased relatives, contact with other-than-human entities, and knowledge of beyond-human intelligences. In brief, expanded states facilitate the development of the ego-Self axis.

In a psychedelic assisted session, the therapist sets aside many conventional therapy interventions typical of psychoanalytic practice, such as interpretation, conversation, or asking the client to analyze their experiences. A therapist who is relating from expanded states during the psychedelic session provides more therapeutic interventions than acting from merely intellectual and cognitive functioning. The expanded states rooted in intuition are more conducive for promoting healing in a psychedelic session. The therapist becomes a conduit. Expanded states centered in a flow of consciousness reveal more dimensions of the physical environment, expanded awareness of the therapist's own sensations and feelings, the therapist's images arising on an inner imaginal screen, perceptions of omens and synchronicities, and the client as a whole. Expanded states are more like a wide-open lens rather than pinpointed focus of the intellect. In the psychedelic session, often dialogue is minimal until the client reaches a psycholytic phase of the session. The psycholytic phase refers to the lowering of the psychedelic effects on the client's consciousness, with the client's state of mind then able to engage with the therapist and external environment in the present moment. In the psycholytic phase, the client is able to engage with the therapist but is still under the effects of the medicine. This is an important phase of the session for reminding the client of their intentions for healing and transformation.

Expanded states allow a unitive sense connecting therapist and client consciousness. The therapist's inner experiences can be a guide to what may be happening subjectively with the client; however, the timing of verbalizing these insights is consequential. During the psychedelic phase of the session, I jot my inner impressions onto paper, waiting until subsequent integration sessions before sharing relevant insights. In some ways, the therapist in expanded states is akin to being in active imagination. In expanded states, one's center is not always within one's own physical body but may float freely throughout the psychedelic field. Healthy dissociability of the psyche (CW 8, §§ 365-366), the ability to expand beyond one's ego complex, is part of the flexibility of moving one's center of consciousness within one's own body, into the client's body, and around the environment. It can be understood that expanded states awakened by psychedelic experiences sometimes do not align with conventional psychology and consensus reality based on a Western paradigm.

I offer an example of my experience of expanded states during a psychedelic session, but my experience stubbornly eludes being conveyed fully in words. Nonetheless, I will try. In expanded states, I can see a ticker tape of my thoughts running above my head while there is a center of consciousness in my chest area connecting to feelings and intuitions. Sinking below my chest, is another center of consciousness concentrated in my lower abdomen, but it expands boundaryless out to the client, throughout the room, and beyond any limits that I can directly locate. Simultaneously, often to my upper left-hand side, witnessing consciousness observes all these distinct centers of consciousness. My ego consciousness is not singular or pinpointed in a stationary location when in expanded states. This is just one way of experiencing expanded states, my personal one, and I offer it as an example and *not* to be generalized as the way to be in expanded states for anyone else.

Here is another example from my psychoanalytic practice. During the psychedelic-assisted sessions, I would open into expanded states, allowing the client's process to unfold without using conventional talk therapy interventions, following prompts from the client during the psychedelic phase, and trusting their inner healer as guide more than my own interpretations. Elias, a pseudonym, gave permission to share his therapeutic process. He is currently 51 years old and was in talk therapy with me for over three years before agreeing to undergo Ketamine psychedelic assisted therapy. He was facing his second divorce, his teenage child whom he loved immensely was in the process of leaving for college, and he was significantly depressed despite his superlative success in business, having retired from work at 32. Elias struggled with alcohol dependency, an incessant racing mind, and loss of purpose in his life. He suffered emotional child abuse, especially witnessing his sister being emotionally and physically abused by their father, resulting in posttraumatic stress disorder. Although having a brilliant intellect, being a highly creative writer, physically fit, and freed from the constraints of having to earn a living, he was deeply unhappy. In my clinical assessment, his typology is thinking-intuitive type, and he was heavily guarded against his feeling function. Talk therapy helped but was not resolving his condition when he agreed to Ketamine-assisted treatment.

Elias underwent six weekly Ketamine-assisted sessions, each lasting approximately four hours. Through intramuscular Ketamine injections at psychedelic dosage levels, he was able to access parts of his personality that were not consciously accessible via talk therapy. In the initial psychedelic sessions, Elias reported that he could see images of his racing mind as shapes in movement. Due to this experience, he has more ego consciousness of and increased healthy dissociation from the obsessive dynamic of racing mind instead of being completely subsumed by the complex. Additionally, Elias directly experienced his feeling function during psychedelic stages of the sessions, accessing self-compassion, and possibilities of life purpose. The following revelatory comments over the course of six weeks of psychedelic therapy suggest how Elias accessed his feeling function, saw the root of his posttraumatic stress complex, and glimpses at a greater purpose for his life:

> I try so hard; my soul is pure. Why do I need to fly this way? I know I'm a good person. I want to help people. That's why I'm here. I'm here to help others. I want to love. I want to be love. Cool … just want to express myself even if I don't know what that means. I have so much love to give. There's vitality to life. Fear, joy, and desire are all dancing. Fear, joy, and desire—chess pieces—coming together, joining, twisted like licorice. Native Americans got it right—Love … your … Mother! The heart is the river! It's like realizing that your parent doesn't love you. If you can't count on your parents (voice breaks off). I don't feel safe in my life. Just live my life!

Over a year later, Elias continues in psychoanalytic sessions to integrate these experiences, having more access to his feeling function, increased healthy dissociation from the racing mind complex, and more insight into his childhood trauma. Elias has conveyed that his psychedelic therapy has changed his perception of the challenges he faces, and he is hopeful that further psychological work will result in deep healing.

Elias was a suitable candidate for psychedelic Ketamine-assisted therapy in part based on his capacity to work with psychedelic experiences. Years prior to entering into Jungian psychoanalysis, Elias participated in healing ceremonies with the psychedelic medicine, ayahuasca-chacruna, with Indigenous healers in the Peruvian Amazon. In talk therapy, he worked on integrating his insights and experiences from his jungle ceremonies. Psychedelic medicine is just one element of the healing process but is inherent in healing traditions of Indigenous healers.

An important differentiation of a Western perspective on psychedelic medicines from that of the Shipibo-Konibo healers is that for the Indigenous healers, psychedelic medicine is not reified as the source of healing. Psychedelic medicine is an energetic portal to receive guidance from other-than-human intelligences which transmit healing energy to the patient for realignment of the patient's physical, emotional, and spiritual components. Moreover, the patient is viewed as a whole, not disparate components, and is interconnected with all levels of being, external and internal. The Shipibo-Konibo healers move into expanded states under the influence of psychedelic medicine, grounded in an animistic and all-encompassing interconnectedness sense of reality. They connect with realms that seem invisible and are in the unconscious from a Western paradigm. The healers, in expanded states, connect to unseen-yet-real intelligences while sitting in front of the patient, paying attention to what they see on their subjective inner screen, (like in active imagination experiences), and transmit healing energy into the patient through their vibrational songs. The Shipibo-Konibo sacred songs, called ikaros, reorchestrate the patient's body, psychology, energy, and spirit much like how one vibrating tuning fork will affect an adjacent tuning fork to synchronize with it. Since 2017, I have watched these three Shipibo-Konibo healers in expanded states transmit healing energy to numerous patients who are now changed fundamentally through their deeply effective abilities for healing.

Another key point to consider for the therapist's development of expanded states is the therapist's own healing. This is primary. Healing does not, however, denote completion of the healing process but is ongoing, in conjunction with, and parallel to the healing processes of the client. The therapist must let go of the stance that the therapist is the agent of healing, imparting healing onto the client. The process is interconnected. In psychedelic-assisted therapy, the therapist's and client's healing processes occur in tandem, paradoxically separate yet intertwined.

Considering the interconnectedness of therapist's and client's processes, the therapist's responsibility is an ongoing, ruthlessly honest self-inquiry into the therapist's motivations for being a psychedelic assisted therapist. Clarifying and being mindful of complexes, such as identifying as the wounded healer or the source of healing for others, the shadow aspects of wanting to raise the client's consciousness, unconscious motivations to enlighten or heal or fix the client, or more destructively, psychological inflation of being a self-identified shaman. Humility is paramount as a psychedelic assisted therapist, trusting that larger forces are in charge beyond the therapist's will and ego complex. As the saying goes in psychedelic therapy circles, "don't get ahead of the medicine" when working with the client in the psychedelic assisted session, meaning to be in service to the mysterious processes of these healing medicines and mind-expanding forces of the Greater Self.

Psychedelic Field Phenomena from a Jungian Perspective

Set and setting is a concept commonly used in the Psychedelic Renaissance, referring to the client's intentions (set) and the environment (setting) where the medicine sessions take place. From a Jungian perspective, phenomena of the psychedelic field include: the conscious levels of set and setting, as well as layers of the personal and collective unconscious—in which energetic fields of both the physical and unseen realms can manifest in the environment of the medicine session. These phenomena of the field also occur outside time and the physical setting where the medicine sessions take place. Phenomena of the psychedelic field begin prior to and after psychedelic sessions through dreams, prescient information, omens, and synchronicities. Importantly, the psychedelic therapist's engagement with the psychedelic field includes careful attention to dreams as guides for the psychedelic process.

Consciously working with the psychedelic field, veritable portals can open to experience the volition of the medicine as an entity per se, in other words archetypes manifesting through to empirical levels. The psychedelic field can be engaged by the therapist moving from an egocentric identity to developing a real-lived ego-Self axis. Moreover, the psychedelic field can be a learning ground for knowing one's personal myth, engagement with living symbols, and conscious reciprocal interaction with the entelechy aiming toward individuation.

Consciously engaging with the phenomena of the psychedelic field includes the following but is not limited to: 1) dyadic exchange between the therapist's and client's conscious and unconscious; 2) neurobiological and perceptible physical effects of psychedelic medicines; 3) perceptible energy exchange between therapist and client; 4) spontaneous and intense emotional states; 5) rapid and radical transformation from deeper than intellectual effort; 6) expanded states beyond the ego complex; 7) experiences of transpersonal levels of psyche and archetypal symbols; 8) phenomena originating beyond the therapist's and client's individual psyches; and 9) sometimes direct experience of deceased relatives or nonhuman intelligences. This field commences prior to, occurs during, and continues after the administration of the psychedelic medicines regardless of the therapist's attention on how the field is manifesting. The psychedelic field of a unitive phenomenon comprised of therapist—client—psychedelic medicine—expanded states, in sum, paradoxically forms a whole simultaneously with its independent parts.

Jung's concept of the psychoid unconscious (CW 8, § 368; CW 14, § 786) may be helpful in understanding a depth perspective of set and setting. The psychoid unconscious may be considered a repository (not to be reified) of all archetypes, not directly perceptible through the five senses, but experienced by how the archetypes in the psychoid unconscious manifest themselves. A fitting analogy is how wind cannot be seen but can be experienced by watching the leaves of a tree move or feeling the sensation of a warm breeze passing over the skin.

The psychoid unconscious manifests simultaneously as empirical, psychological, and ethereal without separation or compartmentalization. Considering this premise, psychedelic expanded states reveal a fallacy in identifying as a being that is a separate self from the whole. The psychedelic experience that all is interconnected, no separate self from the whole, is often precisely the healing experience for depression, anxiety, and trauma. The direct experience of all connectedness—*unus mundus*—is inherently a healing agent in psychedelic treatments.

It is common that the therapist, consciously engaged in the psychedelic field, can perceive information about the client that is not conveyed through empirical means. Aspects of the psychedelic field facilitate portals to the psychoid unconscious in which images and information about the client can appear in the therapist's consciousness, and vice versa. In one of the Ketamine-assisted sessions with Elias, while in a psychedelic stage of the Ketamine session, he looked at me and said that he could see different images of me that were much younger than my chronological age at the time.

The following is an example of the psychedelic field being activated prior to a psychedelic medicine session. My client had been in psychotherapy with me for approximately two years and knew about my work with the Shipibo healers. A couple months prior to this synchronistic event, she had first expressed interest in travelling to the Amazon to work with the Shipibo healers at their healing center. Recently, I walked onto the patio of my house for a quick break immediately prior to her appointment. I noticed something long, wavy, and out of place on the patio. I approached it and realized it was a snake sunning itself. This was the first time seeing a snake on my patio in all the years I have lived here. I admired its beautiful coloring. Then noticing the time, I returned to my computer to meet with the client, not giving the snake a second thought. Halfway through the session, my client mentioned the topic again of wanting to work with the Shipibo healers. We explored her desire, then she disclosed her deepest fear of going to the healing center in the Amazon, previously unbeknownst to me: snakes. The synchronicity of the snake on my patio moments before the session, and her disclosure of her intense fear of snakes gave me clear indication of the psychedelic field being active.

Dreams are another way to access the psychoid unconscious and the psychedelic field. Core to Jungian psychology is dreamwork, and this is no exception in psychedelic therapy. In psychedelic therapy dreams are gateways allowing access to beyond-ego communications between therapist and patient, access to other realms rooted in the psychoid unconscious, and sometimes offering prescriptive information about the client's treatment. Likewise, dreams offer guidance directly to the therapist about the therapist's role in the psychedelic sessions.

A prescient dream happened in 2016 before I knew about psychedelic therapy or Indigenous healing traditions with psychedelic medicines. Briefly, I dreamed of an Indigenous healer who was fed tiny bits of apple carried to his mouth by hundreds of spiders. Since that night, dreaming of this man and his spiders, spiders manifest repeatedly in conjunction with any big event that I undergo with psychedelic medicine, showing themselves to me as allies related to psychedelic medicines. Spiders certainly were not my preference at the start; nevertheless, living with this archetype and its manifestations from the psychoid unconscious, I deeply appreciate its involvement in my life. Apparently, chosen by the spider archetype, spiders manifest themselves consistently throughout my work as a psychedelic therapist and in training with the Shipibo healers. The most recent manifestation of the archetypal spider happened two weeks ago when I presented on Jungian psychology and psychedelic treatments at the C.G. Jung Institute-Kusnacht, Zurich. In the morning of the conference, I woke and the first thing I saw was a spider crawling across the blanket over my chest. At that moment, I knew spirits of the medicine and the psychedelic field were going to be present for the presentation later that day.

Consciously created and genuinely experienced, ritual adds immense value to working with psychedelic treatments. Rituals express through the body, voice, intuition, and movements preconscious intentions and living symbols (CW 14, § 603), connecting image and instinct inherent in the psychedelic field of the client's psychedelic processes. In my practice, I intentionally create rituals to connect with the psychedelic field. The importance of ritual is to honor the client and access the psychedelic field which creates the temenos for the work. When we are mindful of the root from which synchronicity, omens, and prescient dreams appear, the therapist can tap that root directly in service of healing and individuation processes. Before I sit with a client, three to five nights before a psychedelic session, I prepare through ritual, directed intention, meditation, active imagination, song, and prayer to the Greater

Good, asking for insight about the client's process and for humility to be a conduit of healing. Recently during a ritual preparation, three days before holding space for a woman in a psychedelic session, I received what seemed like a directive to go to my nearby woods, meditate, and collect fern fronds growing along the creek. In the morning of the session, I followed that directive completing its instructions in preparation for the psychedelic session. At the beginning of psychedelic-assisted session, I brought out the fronds for the opening ritual of her session. The woman paused, teared up, saying that she was suddenly filled with memories of her childhood growing up among ferns on her grandfather's land. I did not know about this part of her life. She recounted to me the meaning of having these fern fronds in her childhood and in her psychedelic assisted session. This was a clear sign to me that the psychedelic field had been constellated prior to the start of our psychedelic assisted session. The connective psychic tissue between client, therapist, and spirits of the medicines can be consciously accessed and is an important and vital healing aspect of psychedelic treatments.

Conclusion

The value of including Jungian psychology in psychedelic research and therapy cannot be overstated, offering comprehensive psychological maps to understand and navigate expanded states, psychedelic experiences, and integration. Jungian psychology's contribution seems indispensable for making meaning of baffling experiences and inchoate symbols which surface unfiltered from the unconscious during psychedelic sessions. Psychedelic medicines viewed through a Jungian lens can offer more coherent and intuitive understanding of the unconscious—both personal and collective—enhancing the individuation process of conscious integration of shadow, persona, ego, cultural complexes, and dyadic relations with the Self. Psychedelic therapy for some can be an invaluable tool in the individuation process, resulting in reparative brain functioning, living more in sync with *anima mundi,* communicating with invisible-yet-real nonhuman realms, and accessing mysterious intelligences which guide and heal. The *prima materia* that psychedelic therapy uncovers can offer invaluable guidance for the individuation processes of both therapist and patient. Additionally, a Jungian perspective offers a broader way of relating to cultural complexes impacting the psychedelic treatment. Often a patient's psychedelic experiences include archetypal, transpersonal, and ancestral ways of knowing beyond the individual's ego complex and cultural worldview. From a Jungian perspective, navigation of the psychedelic field enhances a living temenos for deep and sustainable healing.

From a post-Jungian perspective, psychedelic therapies go beyond treating illnesses. The legitimacy of responsibly employing psychedelic medicines with well-functioning individuals to assist in self-development, integration, and facilitating individuation processes warrants consideration in the Psychedelic Renaissance by psychedelic researchers and clinicians. From this perspective, psychedelic medicines can be considered entheogens. An entheogen is a psychedelic medicine that produces expanded states specifically for spiritual purposes. Respectfully engaging with these entheogenic medicines as sacraments to connect with Self or Greater Mystery falls squarely in post-Jungian models of treatment. Psychedelic medicines as entheogens hold promise for integral living by deepening psychological wellbeing, healing ailments of our collective Western paradigm, and individuating through direct experiences of *unus mundus*—the interconnectedness of all.

References

Clark, G. (2021). Carl Jung and the psychedelic brain: An evolutionary model of Analytical Psychology informed by psychedelic neuroscience. *International Journal of Jungian Studies,* 1-30.

Edinger, E. (1972). *Ego and Archetype.* Penguin.

Jung, C.G. (1975). *C.G. Jung Letters vol. 2: 1951-1961.* Gerhard Adler (Ed.). Princeton University Press.

Mahr, G., & Sweigart, J. (2020). Psychedelic drugs and Jungian therapy. *Journal of Jungian Scholarly Studies, 15* (1).

Phelps, J. (2017). Developing guidelines and competencies for the training of psychedelic therapists. *Journal of Humanistic Psychology, 57*(5), 450-487.

Prakash, S. (2017). Dreams are Nature, Nature is Eternal: Jung and Individuation in Light of Ayahuasca Shamanism. *Medium.com.* https://medium.com/@SandeepPrakash/dreams-are-nature-nature-is-eternal-jung-and-individuation-in-light-of-ayahuasca-shamanism-8dc22347fdc6 (Last accessed: 14 July 2023).

Singer, T. & Kimbles, S. (2004). *Cultural complex: Contemporary Jungian perspectives on psyche and society.* Routledge.

Swank, M. (2021). Mercurius ubiquitous: A Jungian approach to psychedelic therapy. *International Journal of Jungian Studies,* 13-40.

Are the Use of Psychedelics
Really Necessary?

Deborah Bryon

This paper will examine some of the issues we are facing as Jungian analysts and clinicians regarding psychedelic-induced experiences as to the following:

1. The collective complex constellated in modern culture in response to the use of psychedelics.
2. In contrast to the use of psychedelics in the current culture, similarities and differences between the drug-induced ayahuasca experience and states of ecstasy that shamanic medicine people call *paqos* (Andean shamanic medicine people) facilitate without the use of plant medicine. This will be explored in relation to the individuation process.
3. A description of the re-entry process that often happens after numinous experience and how this experience may hinder or deepen the individuation process.
4. Clinical case material illustrating some of the issues emerging regarding psychedelic-induced experiences within our current mental health paradigm.
5. The validity of current research findings and whether drug induced states are necessary to achieve deeper connection with the cosmos and the Self.

The Current Collective Psychedelic Craze

Lately, it seems that at least once a week an analysand announces during a session that they are planning to participate in a psychedelic experience, sometimes with friends, but recently more often with a practitioner who facilitates psychedelic journeys. Some analysands who are therapists have begun training to become psychedelic practitioners, and report that they have started growing their own mushrooms. There is currently a buzz about psychedelics in the collective milieu, encouraged by the circulating news hype creating an air of *participation mystique*, in which critical reflection appears to be missing.

I notice that I am becoming increasingly wary of this new wave of interest in psychedelics that often borders on a mild state of frenzy set loose in the collective. In our modern Western culture, we appear to have an addiction craving immediacy and intensity, often without deeper exploration into our own psyches. I find myself wondering if the immediate breakthroughs analysands are hoping to achieve using psychedelics are indicative of a cultural complex hidden under the guise of a search for deeper meaning. This approach seems incongruent with the analytic process in Depth Psychology.

The Shamanic Ayahuasca Experience

Obviously, not everyone who works with plant medicine is driven or influenced by a cultural complex. People living in the Amazon jungle of Peru have ongoing relationship with psychedelic plants, which grow in their native environment. The ayahuasca plant plays a significant role in daily spiritual practice and rituals. *Ayahuasqueros* are trained in the ceremonial traditions involving the ayahuasca plant, including the ritual of preparing the plant medicine for sacred ceremonies. They work with the spirit of the plant and facilitate ceremonies assisting people in ayahuasca psychedelic journeys. Aspects of the ayahuasca plant medicine ceremony, referred to by *ayhausqueros* as *the spirit of the jungle*, share commonalities with the individuation process. This is primarily because the ego surrenders to something greater, which in this case is the living cosmos—referred to in the native Peruvian language, Qechua, as *wira cocha*.

While Amazon ayahuasca ceremonies occur in a more indigenous natural setting and the training the *ayhausquero* receives is extensive (passed down through generations and more involved than what psychedelic practitioners in our culture appear to be receiving), these plant medicine experiences are considered by some to be controversial. The late anthropologist Michael Harner, author of best seller, *The Way of the Shaman*, wrote that shamans in the Peruvian Amazon call the ayahuasca medicine "the little death" (Harner, 1980, p. 2). In a personal conversation with Harner several decades ago, he told me that he did not recommend the use of ayahuasca because it was dangerous and not necessary for shamanic journeying.

Based upon my own experience working with plant medicine in the Amazon jungle, I have found ayahuasca to be an interesting teacher in that it forces one to shift between psychic self-states into atemporal dimensions, with the opportunity to transcend into deep connection with *wawira cocha. Pachamama*, the Great Mother in Peruvian cosmology, emerges symbolically in a collective archetypal representation as *Amaru,* the great serpent which brings fertility and manifestation to physical reality. In the ayahuasca journey, the personal shadow is usually confronted, requiring the surrender of one's physical body—and ego—to the jungle spirit. This often occurs in the process of being eaten by the giant anaconda spirit, the giver of life and death, before becoming one with the *ch'askas,* or stars, and *wira cocha*. This can be understood to be a metaphor for the individuation process, with the ego surrendering in service of the Self.

While the ayahuasca experience can be transformative, related to what Harner described, I have also witnessed darker aspects of an ayahuasca experience. In one incident during my time in the Amazon jungle, the lead *ayahuasquero* did not show up to oversee a group ceremony and the event devolved into what felt to me to be like an uncontained psychic meteor shower in the energy field of the group. Under normal conditions, a skilled *ayahuasquero* will actively use their song (a melody that has come to them through working with the ayahuasca plant) to move energy during a ceremony. They also use tobacco smoke to shift the direction of someone's journey the plant medicine may be taking. In the ceremony without the *ayahuasquero*, I witnessed the emergence of unprocessed psychic material (referred to in Qechua as *houcha*) bouncing energetically around a group with many people vomiting for hours. The next day after the ceremony, I observed one woman in a state of extreme anxiety, with symptoms that resembled PTSD. The outcome of this ceremony, lacking the presence of a trained *ayahuasquero*, emphasizes the need for competent guides experienced in actively working with the spirit of the medicine.

Non-drug Induced States in Andean Medicine

While I believe that there is value in the ayahuasca experience, when facilitated by an experienced *ayahuasquero*, the non-drug-induced states of ecstasy I have entered, working with Andean *paqos* (Inca shamans) in the sacred mountains of the Andes, have been more profound for me. In Andean medicine, *paqos* enter states of deep-rooted connection with *Pachamama* and the *apu* mountain spirits, making a shift from physical reality into communion with the spirit world, an atemporal dimension of an energetic collective. Rather than using plant medicine, moving into these states involves working with a *misa* (medicine bundle) made up of *quiyas* (stones) that a *paqo* has collected. The *misa* becomes imbued with energy that serve as a portal between realms.

Deep connection with the *apus* and *Pachamama* in these atemporal states is intentional and focused, and as *paqos* emphasize: *heart-based*. Like individuation, in Andean medicine, the capacity to enter profound energetic states with *wira cocha* usually develops over years of practice; it is not a quick fix. I have heard *paqos* say, "Slow down to move fast." Parallel to the alchemical process of individuation, the psyche needs time to cook for transformation to occur.

Paqos say that they serve numinous experience, and, as Jungians, we acknowledge that we draw meaning from numinous mystical encounters. Both *paqos* and Jungians consciously enter a receptive relationship with the unknowable that is greater than our limited ego perspective. According to the *paqos*, when one is on a spiritual path, an intention is set for spiritual connection, and then the decision is made to act in a way that supports this connection. Similar to what is demanded by the unconscious in the individuation process, *paqos* ask, "What will you die to—and for—in your surrender to the cosmos?" Both individuation

160

and Andean medicine require being in a fluid energetic exchange, which *paqos* refer to as *right relationship* or *ayni* with *wira cocha*, similar to the relationship in the individuation process with the unconscious.

States of Ecstasy in Peruvian Shamanism the Levels of Psychic Engagement

In the ayahuasca experience and Andean medicine, there are four levels of psychic engagement in the transition from physical reality into experiencing numinous states of oneness. They are referred to as the *physical, symbolic, mythic,* and *energetic* (Bryon, 2012). The levels of psychic engagement occur in mystical numinous encounters and in meditative practices, induced with or without the aid of psychedelic substances.

The *physical level,* the first level of psychic engagement takes place from a temporal perspective in physical reality. It is grounded in consensual, temporal experience that is directed toward daily activity and functions solely in the domain of ego consciousness.

The *symbolic level*, the second level of psychic engagement, occurs in dreams and waking states of reverie, and in flow states involving the creative process. It is the psychic entrance into the liminal psychic state that Winnicott (1971) described as the transitional space between creative play and reality.

The *mythic level,* the third level of psychic engagement, is the primordial archetypal realm, which shifts from a personal to a collective perspective. The mythic level is associated with the collective unconscious, universal to mankind, and the source of the common themes and symbols that emerge across different cultures and societies. The mythic level involves a shift into the psychoidal realm of atemporality, where synchronic events occur.

The *energetic level*, is the fourth level of psychic engagement and refers to experiencing psychic states of ecstasy, also referred to as oceanic experience (Freud, 1923-1925): states of oneness. The *energetic* level occurs in an atemporal, non-ego dimension in the objective psyche (Jung, CW 8, § 342), in which physical form, time and space, cease to exist and everything is experienced as happening simultaneously in a state of connection with the cosmos.

Coming Back from States of Oneness: The Re-entry Process

In addition to the need for clear intention before entering deep states of connection in mystical experience with or without the use of psychedelics, another critical factor is creating a safe space for the re-entry process. Re-entry occurs when a psychic shift is made from the atemporal dimension of energetic experience back into the psychic space in temporal reality of daily living. I had a supervisor in analytic training who once remarked, "Anyone can drop a couple of hits of acid and you're in—it's the coming back that's hard." Returning after a numinous encounter with the cosmos can be challenging; it is often both jarring and alienating. The re-entry process after a profound numinous experience in many ways parallels the near-death experiences described by P.M.H. Atwater (2007).

There are parallels in the re-entry process between drug-induced experiences and mystical encounters that occur without the use of drugs (Underhill, 1964). Often, during psychedelic-induced experiences and in non-drug-induced states of ecstasy, one enters an atemporal dimension, creating a feeling of timelessness and universal connection (Hartocollis, 1970; Freedman, 1968).

In quantum physics, a blurring effect is described that happens when moving from atemporal to temporal states. The physicist Carlo Rovelli has written:

> Time determined by macroscopic states having to do with the quantum indeterminacy (i.e. lack of specificity) of things produces a blurring ... which insures—contrary to what classic physics seems to indicate—that the unpredictability of the world is maintained even if it were possible to measure everything that is measurable ... Temporality is profoundly linked to blurring. The blurring is due to the fact that we are ignorant of the microscopic details of the world. The time of physics is, ultimately, the expression of our ignorance of the world. (Rovelli, 2019, p. 123)

Shifting out of an atemporal state of ecstasy into a temporal perspective in physical reality can be both challenging and painful. In *A Hero with a Thousand Faces*, Joseph Campbell (2008) described a phenomenon that can occur after a numinous experience of a deep longing to return. Nathan Schwartz Salant (1998) described this in *The Mystery of the Human Relationship* as moving from a state of *conjunctio,* or connection, into the *nigredo,* in which the darkness of separation is experienced. In her description of returning from a near death experience, P.M.H. Atwater (2007, p. 105) has written, "Once an individual has experienced being one with the universe, little else is of much interest … Frustration is frequently felt after experiencing a deeply moving event that one does not have words for."

After a numinous encounter, the day-world can feel flat in contrast to the sense of aliveness experienced in an energetic state of oneness. This may occur regardless of whether the experience was induced using psychedelics. Initially, what is often acutely missing after such an experience, is knowing how to access and maintain a psychic channel that allows for an active dialogue with the Self, or in the case of *paqos*, the spirit world, to continue.

The physicist Alain Connes (2013) wrote a science fiction story about a woman who had the experience of seeing the world from an atemporal perspective. He has written,

> I have had the unheard of good fortune of experiencing a global vision of my being—not of a particular moment, but of my existence 'as a whole' … And then returning to time, I had the impression of losing all of the infinite information generated by the quantum scene, and this loss was sufficient to drag me irresistibly into the river of time … This re-emergence of time seemed to me like an intrusion. (Rovelli, 2019 p. 123-124)

The late anthropologist who studied shamanism with the Yaqui Indians, Carlos Castaneda, wrote, "No one remembers anything while in a state of heightened awareness" (1984, p. 10). The inability to put something into words often happens after a profound religious experience in a state of ecstasy. Castaneda's description of his own experience with atemporality coincides with the Rovelli's explanation of blurring, when a shift is made from atemporality into temporality, and information is lost. Castanada has written:

> We became cognizant then that in these states of heightened awareness we had perceived everything in one big clump, one bulky mass of inextricable detail. We called this ability to perceive everything at once intensity … Our capacity to remember was in reality, incapacity to put the memory of our perception on a linear basis … The task of remembering, then … was the task of consolidating the totality of oneself by rearranging intensity into a linear sequence. (Castanada, 1981, p. 170)

More important than the analyst being present with an analysand during a psychedelic experience, is the capacity of the analyst to work with the analysand during the re-entry and reintegration process that occurs after such an event has taken place. The return can constellate a sense of deep longing along with an intense grief reaction after leaving an oceanic state of oneness, which is associated with a profound sense of belonging and returning home. It is essential for the analyst to be attuned to the analysand's process with some understanding and familiarity of what they are going through. Different reactions to the re-entry process will be exemplified in the following clinical vignettes.

The Drug-Induced Psychedelic Experience and the Clinical Setting

The first clinical example is an illustration of the difficulty some people actively experience in the re-entry process after returning to their daily life.

Kate's Transition After Undergoing a Psychedelic-Induced Experience

An analysand, whom I will refer to as Kate, is a practicing Buddhist who has grappled off and on with chronic depression. In a session together, Kate informed me she had stopped taking the anti-depressant that she had been prescribed and undergone a psychedelic-induced experience with a practitioner. I was a little surprised that we had not explored her decision together beforehand. Kate said that she had been hopeful that the psychedelic-induced experience might help free her from the fatigue and feelings of dysphoria she had been living with.

As I listened to her describe what had happened, Kate told me that, during the psychedelic experience, she had the sensation of feeling her heart opening, which had been wonderful and life changing. Kate explained that she had moved into a state of union with the plants in the garden where the experience had happened, in awe of the life surrounding her. Kate's demeanor changed as she continued recounting the chronology of what took place. She reported tearfully, two weeks after the experience, that she was trying to deal with the increased sensitivity she was feeling being out in the world, and that she had been too overwhelmed to return to work. Kate mentioned she had not reached out for support from the person who had facilitated the journey afterwards, which apparently was not part of the protocol.

A month after the experience, in tears again, Kate announced that she was still struggling. She said she was not sleeping well and was feeling a lot of anxiety. Kate said she still has not been able to return to work full time. She said that she had become acutely aware that she was not happy in her marriage and was feeling incredibly guilty.

Kate reported to me that she had not been able to access the mindfulness skills she had learned in her Buddhist practice. When I asked her how she currently felt about the psychedelic-induced experience, she replied that she was glad that she had the experience because, "It was so profound. Before I was feeling really constricted and not in touch but I underestimated how much it would blow things up. All the stuff going on before is now no longer being pushed away."

Kate told me that she was considering participating in a second psychedelic experience saying, "I want the mushrooms to work. I still think there's promise." I suggested to Kate that she consider giving herself some time to integrate the first experience, and for us to work with exploring the snake imagery that was emerging in dream states and disrupting her sleep, and she agreed. She also promised to schedule a consultation appointment with her psychiatrist and consider resuming the medication for depression that had helped her in the past. During the session, Kate and I explored finding a middle ground between feeling that her emotions were "flattened and less accessible" and having "no skin" or emotional buffer. We agreed that reaching a balance between the two extremes might make it easier for her to function more comfortably in the world.

As I have reflected on my recent sessions with Kate after her psychedelic experience, I continued to feel uneasy and wondered about the ethics and training in administering psychedelic drugs. I question whether the field of mental health is being somewhat short-sighted in allowing psychedelics to be given to people with little preparation or sufficient screening in advance. As demonstrated in Kate's situation, the way the transition experience after the actual drug-induced experience is supported is an important aspect of protocol. The next case, in which these measures were in place is an example of this, resulting in a more favorable outcome.

Claire's Psychedelic-Induced Experience and the Importance of an Adept Facilitator

Another young analysand, whom I will refer to as Claire, has wrestled with an early trauma history and an eating disorder, and experienced a painful breakup several months ago. She recently participated in a drug-induced experience with a skilled clinician, also trained in somatic processing, with positive results. In the analytic session after the drug-induced experience, Claire reported having a sense of well-being and was feeling more embodied.

Claire said that, before receiving the drug, which in her case was a mild dose of cannabis, the practitioner had spent a couple hours with her, helping her identify the issues she would like to address during the session. This process involved "clarifying the relational patterns that Claire was holding in her nervous system" that became constellated in reaction to the painful breakup she has been dealing with.

Claire said the facilitator had been "very present" and "actively listened" to her while she communicated descriptors of the bodily sensations she was experiencing. The sensations she described included a gentle vibration of energy moving through her entire body, with a more acute sense of color and sound, and a sense of well-being, while at the same time feeling very alive. He then accurately recounted and consolidated what she had shared. Claire's description of the facilitator's skill in mirroring and actively engaging with her reminded me of observing a master *ayahuasquero* track and bend the direction of the movement of energy in an ayahuasca journey. Claire said the session had been extremely beneficial and felt that it supported the analytic work we have been doing.

Claire's response to the initial drug-induced session has continued in our subsequent sessions together. I have observed a greater openness in her to the analytic work. It seems that Claire has shifted from being locked in the trauma vortex she frequently found herself in. After the psychedelic session, it appears there is greater opportunity for us to explore the psychic material emerging from the unconscious in Claire's dreams and waking life reflections, because they have become more consciously accessible.

The difference between the outcomes of my two analysands' experiences is significant. Having a facilitator that can actively engage with psychic content as it arises in the person having the drug experience, rather than sitting as a passive observer, seems paramount. It sounded to me that the facilitator in Claire's experience was an attuned clinician, responsive to her needs. From her account, he appeared to be able to help her work with the unprocessed pain that she previously had been holding in her body that emerged in the energetic field during her treatment.

The outcome of Clair's psychedelic sessions was positive, emphasizing the need for a competent facilitator. Whether the plant medicine was necessary in facilitating her experience of positive therapeutic change is unknown. Unlike Kate, Claire had a lighter dose, perhaps closer to micro-dosing, with a substance that is mood-altering but not necessarily psychedelic. Claire's experience also made me aware that with a competent facilitator, it is possible for drug-induced sessions that take place outside of the analytic container to enhance the analytic process without the analyst being the one that administers the drug.

The Spiritual Complex and the Use of Psychedelics

The underlying motivators of people drawn to numinous experience and psychedelic drug-induced treatment vary, depending on their individual psyches. Some people, who have worked to become conscious of their underlying complexes, want to deepen their relationship with the Self in their individuation process and strengthen their connection with spirituality in their search for meaning in their lives. Consciousness in these individuals tends to grow through exposure to the numinosity of mystical experience. For other individuals, living what Von Franz (2000, p. 60) has referred to as an "unlived life," meaning they have avoided facing outer world challenges by living in a fantasy world of denial, the affinity for mind-altering states can be avoidant and a regression toward "longing to return to the womb" (Edinger, 1985, p. 48).

In shamanic and religious communities there is a phenomenon that can occur, referred to as spiritual bypassing, when the focus is on love and light as a way of sidestepping darker psychic material associated with underlying complexes. As a result of the shadow being avoided and unacknowledged, the subject remains in an unconscious state of denial and may act out or project onto others unconsciously. Sometimes a spiritual complex develops that is a potential byproduct of mystical experience, creating an ego-inflation, a sense of grandiosity. The manic reaction is sometimes brought on by an over-identification with the archetypal energy of the numinous. A manic response can also be a defense of flying high above the discomfort of unprocessed trauma. Both can develop after a psychedelic induced experience and may adversely affect the analytic process. If there is a lack of ego-strength, there can be a compensation against feeling the loss of control, a fear reaction that develops from being taken over by something greater in a mystical experience. This can result in the psychic defense structure becoming more rigid and impenetrable.

The case material of the first two analysands presented demonstrates the importance of receiving support during the re-entry process, as well as during the actual experience, with a trained facilitator. The next vignette is an example of long term effects after a negative drug-induced experience that stresses the need for more in-depth screening beforehand. The psychological stability of individuals wanting to participate in psychedelic drug-induced treatment should be assessed to determine if they are a good candidate.

Analysis After a Negative Psychedelic Drug-Induced Experience

I began working with an analysand, whom I will refer to as Sara, about a year after she had a traumatic psychedelic plant medicine experience with a shamanic practitioner in a Central American jungle. On the phone before our initial meeting, Sara told me that she had sought me out because she had felt "judged" by her previous therapist and wanted an analyst that could help her work through "unresolved issues with her mother." When we met for the first time, Sara said she was still trying to recover from a terrifying fear of "disintegrating into nothing" experienced during the plant medicine ceremony, which she was continuing to have disturbing dreams about. In analysis, Sara resisted exploring the residual fear left over from her plant medicine experience because it felt "too intense," while at the same time seemed driven to speed up the pace of the work. Sara's overwhelming anxiety that sometimes bordered on panic became channeled into a manic response that was an obstacle in the analytic process. During sessions, Sara repeatedly steered away from talking about feelings associated with early traumatic memories and told me that she wanted to focus on what she referred to as "big dreams and archetypal imagery." In conjunction with the analysis, in the year we worked together, Sara was a student in a graduate program in Depth Psychology, began somatic training, and made a trip to Zurich to investigate applying for analytic training.

The avoidance of exploring the uncomfortable feelings emerging often manifested in a defensive quick fix mentality, of wanting something different, better, and more. Like the outcome with her first therapist, Sara unexpectedly ended her analysis with me in a phone call, informing me that she wanted to work someone whom she felt was "better suited" to what she "was looking for."

Sara's attraction to psychedelic plant medicine, which resulted in a traumatic experience of having an overpowering feeling of annihilation, may have been symptomatic of a preexisting condition, rather than caused by the psychedelic-induced event. However, the psychedelic experience did seem to destabilize Sara's already fragile ego even further, creating a stronger rigidity in her psyche, in an attempt at self-protection. The defensive characterological structure that had developed in response to a culmination of parental complexes became more impenetrable. This most likely occurred in reaction to the fear of annihilation brought on by exposure, through the plant medicine, with the manic response intensifying. This fortification of the pre-existing defense system became an additional obstacle, making it very difficult for Sara to tolerate her own vulnerability. I believe this prevented us from moving further in our analytic work together. When her apprehension of becoming lost in a psychotic state, exacerbated by the memory of decompensating brought on by the psychedelic experience, became too much for Sarah to endure, she abruptly pulled away.

The Need for Prescreening and Assessment

Reflecting on Sara's experience and what I have witnessed in others, I have come to wonder if individuals who lack ego strength—and are avoidant of shadow material, causing them to potentially be predisposed to decompensating—are drawn to psychedelic experience as plant medicine as a distraction or a cure. The struggles some individuals face in the re-entry process after a psychedelic induced experience substantiate the need for a more extensive screening protocol by practitioners assisting in psychedelic therapy treatment before it is administered. In addition to a prescreening process, it seems important for analysts to help analysands explore their motivation, intention, and outcome expectations before undergoing a psychedelic experience. Another important consideration is dosage as micro-dosing, as small quantities of mushrooms are very different from an ayahuasca experience.

In countries outside of the United States, more intensive screening processes occur with other types of plant medicine treatment. Before administering the psychedelic drug ibogaine to treat heroin and methamphetamine addictions,[1] in countries where the drug has been legalized, many treatment facilities require an initial process screening including an EKG before an individual is admitted. In the United States, patients are assessed by licensed medical professionals before psychotropic medicine is prescribed, yet there appears to be much less screening on the part of practitioners administering psychedelics, except perhaps in some of the research protocols (which will be described in the next section). In addition, psychedelic practitioners are not required to have a medical license or to be licensed as mental health workers.

The approach to psychedelic induced experiences currently seems to have a bit of a wild west attitude in that it there appears to be a mad rush into uncharted, potentially dangerous territory with minimal regulation. Whether the psychedelic induced experience occurs within our cultural paradigm or in an indigenous setting, as illustrated in the cases I presented, there are similar risks.

Research Findings on Psychedelic-Induced Experiences with Positive Outcomes

Many research studies have reported favorable results on psychedelic-induced treatment in a diverse group of participants. In France, a meta-analysis that included eight studies showed a significant decrease in depressive symptoms the day after the drug was administered (Vruno, 2020). A literature review of twenty-five studies between 1990 and 2020, in which lysergic acid diethylamide (LSD), ayahuasca, or psilocybin was administered, found immediate results lasting several months even after a single dose, suggesting psychedelics appear promising, well-tolerated treatments for anxiety, depression, and addiction (Berkovitch et al., 2020). Other studies have shown similar outcomes (Leger & Unterwald, 2022), with the most favorable results occurring after multiple treatments.

A meta-analysis that surveyed 369 studies, found that specific personality traits, such as self-transcendence, appeared to influence the effects of psychedelics (Bouso, et al. 2018). The research concluded psychedelics administered in controlled settings may encourage personality changes including openness and self-transcendence, and that some individuals may be better candidates for positive outcomes with psychedelic-induced treatments (Bouso, et al. 2018). Psychedelics have also been shown effective in treating conditions common among older adults that include mood disorders, psychological distress associated with a serious medical illness, post-traumatic stress disorder (PTSD), and chronic grief disorder (Bree & Kerr, 2023).

Johns Hopkins (2022) has reported being involved in major research on psychedelic-induced treatment, with over $17 million in funding, to further explore research on psychedelics for illness and wellness. Natalie Gukasyan et al. (2022)[2] found "substantial anti-depressant effects" of psilocybin-assisted therapy may be durable at least twelve months after treatment in some participants. It is worth noting that, in this study, participants were pre-screened by trained mental health clinicians who were present during the session when the psilocybin was administered and provided immediate follow-up support sessions. These factors may have contributed to the success of the outcome, adding further support for greater treatment controls in psychedelic treatment.

The External Validity of Research on Psychedelic-Induced Treatment

While a significant number of studies on psychedelic-induced treatments have reported positive outcomes, many scientific critiques have been published regarding the questionable validity of clinical studies on potential therapeutic benefits of psychedelics; some of these studies also report on the many difficulties obtaining regulatory approval (Sellers, 2017; Sellers & Leiderman, 2017; Bouso et al., 2018; Sellers et al., 2018; Yaden, et al., 2022; Light et al., 2022).

Aday et al. have studied the internal validity of research results reported on the efficacy of psychedelic drugs. They have written:

> Although some challenges are shared with psychotherapy and pharmacology trials more broadly, psychedelic clinical trials have to contend with several unique sources of potential bias. The subjective effects of a high-dose psychedelic are often so pronounced that it is difficult to mask participants to their treatment condition; the significant hype from positive media coverage on the clinical potential of psychedelics influences participants' expectations for treatment benefit; and participant

unmasking and treatment expectations can interact in such a way that makes psychedelic therapy highly susceptible to large placebo and nocebo effects. (2022, p. 2)

The research indicates a need to more closely examine the criteria being used to determine the efficacy of psychedelics, and whether a distinction is being made between microdosing and a psychedelic trip as they are very different experiences with diverse outcomes. The analysand that I described who terminated analysis unexpectedly may have shown up as a success if criteria were based upon self-report measures and level of engagement in the world. Some mental health symptoms may be missed in the measurement criteria of studies reporting a favorable outcome. As study participants are all volunteers, if they are those drawn to psychedelics and who use defenses such as spiritual bypassing and denial to manage anxiety and avoid shadow material, self-reporting may not be an accurate way of measuring the outcome. In many of the studies, the measurements used to evaluate the treatment success was not reported in the methodology. Because subjects are volunteers, there is no random sampling, which potentially skews the results.

Are the Use of Psychedelics Really Necessary?

Jung wrote, "The shaman's experience of sickness, torture, death, regeneration implies, at a higher level, the idea of being made whole through sacrifice, through transubstantiation and exalted to the pneumatic man in a word, of apotheosis" (CW 11, § 448). This relates to the psychological experience that happens for shamans reaching the atemporal states of ecstasy that involve the surrender of the ego in connecting with something greater—*wira cocha* and the Self. *Paqos* have demonstrated that this state can be reached either with or without the use of plant medicine or psychedelic substances.

As I have contemplated my own experiences working with analysands who have undergone psychedelic induced treatment and considered the methodology flaws in much of the research, particularly the lack of random sampling and the ways the treatment outcomes are being measured, I find I am less enthusiastic about psychedelic induced drug experiences. My own experiences working with *ayahuasqueros* and the Andean *paqo* in Peru has made me aware that psychedelics are not necessary in achieving energetic states of connection with the cosmos.

Personally, I believe there is great benefit in learning how to traverse between levels of psychic engagement intentionally, without the use of psychedelics or plant medicine. For individuals who have never experienced spiritual connection, and are locked in an ego-driven narrative, psychedelics may be instrumental in opening neural pathways and potentially establishing a conscious connection with the Self. However, for individuals who are already actively engaging with the unconscious, who have experienced numinosity, developing a deeper connection with *wira cocha* or the Self through the process of individuation without relying on mind-altering substances seems more congruent with the analytic process in Depth psychology. *Paqos* achieve states of ecstasy by learning how to move into a relationship of connection with the cosmos, making themselves available by opening their hearts and minds in a deliberate act of submission. Like the individuation path described by Jung (CW 9, § 73), a spiritual path involves a commitment that deepens over time through devotion.

Achieving a higher state of consciousness that is not drug-induced requires discipline and is not the result of entering a regressed state of ego-detachment through a dissolution process, referred to in alchemy as *solutio* (Edinger, 1975, p. 47). According to Ram Dass, becoming reliant on psychedelics to connect with the cosmos does not produce lasting results. In *The Only Dance There Is*, Ram Dass has written:

> My guru, in speaking about psychedelics, said: 'These medicines will allow you to come and visit Christ, but you can only stay two hours. Then you have to leave again. This is not the true samadhi. It's better to become Christ than to visit him—but even the visit of a saint for a moment is useful.' Then he added, 'But love is the most powerful medicine.'[3] (1974, p.112)

174

Achieving states of ecstasy independent of substances suggests a familiarity with the pathway of the ego-self axis, indicating that a receptive attitude toward the unconscious exists and that a strong relationship between the ego and the Self has been established. Developing the awareness of how to embody a submissive stance of surrender toward the unconscious requires a certain degree of ego-strength and consciousness. Understanding and accepting the totality of the Self as the center of the psyche is in alignment with the *paqos* premise that following a spiritual path involves intention and decision. Adopting a conscious position in service of the Self by coming to terms with the realization that it is the center of the psyche enables the ego to maintain a more receptive perspective, allowing greater access to receiving wisdom and direction from the Self.

References

Aday, J.S., Heifets, B.D., Pratscher, S.D., Bradley, E., Rosen, R., & Woolley, J.D. (2022). Great expectations: Recommendations improving the methodological rigor of psychedelic clinical trials. *Psychopharmacology*, *239*(6), 1989-2010.

Atwater, P.M.H. (2007). *The big book of near-death experiences*. Rainbow Ridge Books LLC.

Bae, H., & Kerr, D.C.R. (2020). Marijuana use trends among college students in states with and without legalization of recreational use: Initial and longer-term changes from 2008 to 2018. *Addiction*, *115*(6), 1115-1124.

Berkovitch, L., Roméo, B., Karila, L., Gaillard, R., & Benyamina, A. (2020). Efficacité des psychédéliques en psychiatrie, une revue systématique [Efficacy of psychedelics in psychiatry, a systematic review of the literature]. *Encephale*, *47*(4), 376-387.

Bouso, J.C., Dos Santos, R.G., Alcázar-Córcoles, M.Á., & Hallak, J.E.C. (2018). Serotonergic psychedelics and personality: A systematic review of contemporary research. *Neuroscience Biobehavioral Revews*, *87*, 118-132.

Bryon, D. (2012). *Lessons of the Inca shamans, part I: Piercing the veil*. Pine Winds Press.

Campbell, J. (2008). *Hero with a thousand faces*. Princeton University Press.

Castaneda, C. (1981). *The eagle's gift*. Simon & Schuster.

Castaneda, C. (1984). *The fire from within*. Pocket Books.

Connes, A., Chereau, D., & Dixmier, H. (2013). Le Theatre quantique, Odile Jacob, Paris. In C. Rovelli, *The order of the universe*. Penguin Books.

Edinger, E.F. (1985). *Anatomy of the psyche: Alchemical symbolism in psychotherapy*. Open Court Publishing.

Freedman, D.X. (1968). On the use of abuse of LSD. *Archives of General Psychiatry*, 18330-18347.

Freud, S. (1923–1925). *The ego and the id and other works* (Standard Edition, vol. 19).

Gukasyan, N., Davis, A.K., Barrett, F.S., Cosimano, M.S., Sepeda, N.D., Johnson, M.W., & Griffiths, R.R. (2022). Efficacy and safety of psilocybin-assisted treatment for major depressive disorder: Prospective 12-month follow-up. *Journal of Psychopharmacology, 36*(2), 151-158.

Hartocollis, P. (1972). Time as a dimension of affects. *Journal of the American Psychoanalytic Association, 20,* 92-108.

Jacobs, A. (2021). The psychedelic revolution is coming: Psychiatry may never be the same. *The New York Times.* https://www.nytimes.com/2021/05/09/health/psychedelics-mdma-psilocybin-molly-mental-health.html?action=click&module=Top_Stories&pgtype=Homepage (Last Accessed 2 August 2023).

Koenig, X., & Hilber, K. (2015). The anti-addiction drug ibogaine and the heart: A delicate relation. *Molecules, 20,* 2208-2228.

Koval, A.L., Kerr, D.C.R., & Bae, H. (2019). Perceived prevalence of peer marijuana use: Changes among college students before and after Oregon recreational marijuana legalization. *American Journal of Drug and Alcohol Abuse, 45*(4), 392-399.

Leger, R.F., & Unterwald, E.M. (2022). Assessing the effects of methodological differences on outcomes in the use of psychedelics in the treatment of anxiety and depressive disorders: A systematic review and meta-analysis. *Journal of Psychopharmacology, 36*(1), 20-30.

Light, N., Fernbach, P.M., Rabb, N., Geana, M.V., & Sloman, S.A. (2022). Knowledge overconfidence is associated with anti-consensus views on controversial scientific issues. *Science Advances, 8*(29), eabo0038.

Myran, D.T., Tanuseputro, P., Auger, N., Konikoff, L., Talarico, R., & Finkelstein, Y. (2022). Edible cannabis legalization and unintentional poisonings in children. *New England Journal of Medicine, 387*(8), 757-759.

Nielsen, S., Larance, B., Degenhardt, L., Gowing, L., Kehler, C., & Lintzeris, N. (2016). Opioid agonist treatment for pharmaceutical opioid dependent people. *Cochrane Database of Systematic Reviews, 5*, Article CD011117. Update in: Cochrane Database of Systematic Reviews, 2022 Sep 5;9:CD011117. PMID: 27157143.

Johnston, B., Mangini, M., Grob, C., & Anderson, B. (2023). The safety and efficacy of psychedelic-assisted therapies for older adults: Knowns and unknowns. *The American Journal of Geriatric Psychiatry, 31*(1), 44-53.

Pollan, M. (2018). *How to change your mind*. Penguin Books.

Ram Dass (1974). *The only dance there is*. Random House.

Rovelli, C. (2019). *The order of the time*. Penguin Books.

Schwartz-Salant, N. (2007). *The black nightgown: The fusional complex and the unlived life*. Chiron Publications.

Sellers, E.M. (2017). Psilocybin: good trip or bad trip. *Clinical Pharmacology and Therapeutics, 102*(4), 580-584.

Sellers, E.M., & Leiderman, D.B. (2017). Psychedelic drugs as therapeutics: No illusions about the challenges. *Clinical Pharmacology and Therapeutics, 103*(4), 561-564.

Sellers, E.M., & Romach, M.K. (2023). Psychedelics: Science sabotaged by social media. *Neuropharmacology, 227*, Article 109426.

Sellers, E.M., Romach, M.K., & Leiderman, D.B. (2018). Studies with psychedelic drugs in human volunteers. *Neuropharmacology, 142*, 116-134.

Underhill, E. (1964). *The mystics of the church*. Schocken Books.

Von Franz, M.L. (2000). *The problem of the puer aeternus*. Inner City Books.

Vruno, R. (2020). *Department of Psychiatry and Addictology*. APHP, Paul Brousse Hospital, Villejuif, France.

Winnicott, D.W. (1971) *Playing and reality*. Penguin Books.

Yaden, D.B., Potash, J.B., & Griffiths, R.R. (2022). Preparing for the bursting of the psychedelic hype bubble. *JAMA Psychiatry, 79*(10), 943-944.

Endnotes

[1] Ibogaine is a drug that has been shown to have a high efficacy rate in treating addiction that is still illegal but in trial in the United States

[2] In the study conducted by Gukasyan et al. (2022) the participants went through an initial screening and were accessed as being "mentally stable" and met criteria for moderate major depressive disorder. After participants entered the intervention period, they were provided with 6-8 hours of preparatory meetings with two facilitators, with at least one facilitator with master's level or doctoral level training in mental health. There was also follow-up visit with at least one of the facilitators for 1-2 hours at one day and one week.

[3] https://www.ramdass.org/the-trap-of-psychedelic-experiences/ (Last accessed 31 July, 2023)

Ayahuasca and Amerindian Perspectivism: The Shamanic Emergence in the Jungian Clinic

Walter Boechat & Ana Luisa Teixeira de Menezes

Introduction by Walter Boechat

It was a unique experience for me to be Ana Luisa's advisor on her graduate thesis as a Jungian analyst at the Jungian Association of Brazil (AJB). In a very personal tone, but with an admirable theoretical rigor, Ana Luísa explored the paths of her inner discoveries through her fieldwork with different ethnic groups from southern Brazil, the Guarani, the Kaigang, and also the Inga from Bolivia. In these groups she had close contact with shamans, their healing techniques, and spiritual search. In her thesis, the author sought to establish bridges between the healing methods of these indigenous peoples and western psychotherapy. In her fieldwork, Ana Luisa had contact with the various ritualistic practices by which the indigenous people reach their altered states of consciousness, aiming for the therapeutic benefit of their patients and a greater spiritual development. On some occasions, the author herself made use of Ayahuasca, giving very rich tones to her monograph. Certain passages are illustrated by the author herself with paintings that express all the richness of the ecstasy caused by the Ayahuasca experience. Some of these paintings are reproduced in this work, with psychological comments.

The paintings make clear how the ritual use of Ayahuasca puts the patient and therapist in contact with images from the collective unconscious, which have special relevance in the therapeutic process. These images occur in the interactive field of the therapeutic process. When shared, they have special importance in the process of psychological transformation.

181

This chapter is structured in the form of a dialog similar to the conversations Ana and I had during the development of her monograph. Ana's fieldwork, the work with her patients in her Jungian therapeutic clinic, her drawings full of symbolism and mystery, the transferential field with her patients, the silent mediation of Ayahuasca, and my observations and comments all weave together to create a rich embroidery of experiences.

In Ana Luísa's work, the Myth of the Guarani Twins was given special emphasis. This was so because this myth guides the whole thread of the narrative and the imagery experiences.

Walter: Ana, maybe you should try to describe in general terms your experience with the indigenous ethnic groups, the use of Ayahuasca by certain groups, and how you personally encountered the plant.

Ana: Walter, my most remarkable experience with Ayahuasca was with the Colombian Ingas Indigenous People, with the *taita*, a shamanic leader, in Pontumayo. It was a rainy night and we went up the mountain carrying blankets and mattresses to spend the night, opening the paths for this journey with Ingas' ancestral medicine. This experience was part of an exchange in the postdoctoral research called *Shamanic epistemology and the childhood experience in Indigenous Autoethnographic Studies in Education*, carried out at the Federal University of Rio Grande do Sul. We spent the whole night on top of the mountain, experiencing ancestral medicine. Among the Ingas, Ayahuasca or *Yagé*, as it is called in Colombia, is used as a medicine for spiritual illnesses and as a process of self-knowledge. This is a widespread practice among the Ingas and Colombian indigenous communities. There are different intensities of plants that vary in the effects they produce. A leader told us that there are six types of Ayahuasca.

The memory of the emerged images is striking and opened a path for dialogue with Colombian indigenous mythologies, based on the image of the serpent and ancestral bones. The experience was one of death, and the desire I had was to turn back time so as not to face what was coming, just as Jung describes in *The Red Book*: "You cannot at the same time be on the mountain and in the valley, but your way leads you from mountain to valley and from valley to mountain. Much begins amusingly and leads into the darkness. Hell has levels" (Jung, 2009, p. 265).

Walter: It is fascinating to see how we can learn more and more from the Indigenous People at a time when the western culture is seriously threatened to collapse. The Brazilian ethnologist Eduardo Viveiros de Castro became internationally known for proposing the concept of *Amerindian perspectivism* (2002). Castro noticed how South American tribal societies, and also some Asian tribal societies, have a perception of the universe that is opposed to the dichotomized vision of the Western man, who perceives human culture as dissociated from nature and the latter as a source (in his fantasy, an inexhaustible source) of raw materials. According to the Amerindian perspectivism, spirits, ancestors, human beings, animals, plants, and even mountains and rocks are interconnected and part of an inseparable Whole. This is a perception of an absolutely integrated and harmonious universe, a true *Unus Mundus*.

It calls my attention that you are drawing parallels between the experience of death, the descent you have experienced with Ayahuasca, and *Liber Novus*. Jung, upon realizing the dead-end of modernity, during the crisis of the 1st World War, took a true *reculler pour mieux sauter* (a step back in order to jump better, as Pierre Janet would say), revisiting a medieval epistemology, basing himself in Gerard Dorn (early 16th century), disciple of Paracelsus, to propose the model of *Unus Mundus* to escape from the dissociations of modernity. And how this *alchemical perspective* of Unus Mundus resembles the Amerindian perspectivism of our Latin American Indigenous People!

Ana: Yes, being on the mountain, drinking Yagé, led me to what Jung warns us about the identification we feel in being "a frog among frogs, a fish among fishes," (Jung, 2009, p. 266) and in this case, a serpent among serpents:

> Your heights are your own mountain, which belongs to you and you alone … There you live the endlessness of being, but not the becoming. Becoming belongs to the heights and is full of torment. How can you become if you never are? Therefore you need your bottommost, since there you are. But therefore you also need your heights, since there you become. (Jung, 2009, p. 266)

Being at this altitude, with the Indigenous People and the Yagé, enabled an intense experience of imagination, enigmatic; according to Jung and the Ingas it brings a clarity of ourselves. However, I wanted to go down and spend the day sleeping, in order to appease this depth. But, instead, we spent the day going up and down mountains, dialoguing with other spiritual leaders. Everything was enigmatic but extremely simple, like a Shaman's teaching when he said that he discovered his vocation as a taita when he found clay pots on the mountain, then he felt that this was his path.

In the period of six months, from research studies, experiences with the Mbya-Guarani[1] indigenous people in Brazil, and participation in Santo Daime[2] rituals, the relationship with the animals intensified. I emphasize that it was a process that went beyond the *mirações*[3] in the rituals. I dedicated myself to being beside a waterfall at dawn, and I felt in a very real way the strength of the animals acting within my body and so I came to viscerally understand that the words act creatively in the spirit and life can flow along unlimited paths.

Walter: Yes, Ana, how fascinating is this interconnected universe, the world of the psyche and material things in constant meaningful dialogue. Being on the mountain, finding clay pots, and the emergence of the taita vocation! Jung's late ideas of psychoid and synchronicity are a way to rescue these important lost references. But we are no longer indigenous, it is no longer possible to return to this worldview concretely. We would be falling into what Bauman (2017) called "retrotopia." Jung's proposal of a worldview with a search for meaning and a symbolic attitude within contemporary complex thought is a post-modern way out of the dichotomies of modernity. Ayahuasca, when combined with an appropriate moment and a specific ritual, seems to facilitate the emergence of symbols from the cultural unconscious with great intensity. This emergence constellates a "shamanistic complex," as Eliade (1974) called it. But, according to your personal experience, what is the role and relevance of Ayahuasca in the therapeutic situation?

Ana: I realized that Ayahuasca produces an affective overload in the activation of unconscious material constellated as natural elements in the psyche, as we shall see below. Through this activation one can transcend the duality of human/nature. I experienced an image with a patient in which he was at the bottom of the water, he emerged from the water and a serpent coiled him, first he became tense, and then he opened his arms and chest surrendering himself to a connection with a vital energy. I looked at him and realized that this was his healing process. In the next session, he described a dream that had the same structure as the one I had visualized: he was in the water, at the bottom, drowning, when he saw two deflated basketballs, and so he realized that they could inflate and help him to rise from the bottom. One of them inflated and he started rising along a thread. He came across a cement ceiling that a woman was breaking through and so he managed to stand up, met that woman, and hugged her.

The image of the snake and the patient, besides the possibility of healing, brings the image of the masculine and feminine, the numinous and the dark. The serpent Anaconda is considered "the Mother of water," as an original matrix that contains and transforms the germinative power of the sun to give light to humanity, a cosmic deity and the first ancestor in the Amazon religious cosmovision (Gutiérrez & Torres, 2011, p. 93).

We can interpret the appearance of the serpent, expressed in painting 1 (Figure 1), as having an effect for this patient similar to Anaconda's function as a feminine element, a womb that promotes the procreation of fishes and other water creatures, in its germinal and seminal properties. Furthermore, one can perceive that life is compared to the ascent of the river and its mouth, its descent into the headwaters which is experienced as a spiritual rebirth, as a new life in another dimension.

For Letuama mythology, the first ancestors were transformed from the Great Anaconda:

> Ahora bien, los matices sonoros de las flautas, trompetas y demás instrumentos musicales que se identifican con los ancestros míticos y se inspiran en las voces de los animales (cantos, silbidos, zumbidos, percusión) que emiten los pájaros, los monos, los jaguares, los tapies, las anacondas, participan de un alto potencial fertilizador.[4]
> (Gutiérrez & Torres, 2011, p. 96)

The healing experience goes through an intertwining, allowing oneself to be captured in order to be transformed, allowing oneself be swallowed in order to also swallow and vomit, allowing oneself to suffer a metamorphosis, as suggested by the mythology of the great serpent in the encountering spiritual sounds. The bird has a sound, the snake has a dance, the jaguar has a movement, and humans can learn about this, this cyclical and cosmic universal greatness.

At this time [when the painting was created], I was under the effect of Ayahuasca and began to apprehend the symptoms of some patients, in a more symbolic language, which I could better express only through nonverbal techniques through the use of paintings. There is an intensification of the analyst-patient interaction, with the activation of the healing field of the analysis.

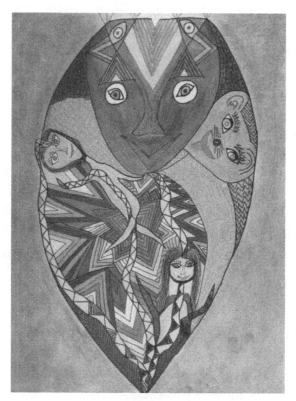

Figure 1

Walter: In what sense are you using the concept of *field*? Indeed, the notion of *interactive field* has increasingly appeared in Jungian writings and psychoanalysis in general. Jung (CW 16) more poetically described it alchemically in his study of the *Rosarium Philosophorum*. The interactive field appears there prefigured as the alchemical mercury that provides the transformation of metals, the mutations of the Sun and Moon, the King and Queen. A few years later, in the early 1950s, texts by psychoanalytic authors such as Heimann (1950), Ogden (with his concept of the *analytical third)* and Bion were published, with very similar ideas, but well tied within a psychoanalytic theoretical structure. Among the Jungians, Jacoby (1995), Schwartz-Salant (1995) and Carter (2010) were some who used the concept of interactive field in analysis. The interactive field constellates unconscious elements with greater or lesser intensity in different situations. It can be observed that without the emergence of the interactive field, the transferential phenomena and the analysis itself are impossible. I noticed the subtle emergence of the interactive field even in online analysis during the Covid-19 pandemic. In this case this emergence takes place in the virtuality of the internet. Conolly (2015) mentions the presence of paranormal phenomena such as telepathy and others in the interactive field already attested since Freud. The dreams, with shared elements that you and your patient have, belong to this kind of emergence in the interactive field, no doubt greatly intensified by Ayahuasca. It is intriguing the presence of water or mercury as a shared element between the two dreams, and the anaconda serpent as a healing and transforming element. In figure 1, I see the expression of a great dream of archetypal transference activated by Ayahuasca, in which the therapist is called to contain and cultivate, keeping these strong symbols alive for the patient. The analyst appears in this watery environment, joined to the patient by the serpent. Other mysterious entities are constellated in the interactive field, figures of the objective psyche acting to promote the healing process with autonomy.

Ana: Ayahuasca helped me to amplify a relationship between synchronicity and emergence developed by Cambray (2013). I think that the plant activates a field of synchronicities with emergence of nature in the psyche, similar to the understanding of the *vital image* in Yanomami cosmology (Kopenawa & Albert, 2015), as a materiality of image and energy experienced in the body. The paintings which I bring in this dialogue with you, Walter, are the condensation of voices, energies, experiences with spiritual beings materialized in these images, experienced as the emergence of connections that shamans mediate and express through dances at the shamanic rituals.

Walter: No doubt, Ana, I consider important to bear in mind this emergence constellated by Ayahuasca within a shamanic ritual. We may employ Cambray's notion of *emergence* to a dimension of what Eliade (1974) calls the shamanistic complex. Eliade differs the shaman from other medicine-men in preliterate societies in particular in relation to his initiatory process, and in his therapies. He uses the resource of altered states of consciousness, or *shamanic ecstasy*. For this, he uses certain herbs, such as Ayahuasca, the dance, the sacred drum, the rhythm, the cigar and the blown smoke, as seen among Brazilian shamans. That is why Eliade defines shamanism "as a technic of ecstasy." In my graduate thesis at the C.G. Jung Institute in Zurich, I tried to establish connections between shamanistic healing and modern psychotherapy as conceived by Freud and Jung (Boechat, 1979). Ana, your fieldwork, as well as your work with your patients are a constant affirmation of the emergence of the shamanistic complex in contemporary Jungian clinics. There are some other works highlighting this emergence such as Murray Stein's (1992).

Ana: The relation you make in your work on shamanism and psychotherapy expands the notion of Jungian clinic. We can think of the relationship between patient and analyst as a state of connection, in which patient and therapist are healed in a process of identification, whereupon "the analyst reflects the illness of the analysand ... as the illness is assimilated and suffered, the analyst begins to seek healing" (Stein, 1992, p. 74, my translation). This relationship is similar to the healing rituals among the Guarani, in which the community needs to legitimize the *karai* (shaman) as the person who heals. Likewise, it is the patient's healing that will confirm the therapist. I think of a therapeutic relationship as twinning that makes us expand symbolic perceptions of the patient's own speech and the therapist's perception. As you stated in our conversations, Walter: The sun as a patient, and the moon, the analyst, being able to reflect the unconscious contents.

When we think about the possibility of an analytical field triggered by Ayahuasca, we realize how much this plant can facilitate the emergence of new psychological and mythical realities or the encounter with other spiritual entities. We are in contact with a kind of self-organizing movement of life, as a trigger of dissipative structures capable of initiating personality changes (Cambray & Carter, 2014). Perhaps we can conceive the action of a guiding principle in nature, promoting a symbolic elaboration in humans.

In figure 2, I saw myself entering the stem of the tree and going inside the soil, through a vaginal channel, as if the earth was a womb that received me and there spoke to me about spiritual life. At first, the tree leaves emerged as fractals and connected me to thoughts, as if they were particles of neurons acting in new neuronal connections on my mind. Sometimes I felt that I was the leaves and that they were acting within me.

A forest based on the thought of land-forest is designated by the Yanomani shaman *Kopenawa* as *urihi* (2015, p. 480). In indigenous language, we can imagine that the thought can be a tree, can be transformed into a tree, with the branches being a network. Birds perch on the interconnected tree-mind.

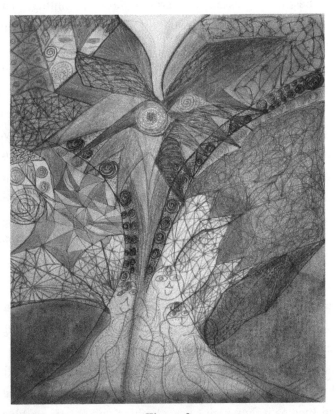

Figure 2
Painting *The tree is a mind of the universe*

Walter: Yes, Ana. In figure 2 it is possible to see a deep integration between mind, body and nature. Indigenous People have this state of integration and communion with nature that Western societies have lost with modernity. New epistemologies of complexity have been discovering these already trodden paths, as in Mancuso (2019), who works with the importance of plant consciousness for the maintenance of life across the planet. Or like Wohlleben (2017), who describes in the now famous *The Hidden Life of Trees,* how trees have an organized social life. This image of the tree as the mind of the universe confirms this deep identity of plants with the human beings. We are encountering here the ancient aphorism of Gnosticism: *God sleeps in the mineral, breathes in the plants, dreams in the animal, and awakens in man.*

You are creatively experiencing inexpressible boundary states, which can best be expressed non-verbally through paintings. This non-verbal resource was also used by Jung in the creation of the calligraphic copy of *The Red Book.* In crucial passages, as in the moment of near-death of the hero Izdubar in *Liber Secundus,* Jung interrupts the automatic flow of his writing and resorts to the use of several paintings of great beauty. In them, the whole mysterious process of the hero's near-death and resurrection from the Egg in the form of the god Phanes, is portrayed. The restoration of Izdubar in a new form is facilitated by equally mysterious Eastern songs to restore the hero's virility. Such a process of rebirth cannot be rationally explained, nor even described, it can only be alluded to by the mysterious illustrations. This method to better promote imagination places Jung as one of the great pioneers of non-verbal techniques in psychotherapy. Also, the synchronistic states of emergence experienced here cannot be rationally expressed, only alluded to by the use of images.

Ana: Walter, it's curious that you are mentioning this passage from *The Red Book* in which there is the experience of Izdubar and the Egg. I also had a shamanistic experience with Ayahuasca in which the Egg plays a fundamental role. I illustrated this experience in figure 3. It was like this: Suddenly, I felt that I was entering a mythical, ancestral indigenous space, like on an Inca path, in which I was climbing and entering a blue Egg. I heard an Indigenous person talking to me about an awareness that there is

190

an ancient knowledge and that the land is ancestral. I felt I was walking through an Indigenous archaic labyrinth, a *Unus Mundus*.

Although I have had many experiences with Indigenous People, this dimension is different because it acts directly in a field of emergence of new realities of thought and feeling. The paintings brought in the text, they speak of an emergence of something not conscious that I needed to touch, so new and overwhelming, like something born and that needed to be materialized. I compare it as a new life, a new consciousness that sprouts, a new way of giving materiality to the mysterious *new* that emerges in the interactive field.

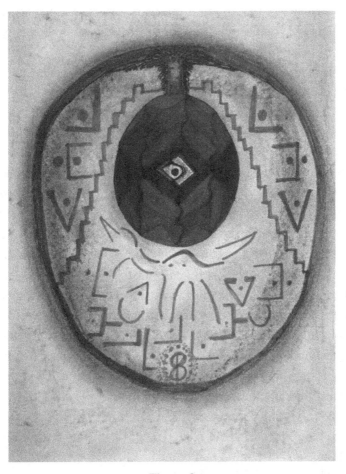

Figure 3
Painting *Indigenous Ancestral labyrinth*

191

Walter: Ana, what a fascinating image! It portrays really your entrance into a new spiritual world, into a new unknown sphere represented by this Cosmic Egg. The Egg has a dark blue center, the color of the spirit, the periphery with characters similar to unknown inscriptions. These inscriptions remind me of Jung's *Black Books*, in particular the *Black Book, Volume 7* which describes the encounter with the Black Magician Ha. This intriguing figure narrates to Jung's soul a whole cosmogonic myth through mysterious runes. The translators of the *Black Books* (Shamdasani, Liebscher & Peck, 2020) are emphatic in saying that the runes of Ha are original expressions of the unconscious, having nothing to do with hieroglyphics or Nordic runes. Also here, Ana, I think that this mysterious writing is an expression of the indigenous cultural unconscious, with which you are at this moment in communion, bringing an ancestral knowledge to be rescued.

It is an evident phenomenon that Ayahuasca plays an essential role in these altered states of consciousness. In Western psychotherapy we already have a predisposition for these anomalous states of consciousness occurring in the interactive field. This field is constellated at the boundaries of the mind-matter duality, in the psychoid universe. Jung and Wolfgang Pauli sought to systematize theoretically these states. Atmanspacher & Fach (2013), in a series of articles in the *Journal of Analytical Psychology*, raised important questions about the mind-matter duality. According to these authors, Pauli and Jung approached mind-matter duality from the perspective of a dual aspect monism, that is, underlying the apparent mind-nature duality is the subtle unity of the *Unus Mundus*. The great novelty that emerged from Pauli and Jung meeting is that two apparently separate universes, the material universe and the psychic universe, could be intimately related, according to what Atmanspacher calls "the Pauli-Jung conjecture" (2013, p. 221). The term *conjecture* is used here because the unique spirit-matter reality cannot yet be demonstrated with scientific rigor. Only the manifestations of a single reality behind the apparent duality are perceptible, which leads to the formulation of a dual-aspect model of monism. The subtle *Unus Mundus* is this monistic reality that underlies the apparent mind-matter duality.

The term *model* is used by Jung in several moments of his work, as in the formulation of a model for the archetype theory, for instance. An example of a model can be found in Niels Bohr's theoretical construct to explain the structure of the atom. According to this model, the atom would consist of a nucleus with protons and neutrons, and with electrons circulating around the nucleus in various orbits. However, since the new findings of the new physics, the traditional model of the atom no longer accounts for the new discoveries. If in essence we do not know what matter is, much less do we know ultimately what the psyche is. We can only rely on models that work in the clinic and are operative within a certain theoretical construct. In this respect Jung and Pauli launched new models of the psychoid, synchronicity, and the *Unus Mundus*. This is the operative model we are using here to try to approach these subtle phenomena that emerge in the interconnected field of nature, body and psyche.

Ana: Walter, this is exactly where we start from, a place of not knowing about the matter, nor the psyche, in a movement towards the new models of the psychoid, in which matter and spirit converge. Do you remember when I told you about the images that were emerging and I was trying to disguise these states from the everyday world, because I was strongly experiencing these imaginative states? Figure 4 shows the moment when the jaguar emerged, as in other paintings, without my control of the process. I was taken aback by its appearance, followed by an awareness of a new reality, absolutely real, imaginative and spiritual. These two dimensions came together. The jaguar and a spiritual guide (the image of the jaguar in the background) were guiding me, as two beings that seemed distinct, but represented two faces, as the realization of instinctive nature in its divine force. Therefore, the jaguar and the spiritual guide are perspectives of the animal and the divine, walking together towards psychic totality. I realized that I was entering the mythology of the Guarani twins, as a character who enters and dialogues with instinct and spirit, with danger and divine protection.

Walter: This emergence of the jaguar seems very significant to me, because it speaks of the importance of the connection with the Latin American cultural unconscious and its rich imagery. We, Jungian analysts of Latin America, must be aware of the rich mythological imagery of the Indigenous and Black cultures in our cultural unconscious. We have

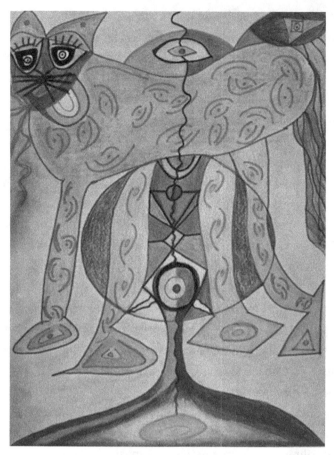

Figure 4
Painting *The jaguar in a movement of totality*

observed in our clinic the importance of these images for the understanding of our patients. Animals have an important presence in this mythological process, and probably the intense presence of zoomorphic symbols is associated with the particular development of consciousness in these cultures, where there is no dissociation of instincts and life in general. The jaguar is one of the most important animals in this mythologization. Representative of fire, bearer of new consciousness is a true Promethean element in Indigenous myths. Galdino (2011), in his extensive research on Brazilian indigenous myths demonstrated their universality, finding the same patterns of the great universal myths: stories of creation from a primordial ocean, the flood, the creation of man from a breath of the creator, the loss of paradise, etc. The jaguar can be understood in a Promethean context bringing the fire of the new consciousness, represented in this case by the spirit that accompanies it. But this significant manifestation of these symbols seems to occur within a context of the Guarani twins' myth, Ana. Could you tell us a little more about this myth?

Ana: In dialogue with Vherá Poty, a Mbyá-Guarani Indigenous intellectual (2015), the myth of the Guarani twins was expanded as the journey of Nhamandú (Guarani deity). Papa Tenondé, the first great Guarani deity, is a little child that was born out of nothing. It is the end and the beginning of everything, like the existence of night and day, like the opening and closing of eyes, as creation and imagination. We can think of the psyche as a producer of images, as creation and imagination, in which we can generate and be born from ourselves. Thus, the child is born from the jaguar and becomes humanized in the womb of the ancestral goddess.

Vherá Poty (2015) warns that what we call myth is the story of the beginning of Guarani life, and also warned that one of the most fearful things for the Guarani, is the transformation into a jaguar. This can be fatal. The connection with the jaguar symbolizes the encounter with the transformation of people into animals, with *tekoachy*, the Guarani term for imperfection.

The encounter with the jaguar is a connection to a world of unconscious, shadowy images, as an instinctive and spiritual force. How can one feel voices of God and the Devil? Jung (CW 9i) warns us about the process of unconsciousness we experience, a demonism that takes hold of us when we allow ourselves to be fixated on an idea of a human spirit that is considered harmless, ingenious, inventive, and sensible and we are at the same time unaware of the demonism inherent in it. It is what you say, Walter: voices of the unconscious speak to us, and it is necessary not to remain in the literalization. They are emerging images that lead us on a journey to the mandalic center.

Looking at the jaguar means an approach to facing difficulties, to an encounter with courage. This has nothing to do with the intellect, but with existence itself, with expanded thinking, at various levels of connection.

The paths of Jungian clinical practice strongly emphasize the value of unconscious processes experienced through images. They are like symbols that bring creative solutions for our impasses, they value the creative dimension as a space for elaborating and overcoming one's sufferings. For Jung (2009), this image is absolutely real and autonomous. It has a life of its own. At the same time, the experience of the world happens, inside each one and in the way each person is subjective, based on this vital force.

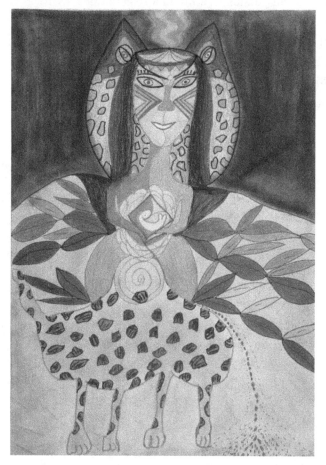

Figure 5
Painting *Humanization of the jaguar in the womb of the ancestral goddess*

Walter: Yes, when Vherá Poty warns us to be careful when approaching the jaguar, about the danger of the transformation into an animal, this reminds me of the attention we analysts must have with the possibility of psychotic processes in analysis. The image of the jaguar is fascinating, numinous, enclosing powerful opposites. It devours, thus representing the painful entry into the unconscious, and the sufferings of the hero, but it also delicately protects the fragile divine child, being a facilitator of its mystical birth. The ancestral images have all the power of fascination (in Latin: *fascinans*, to bind, to hold), but they also have their *mysterium tremendum* as Rudolph Otto pointed out (Otto, 2010). Jung (1919, CW 8) in the essay *Instinct and the Unconscious,* linked the archetype-in-itself with patterns of behavior in animals (Konrad Lorenz). So, perhaps we can see this association in the image of a spiritual presence associated with the jaguar. No doubt, Ana, what you raise about the autonomy of these images is pertinent. They occur by themselves, they belong to the objective psyche, as Jung called it. Philemon's poetic expression in *The Red Book*, "you are not the author of the psyche play" finds a vibrant echo in Elijah' warning to Jung still in *Liber Primus*: "You may call us symbols for the same reason that you can also call your fellow men symbols, if you wish to. But we are just as real as your fellow men" (Jung, 2009, p. 249). Paintings 4 and 5 seem to reflect a gradual process of a *hypostasis* (an evident manifestation of a god by an equivalent representative); in this case, the jaguar, manifestation of the divine Fire that transforms spiritually, but can also burn or swallow. From this initial hypostasis, the content of the collective unconscious is gradually assimilated. In figure 4, the jaguar, representative of instinct, floats, while the spiritual entity hangs by a mysterious umbilical cord to the earth, acquiring a chthonic quality. Here one can see a clear complementarity. In figure 5, the jaguar and the spirit, represented by a shaman-like figure of magical power, are united by a beautiful spiral mandala, signaling that the integration of instinct and spirit has advanced. At the height of his abdomen, the karai holds a wrapping, inside a numinous embryo, similar to a *homunculus,* the new personality being gestated.

Ana: The Guarani child's journey begins in his/her mother's path, which I relate to the symbology of the child archetype in the individuation processes (Jung, CW 9i). According to Jung, the mythologem of the miraculous birth of the child, always exposed in nature and protected by animals, like Jesus in the manger or Moses in the stream and many others, describes psychologically the birth of the true Self, the path of self-realization. Among the Guarani this motif reappears, the Guarani twins are menaced and at the same time protected by the jaguar, a numinous representative of nature.

On the child's journey, the mother is devoured by the jaguars and the sun (*kuaray*) survives by overcoming its obstacles. The mother was swallowed, the child survived and was cared for by the jaguar, which expresses well the meaning brought by Jung: "this is why nature, the very world of instincts, takes care of the 'child,' who is fed or protected by animals" (Jung, CW 9i, § 286). The child, in a Guarani view, is accessible to the worlds of animals and instincts and the desire of the deity was to create something that is opposite to it (Poty, 2019).

Kuaray, son of the sun/Nhamandú, created the moon *Jaxy*, because he felt lonely, and created him as a being opposite to him. This factor helps us think about how much we need opposition in order to follow our path. Nhamandú's path is conceived from the ingestion of the mother by the jaguar. The divine child is born with the death of the mother. The jaguar and the divine child get closer, still in an unconscious way. It is by going through this path that the Guarani turns his word sacred, stands on his own feet, takes possession of the earth.

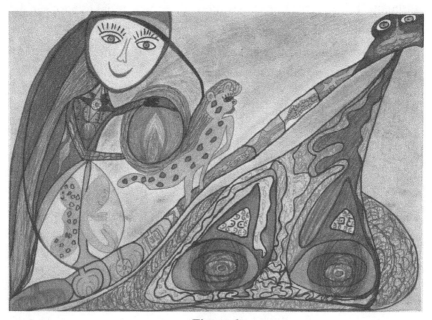

Figure 6
Painting *The humanization of the jaguar on the ascent of the woman's path*

Walter: Ana, it is remarkable how the mythology of the child archetype emerges with symbolic clarity in the Guarani myth. Initially the theme of *exposure,* so common in Greek culture, is evident there. Brandão (1987), Kerényi (1968) and others mention the ritual of child exposure in mythological Greece: Perseus thrown in the sea together with his mother, Atalanta abandoned in the forest, Oedipus hanged by the foot on the mount, Psyche exposed on the rock are just a few. Several of these exposed children are protected and fed by animals: Romulus and Remus by the female wolf, Atalanta by a female bear (Brandão, 1987, p. 77). What does this mean, from a psychological perspective? That the psychic development within the canons of the biological family does not favor individuation. This can only occur when the individual seeks contact with his or her innermost instinctive nature, thus transgressing the common social values given by the environment. It is very interesting to see this mythologem reappearing at the Guarani culture in such a clear way. And this process emerges within the context of the use of Ayahuasca, which, in many cases can be a catalyst of individuation. Figure 6 speaks of this emergence within the archetype of the Way, the long journey, (the *Longissima Via*) of the medieval alchemists, which dominates the painting. The path of transformation crosses the picture, starting from the quadrant of the archetypal Mother, place of origin and beginnings, and ending in the quadrant of the personal Father, place of becoming and future achievements. The figure in animal skin symbolizes the completion of the jaguar's humanization. She walks along this path of transformation paved by the serpent, the healer that changes skins. A numinous figure of a woman watches over the instinct-spirit duality contained in dual form within a uterine continent.

Ana: It is interesting, Walter, that the centrality is not the human, not the person, but the universe in which the Guarani lives as a principle of life, enlivened by the narrative and journey of the twins. Thinking about the path of sun and moon, I highlight four spaces of connection in the psychic transfigurations: the encounter with the jaguar in the act of the mother being devoured and the learning of the sun and moon, as a divine child, in dealing with the jaguar; the encounter with the bird that reveals the origin and enables them to fly; the frog that guards the fire and also gets burned; and the serpent that kills the sun and makes them learn to live new cycles of death and rebirth.

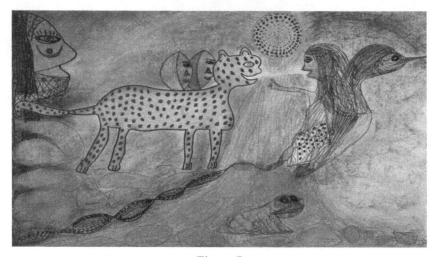

Figure 7
Painting *Myth of the Guarani twins – end of a cycle*

In the mythological version (Clastres, 1990), the Guarani twins did not know their mother. And in this way, the future sun and moon emerged.

The Myth, according to the shaman Vherá Poty, is not a story to be told, simply, with beginning, middle, and end, but a field to be crossed in an intrapsychic movement, as something that is part of each one of us. We are crossed by dualities, sun and moon, night and day, visible and invisible, good and evil, light and shadow.

The psyche is a cosmos, and the myths offer us this learning, approaching the idea that the elements of nature have personalities and as stated by the anthropologist Viveiros de Castro (2002, p. 335, my translation): "The Myth speaks of a state of being where bodies and names, souls and actions, the self and the other interpenetrate, immersed in the same pre-objective and pre-subjective." The Myth of the twins does not speak of a differentiation of the human from the animal.

Walter: Yes, Ana, the complexity of the myth of twins among the Guarani is amazing. We know that the karai are the guardians of tradition and the sacred myths of the ethnic group, as opposed to fables and legends, which fall into the profane domain (Galdino, 2016). The Myth, on the other hand, is told within the ritual by the karai. I imagine the myth being told by the shaman, within the specific ritual. These primordial images really point to a path of spiritualization. You mentioned the presence of the opposites good and evil in search of a greater integration in this path. The twin mythology seems to have a very particular characteristic among Indigenous groups in general. The brothers are closer and work together for a common goal. In other mythological traditions like the Greek (Castor and Pollux), Egyptian (Horus and Seth), and Hebrew (Cain and Abel) there is an opposition between brothers, which can be interpreted as a necessary opposition for the building up of consciousness, the ego complex differentiating itself from the shadow, which personifies instincts, the body and nature. In Guarani and other Indigenous groups, twins collaborate in their cosmogonic work in a joint manner, without necessarily being opposed. This seems to point to a model of development of consciousness and culture without significant dissociation from nature and the instincts.

Figure 7 seems to show the culmination of this whole process, with the participation of the four animals, personifying the four elements, the four psychological functions: the serpent, the rooting in the Earth, illustrates the path to be traveled; the hummingbird, associated to Air, represents the spiritual movement that points to the future; the frog, the Water that devours the Fire, represents the necessary psychological balance against psychic inflation; the jaguar, centralizing the entire image, like Fire, devouring, transforming, the instinctive and at the same time the spiritual element. On the back of the jaguar the twins sun and moon, representing the integration of opposites, assist the process. The woman, personifying consciousness, dialogues with the jaguar, after assimilating the whole process of psychological transmutation. The whole process is observed by the mysterious female face on the left, also present in figure 6, representing the activation of the archetype of the Self.

Final conclusions

Walter: Ana, after revisiting your journey activated by Ayahuasca in your fieldwork with Indigenous groups, I see a strong interactive field activated. In this field there is a visible emergence of contents from the Guarani cultural unconscious linked to your own process of individuation. This process influenced your own work as a Jungian analyst, as your clinical example illustrates. The emergence of the Twins Myth affects you and your work as an analyst. As you well remembered, the twins constellate strongly in the dyad analyst-analysand, where the analyst embodies the moon, promoting the emergence of his twin brother, the sun, within the patient, who gains more insights and develops his consciousness. All your work is a continuous evidence that the shamanistic complex emerges in our daily work as analysts. You chose seven paintings to illustrate this work, but we know there are many more. I consider these paintings as a spontaneous sprouting of the self-healing forces of the collective unconscious mediated by Ayahuasca. We still have a lot to say about this plant and its therapeutic power. But a very important issue is that, in my opinion, one can observe these very positive effects of Ayahuasca in psychotherapy only when there are the ritual and spiritual elements associated with its use.

Ana: Walter, as the Guarani teach us, the journey doesn't stop. Also, I think that the paintings will tell us more. What I feel is a deep gratitude for reliving Nhamandú's path, together, in an interpersonal and collective dialogical dimension, in a perception of being on Amerindian trails, recalling the power of these Indigenous memories, understanding the strength of mythological narratives, of Ayahuasca, in approximation with Jungian psychology.

References

Atmanspacher, H. & Fach, W. (2013). A structural-phenomenological typology of mind-matter correlations. *The Journal of Analytical Psychology, 58*(2), (219-244).

Boechat, W. (1979) *Shamanism and Psychotherapy*. Diploma thesis at the C.G. Jung Institute. Thesis advisor: Mario Jacoby.

Bauman, Z. (2017). *Retrotopia*. Polity Press.

Brandão, J. (1987). *Mitologia Grega* (Vol. 3). Editora Vozes.

Cambray, J. (2013). *Sincronicidade. Natureza e psique num universo interconectado*. Editora Vozes.

Cambray, J. & Carter, L. (2020). Métodos analíticos revisitados. In Cambray, J. & Carter, L. (orgs.). *Psicologia analítica. Perspectivas contemporâneas em análise junguiana*. Editora Vozes.

Carter, L. (2010). Countertransference and Intersubjectivity. In M. Stein, M. (Ed.). *Jungian Psychoanalysis. Working in the Spirit of C. G. Jung*. Open Court.

Conolly, A. (2015). Bridging the Reductive and the Synthetic: Some Reflections on the Clinical Implications of Synchronicity. *Journal of Analytical Psychology, 60*(2), (159-178).

Eliade, M. (1974). *Shamanism: Archaic Techniques of Ecstasy* (2ª ed.). Princeton University Press.

Galdino, L. (2016). *Mitologia Indígena*. Editora Nova Alexandria.

Gutiérrez, L.M. & Torres, M.A. (2011). *Vuelo Mágico de Orión y los animales mitológicos. Un estudio del arte simbólico pré-colombiano de Colômbia*. Ventos Ediciones.

Jacoby, M. (1995). Supervision and the Interactive Field. In P. Kugler, (Ed.). *Jungian Perspectives on Clinical Supervision*. Daimon Editor.

Jung, C.G. (1919/1972) *Instinct and the Unconscious*. CW 8. London: Routledge.

Jung, C.G. (1946/1970). *The Psychology of the Transference.* CW 16. London: Routledge.

Jung, C.G. (1951/1975). *The Psychology of the Child Archetype.* CW 9-1. Princeton: Princeton University Press.

Jung, C.G. (2009). *The Red Book. Liber Novus.* General edition and introduction by Sonu Shamdasani. New York and London: W. W. Norton.

Jung, C.G. (2020). *Os Livros Negros.* [The Black Books]. Editora Vozes.

Kerényi, K. (1968). L'enfant Divin. In: Jung, C. G. & Kerényi, K. *Introduction a l'Essence de la Mythologie.* Payot.

Kopenawa D & Albert, B. (2015). *A queda do céu: palavras de um xamã Yanomami.* Editora Companhia das Letras.

Mancuso, S. (2019). *A revolução das plantas.* [The plant Revolution]. Editora Ubu.

Otto, R. (2010). *The Idea of the Holy.* London: Martino Books.

Shamdasani, S., Liebscher, M. & Peck, J. (2020). Traduzindo as Runas de Jung. In Jung, C.G. Os Livros Negros. [The Black Books]. Editora Vozes.

Schwartz-Salant, N. (1995). On the Interactive Field as the Analytic Object. In M. Stein, (Ed.) *The Interactive Field in Analysis.* Chiron.

Stein, M. (1992). Power, Shamanism and Maieutics in Countertransference. In: M. Stein, & N. Schwartz-Salant, (Eds.). *Transference Counter-transference.* Chiron.

Vherá, P. (2015). Entrevista. In Bergamaschi, M. A. & Menezes, A. L. T. de. *Educação ameríndia: a dança e a escola ameríndia* (2ª ed). Editora EDUNISC.

Viveiros de Castro, E. (2002). *A inconstância da alma selvagem.* Editora Cosac Naif.

Wohlleben, P. (2017). *A vida secreta das* árvores. [The Hidden Life of Trees] Editora Sextante.

Endnotes

[1] We highlight that the experiences with research in Guarani villages last 23 years, but it was in 2017, at the time of the exchange program in Colombia with the indigenous Ingas, during the post-doctorate in Education and later, during the supervision period with Walter Boechat, step for the completion of the monograph on the Jungian training at the Jungian Institute of Rio Grande do Sul, that the experiences became more intense. During that period, I had contact with Santo Daime, and I drank ayahuasca a few times.

[2] Santo Daime cult is a religion based on the ritualistic use of Ayahuasca developed at Amazonian State of Acre, north of Brazil, since 1930. Its founder was Raimundo Irineu Serra, a grandson of slaves. Santo Daime is an ecumenic practice, with Christian and indigenous elements.

[3] Mirações is the name given to Visions provoked by Ayahuasca during Santo Daime ritual.

[4] The sonorous nuances of flutes, trumpets and other musical instruments identified with mythical ancestors and inspired by the voices of animals (songs, whistles, buzzes, percussion) emitted by birds, monkeys, jaguars, tapirs and anacondas, have a high fertilizing potential (Gutiérrez & Torres, 2011, p. 96, my translation).

Establishing
Intentions

Search for Connection
through Microdosing

Marcel van den Akker

Models of psychedelic assisted psychotherapy are primarily distinguished according to the dose of the psychedelic substance. Research in this field to date—including psychoanalytic approaches—has mainly focused on doses that would facilitate either psycholytic (soul-loosening) or psychedelic (mind-manifesting) experiences. Although it is argued that psychedelics in medium or high doses have the capacity to effectively contribute to the analytic process, the benefits of a low dose of psychedelics have received less attention during the second wave of psychedelic research. In this chapter the use of low dose psychedelics, popularly known as microdosing, will be explored in relation to the analytic process.

The benefits of low dose psychedelics were explored during the first wave of psychedelic research in the 1950s and 1960s, and mainly in a therapeutic setting (e.g., Sandison, 1954; Abramson, 1956; Leuner, 1967). Following James Fadiman's 2011 book, *The Psychedelics Explorer's Guide*, which has a chapter on microdosing, a renewed interest has developed in the use of low dose psychedelics. This interest was further prompted by articles in popular magazines and papers like *Rolling Stone* (Leonard, 2015), *Forbes* (Glatter, 2015), *Wired* (Solon, 2016) and *The Times* (Karim, 2017). Microdosing has subsequently become increasingly popular and nowadays large numbers of people take to microdosing as a new way of self-medicating.

As the detectable microdose differs among people, a microdose can usually range from 5-50 micrograms Lysergic acid diethylamide (LSD).

As people react differently, most microdosers tend to experiment with doses to find the amount that produces low detectable sensations. Passie (2019) found that most studies are conducted in the 25-50 microgram LSD range, although some studies mention doses as low as 5 micrograms LSD (Yanakieva et al., 2019). A microdose is sometimes called a *sub-hallucinogenic*, *sub-threshold*, *sub-sensorium* or *sub-perceptual* dose, which means that the person will not feel a high. It does not generate profound perceptual experiences or overwhelm consciousness with unconscious content. A microdose will only activate minimal identifiable drug effects, leaving the ego functions intact to a large degree. Some prefer to integrate microdosing into their life intuitively, while others consider the benefits in certain situations. Most research on microdosing focuses on microdosers who will normally dose one to three times per week. The practice is often regarded as a cyclic activity, with microdosing periods lasting from a few weeks to a few months (Johnstad, 2018, p. 44). Different substances can be used for microdosing, although LSD and psilocybin are the most common choices. The incentives to microdose are mostly related to the treatment of mood and anxiety problems, as well as enhancing creativity and everyday functioning. Microdosing is also recommended for the enhancement of spiritual practices, such as prayer and meditation (Van Dusen, 1961; Stolaroff, 2015, p. 336).

How does microdosing effect the soma and psyche? It is necessary to more thoroughly investigate many aspects of microdosing regarding definition, potential mechanisms, health risks, difference in substances and their effectiveness. Some preliminary findings suggest that, overall, microdosing appears to have no health risks, although further research is required (Kuyper, 2020). Regarding the effects on mental health, studies have found that microdosers report a decrease in anxiety and mood related problems (Cameron et al., 2020; Lea et al., 2020a; Rootman et al., 2022). Furthermore, results to date suggest that microdosing leads to improvements in cognitive or mental flexibility (Prochazkova et al., 2018; Rifkin et al., 2020; Petranker et al., 2022), creativity (Johnstad, 2018, p. 45; Anderson et al., 2019, p. 739; Fadiman & Korb, 2019; Rootman et al., 2021), and connectedness with oneself, others and nature (Carhart-Harris et al., 2017; Forstmann & Sagioglou, 2017). There have also been indications that microdosing alleviates symptoms of migraine headaches, pre-menstrual discomfort, and traumatic brain injury (Fadiman & Korb, 2019). Undesired effects that are mentioned range from insomnia, feelings of overstimulation (Johnstad, 2018, p. 47), to increased anxiety and physiological discomfort (Bornemann, 2020, p. 300). Results from scientific research also raise doubts about the effectiveness of microdosing, with several studies concluding that positive expectations cause, at least, some of the subsequent improvements, suggesting a significant placebo response (Kaertner et al., 2021; Szigeti et al., 2021; Cavanna et al., 2022).

The psychological benefits produced by psychedelics are most often explained in terms of an increase in mental flexibility. Altered states of consciousness caused by the substance lead to regressive conditions, during which the ego functions are loosened, or in high doses may lead to ego dissolution (Millière et al., 2018). This is confirmed by neuroscientific research finding that psychedelics may undo fixated and conditioned cognitions and psychological habits. Indeed, Swanson (2018) states, "psychedelic drugs perturb universal brain processes that normally serve to constrain neural systems central to perception, emotion, cognition, and sense of self." It has been suggested that the reduction of activity in the default mode network (DMN) can explain this to a certain degree. The DMN is, "a network of brain regions thought to support general background activity associated with the functions of normal waking consciousness, such as metacognition, social attributions and self-reflection" (Polito and Stevenson, 2019). In general, it can be stated that we develop habitual pathways of communication between brain regions. Over time, these routes become confined to specific pathways, leading to a constrained and sometimes rigid way of cognitive functioning. These restricted paths of communication between different parts of the brain come to constitute the default mode of operating. Gattuso et al.'s systematic 2022 review "provides evidence to support the notion that classical psychedelics are capable of modulating the DMN, which is correlated with ego dissolution, increased brain entropy, and improved mental health and well-being." This reduction in typical neural activity might explain an increase in mental flexibility, as well as creativity, as it is accompanied by an increase in connectivity between more independent brain regions. It is suggested that free association, as part of the Freudian practice of psychoanalysis and meditation, has a similar influence on the DMN (Novac & Blinders, 2021). Gattuso et al. (2022) suggest that there are indications that low dose psychedelics also cause a decline in DMN activity, although it is not yet fully understood how microdosing influences the DMN.

If the use of psychedelic substances inhibits normal mental functioning and creates a situation where people can divert from their default mode of operating then, as a result, mental rigidity can be overcome. Mental flexibility is generally understood as a collection of dynamic psychological processes concerning a person's relationship with the world around them, reflecting their capacity to meet the challenges of life and navigate through conflict and suffering with resilience and adjustments. It has been associated with psychological dynamics such as personal growth, social interaction, and stress management. It can be stated that mental flexibility is the cornerstone of healthy personal and social functioning (Kashdan and Rotterberg, 2010).

Viewed from a depth psychological perspective, not only the focus of an individual's coping with challenges in the outer world but also the ego's relationship with the inner world are considered to be vital for development. Jung viewed the rigid one-sidedness in ego-consciousness, by which unconscious content is defensively and systematically excluded from consciousness, as the condition for neuroses. Rigidity is what keeps neuroses from being a means to develop our personality (CW 10, § 359). Jung writes about rigidity and narrow-mindedness in relation to the fear of the problem of opposites. Mental flexibility means that the apparent security of a rigid mindset must be exchanged for a "condition of insecurity, of internal division, of contradictory convictions" (CW 7, § 116). Jung states that, "conviction easily turns into self-defence and is seduced into rigidity, and this is inimical to life" (CW 16, §180). Moreover, he relates narrow-mindedness to, "poison and destruction" (CW 10, § 731). From a Jungian perspective, a static state of mind is an obstruction; thus, the psyche in general should have a certain fluidity to it. This fluidity can only be supported by a lowering of rigidity in defense barriers, a lessening of resistance, and allowing for old fixations and convictions to loosen their control.

It has been found that microdosers experience an increase in creativity. This suggests that people on low doses of psychedelics feel an increase in this domain and an openness to the unconscious. It could indicate an increase of fantasy and symbolic thinking and a decrease of one's defenses against emotional depth. A central feature of Jung's work is the importance that he ascribes to one's drive to create. However, to connect to the inner source of creativity, it is necessary to soften one's defenses and face the consequences of opening up to the weight of unconscious material. For Jung, connecting to the source of creativity means going beyond the discovery of one self, "into the sphere of the collective psyche, he will first enter into the treasure-house of collective ideas and then into creativity" (CW 16, § 64). He suggests that for creativity to be true creativity, the drive to create should be "mightier than its possessor" (CW 17, § 206). Creation means allowing something other to express itself. To be truthful to creation, we need to allow something in us to take over. If this condition is supported by a low dose of psychedelics, if embracing and allowing things to crystalize without excessive involvement of our ego control, it could well be argued that psychedelics support creativity and therefore assist the individuation process.

Apart from an increase in mental flexibility and creativity, research has also found that microdosers often report a deeper connection with themselves, others, and nature (Griffiths et al., 2011; Schmid et al., 2015; Lea et al., 2020b). We can speculate that again the effect of microdosing on the defense mechanisms plays a significant role in this domain. From a depth psychological perspective, most psychological suffering in terms of neurosis comes from a faulty relationship between the conscious and unconscious. If the censorship of the defense mechanisms is lowered and the barriers between the conscious and unconscious are dissolved, then this would allow for a more meaningful relationship with unconscious life. Furthermore, impressions of the world around us might have more direct effects on us. Lowering the defenses in this way appears to facilitate a deeper experience of life through feelings of being connected to the inner and outer world. Instead of being flooded by impressions during a full psychedelic trip, microdosing facilitates a lowering of defenses in a much more controlled and secure way.

For Jung, the restriction of consciousness, reduction of attention, or weakening of ego control would be an *abaissement du niveau mental*, the lowering of the threshold of consciousness. In this state, unpredictable contents may emerge from the unconscious. Jung states: "When consciousness 'disintegrates' (*abaissement du niveau mental* apperceptive weakness), the complexes coexisting with it are simultaneously freed from all restraint and are then able to break through into ego-consciousness" (CW 3, § 59). The weakening of the ego often happens spontaneously; for instance, when we are tired or emotional. However, it can also be deliberately produced during a creative process, or active imagination. From the above, it can be concluded that microdosing also produces a low level of *abaissement du niveau mental* in a secure and controllable way and might therefore be considered a valuable collaborator for certain analytical cases.

Intention

When considering the benefits of microdosing for the analytic process, the first thing to contemplate is the intention for microdosing. Many microdosers might be too caught up in the intentions of the ego, being overly enmeshed in its striving. Microdosing appears to be another attempt to satisfy the search for happiness and health. Microdosing could be the next substance in the line of all sorts of psychopharmaceuticals like Adderall, Ritalin, Modafinil and Benzodiazepines. An increasing number of people are looking to self-medicate on substances to enhance their performance or essentially endure life rather than grow psychologically. If the intention for microdosing is primarily linked to striving to cure anxiety or depression, search for happiness or enhance performance, these may be very understandable goals. However, microdosing psychedelics might therefore contribute to regressive tendencies and dependency issues. This will make microdosing an addition to a culture complex that might be called *psyche and substance*, where large groups of people are seized by the idea that relief or even salvation can only be found in the use of a substance. Understood in this way, the use of microdosing will only contribute to misunderstanding of the social meaning of substances.

From a Jungian perspective, we cannot avoid the work that is needed for individuation. There is no shortcut to self-realization. In this sense, microdosing is not a way to skip parts of the journey of becoming. Having an experience of the new does not in itself bring growth. For Jung, becoming conscious and the discovery of new things is an active process and psychological growth is often defined by work and accompanied by suffering. Confrontation with the unconscious is often experienced as unpleasant, even threatening to the ego. This is why it is important to emphasize that the psychedelic journey should be taken for the sake of the soul rather than for the sake of the ego.

However, the intention to microdose might be fueled by different intentions. Many people experience meaninglessness and feel spiritually barren. It is unsurprising that in this secular age with its loss of religious and spiritual perspectives, people tend to seek new ways to find connection, meaning and a re-enhancement of life. An increasing number of people feel the need to seek a deepening of experience. Microdosing seems to promise this by strengthening the connection between consciousness and the world, both inner and outer.

Microdosing as an Indirect Influence on the Analytic Hour

Research has found that with microdosing, "the alternations in conscious are barely detectable, yet it appears to have significant psychological benefits" (Polito & Stevenson, 2019). In places where this is allowed by law, would it be appropriate for the analyst to start suggesting microdosing as a way of self-medicating to his patients? Microdosing certainly has some advantages over other doses. For instance, the use of a minimum effective dose is likely to cause fewer challenges to both the patient and the analyst compared to the use of a medium or full dose. Moreover, the analyst does not have to be involved in the administration and monitoring of the microdose process outside of the analytic hour, nor does he have to be concerned about the setting, as the process is primarily determined by the integration of psychedelics in everyday life. Instead of being in a room with the analyst or assistant having sometimes profound experiences, an analysand microdosing may gain the opportunity to not only focus on the inner processes but also be more affected by the outside world.

In the case of an analyst suggesting microdosing to his patient, there are some important aspects to consider. Next to the responsibility involved when the analyst proposes to his patient to consider taking a substance regularly, suggesting microdosing will have influence on the analytic relationship and the patient's perception of himself. The patient might be under the impression that he is unable to undergo an analytic process without a drug. Thus, it is important to clarify the intentions. These intentions are to help the patient to loosen the rigidity in his cognitive functioning, undo extreme defenses, support his creativity or (as I personally notice while microdosing) achieve a better recall of dreams. Patients who tend to be fixated or obsessive and who present a certain stuck-ness that hinders the progression might benefit from microdosing. If carefully introduced, the analyst and the patient might come to a good understanding about why the analyst brings microdosing to his attention. However, most preferably, microdosing would be initiated by personal motivation of the patient.

Outside of the analysis, as well as during the sessions, microdosing could support a stronger bridge between unconscious and ego-consciousness, furthering the process of development. The use of microdosing seems well suited to support the process of active imagination, which can happen spontaneously but, as a therapeutic technique, is often artificially induced. This process requires a mental state during which the unconscious contents are invited while consciousness is largely intact. The process starts with an attempt to reduce the ego's critical attitude, allowing fantasy images to arise. During this process, the unconscious movements are central while the ego is observing, playing witness to the unfolding story. During the second stage, ego-consciousness becomes actively involved with the unconscious images and affects that flow into awareness. So, the ego actively enters into the experience. For patients who are familiar with active imagination, microdosing could be a supportive enabler for this process outside of sessions. Active imagination is one of the pillars of Jungian analysis and according to Chodorow (1997, p. 13) "is a way to gain independence by doing your own inner work." It is a method that can free the patient from his dependence on the analyst.

Low Dose Psychedelics and the Analytic Hour

I believe it is worthwhile to consider a more immediate way of influencing the psychodynamics during the analytic hour by suggesting to the patient to take a low dose of psychedelics before the session starts as a way to influence the conscious position of the patient. To affect the analytic hour in a more direct way, the dose used will be slightly higher than the regular microdose and the patient will notice the effects. Some have referred to this use of low dose psychedelics as a mini dose (Johnstad, 2018, p. 44), or threshold dose (Vojtěchovský et al., 1972). It is suggested that a mini dose (up to 50 micrograms LSD) makes a significant difference as it has the potency to alter psychological functioning in such a way that it might interfere with normal everyday activities. It is worthwhile to ask the patient to detect his own individual *ego-threshold*, meaning the dose that is detectable but only slightly interferes with general functioning.

The use of pharmacological substances in service of a therapeutic process is not new and dates back to the turn of the 20th century, when attempts were made to influence the state of consciousness by using ether, chloroform, and hashish. Later in the 1920s and 1930s, sub-narcotic doses of barbiturates were used to intensify the psychotherapeutic treatment, in a process that became known as narcoanalysis (Horsley, 1943). German psychiatrist Walter Frederking pioneered with microdosing psychedelics in psychoanalytic therapy in the 1950s. According to his studies, the procedure is indicated, "when it is desirable to shorten a course of therapy, reactivate a stalled treatment of a neurosis, and for the purpose of breaking down affect or memory blocks" (Frederking, 1955, p. 265). Other clinical experiments that followed using lower doses of LSD revealed the usefulness of psychedelics in arousing unconscious material. Stoll (as cited in Passie, 2022) argued that 10 to 50 micrograms of LSD is sufficient to evoke psychodynamic material in "psychologically minded" people.

In the 1960s, psychoanalytically-oriented therapists developed two basic approaches to low dose psychedelic assisted analysis, whereby the patient would be under the influence of a psychedelic substance either before or during the session (Passie, 1997, p. 11). Both approaches support the activation of unconscious material like repressed memories, emotional impulses, and conflicts. However, as this approach involves only a low dose of psychedelics, the purpose is to loosen the rigidity of the psyche, and thus the results largely depend on the patient's willingness and ability to tune into inner experiences. This seems to fit the Jungian viewpoint on the analytic process much better than a full dose. The intention of analysis is first and foremost to let the individuation process unfold, working through the resistance rather than breaking it down. I believe there is a danger that psychedelics can become a form of ammunition by the uninformed analyst, destroying the sometimes carefully built-up resistance serving as protection against the dangers of unconscious material.

It is suggested that during the first approach the patient has experiences induced by the psychedelic substance while being with an assistant or trip sitter (Passie, 1997, p.11). The patient is in a relaxed position and encouraged to turn his or her focus inward to allow a dream-like state to manifest while remaining in communication with the assistant. It could be approached as an active imagination exercise or, for those who are not familiar with this technique, a more passive inner experience. The patient is encouraged to let the inner process unfold, not resisting any material that reveals itself. A receptive awareness should be cultivated, allowing both disturbing and positive images to emerge. The information given to the assistant will be recorded and given to the patient to prepare for the analytic hour. During the analytic hour, the patient can explore the induced experiences, interpret, and work through them. The experience itself only supports the analytic process during the session with the analyst but does not influence it. This approach has several advantages as it allows the patient to go through the process in a safe space with a trained professional. He can let the flow of experience unfold without interruption, without concern for transference issues and hopefully with fewer concerns about a timeframe. If needed, the patient can receive help in preparing before the administration of the substance and additional care can be provided after the psychedelic experiences. One of the disadvantages of this approach is the reoccurrence of resistance during the analytic hour. As the ego is likely to be less vulnerable during the analytic hour in comparison to the experience itself, anxiety, shame, guilt, etc. might prevent the benefits of the experiences from being fully realized.

The second approach is more in line with the psycholytic approach as suggested by Sandison (1954), Abramson (1956) and Leuner (1967). The patient can be asked to take a low dose of psychedelic substance before the analytic hour. According to Passie (1997, p. 12), this offers, "special opportunities to overcome strong and consolidated defense structures in patients who had been previously considered to be resistant to therapy." He found that low dose psychedelic assisted therapy had low risk, improved effectiveness, and the tendency to shorten treatment for less severe neurotics (Passie, 1997).

One of the first Jungian-oriented psychiatrists who researched the influence of low dose psychedelics and psychodynamic work was Ronald Sandison. He became increasingly enthusiastic about low dose LSD as abreactive memory actualizations triggered by the substance led to a significant improvement in neurotic patients (Sandison et al., 1954, p. 498). Sandison et al. found that the experiences produced by LSD can be divided into three types.

> First, generalized non-specific images such as a sense of lightness of the body, changes in the surroundings giving them plasticity and fluidity, the appearance of coloured patterns and other hallucinatory experiences of a non-personal kind. Second, the recall and re-living of forgotten memories and experiences of childhood. Third, the experiencing of archaic impersonal images in terms of images or hallucinatory pictures exactly similar in nature to those experiences of the collective unconscious which patients undergoing deep analysis experience in their dreams, visual impressions, and fantasies. (1954, p. 508)

Low doses will, most likely, facilitate a confrontation with the personal layers of the unconscious and Sandison is adamant that coming to terms with repressed emotional life by re-living forgotten memories is facilitated by low dose psychedelics, and beneficial to the patient's mental health. However, he also argues that for some patients it is crucial to consider the conscious relationship with the more "universal aspects of psychic life" (Sandison et al., 1954, p. 508). It remains unclear whether low dose psychedelics are able to activate these depths of the psyche. A combination of low dose psychedelics and active imagination might strengthen the experience, and make access to the collective realms of the unconscious possible in a more controlled way.

In the 1950s and 60s, not every Jungian analyst was comfortable with the use of psychedelics as a collaborator in Jungian analysis. Scott Hill (2019) addresses the tension between the use of psychedelics in analysis suggested by Sandison as opposed to conventional Jungian therapy. In reaction to Sandison, Jungian analyst Michael Fordham (1963) argues that it is necessary to distinguish between the passive process of psychedelic assisted analysis and the active process of conventional Jungian analysis. Apart from analysis being an intentional activity instead of a passive process induced by biochemical means, Fordham argued that it remains the therapeutic relationship that determines the outcome of analysis rather than the psychedelic experience (Hill, 2019, p. 25-26). When Hill asked Sandison in 2009 about this, Sandison acknowledged that Fordham's criticism was to some extent valid. However, he felt that only a small proportion of patients had the opportunity to undergo analysis and that LSD was available and effective (Hill, 2019, p. 26).

Sandison's colleague, Jungian analyst Marion Curtner, seems to agree with Fordham and expressed her concerns about the use of psychedelics. She writes, "[My] aim has always been to use it as sparingly as possible and to keep the main accent on analysis itself" (Curtner, 1959, p. 716). She resorts to using psychedelics, "when the patient's material is not coming forth sufficiently for the work to proceed" (Curtner, 1959, p. 717). She is aware that different aspects in the analytic process may stall the psychological material, like a hindrance in the transference and periods that feel unproductive but are devoted to the process of integration. Therefore, before considering the use of a substance, the analyst is encouraged to explore reasons for the suspension, whether it is beneficial or detrimental, and consider alternative approaches. Furthermore, Curtner found that although the psychedelic experiences show unpredictable and astonishing variations, they appear to follow psychological laws. She states, "it is surprising to find that unconscious activity observed under the influence of the drug reveals the compensatory character" (1959, p. 720). She continues, "there seems to be an autonomous selective process is at work, determining the sequence of the emerging material in a purposive way" (1959, p. 720). In this, Curtner found confirmation of Jung's ideas about the self-regulating system, "in which unconscious activities function as compensatory factors in the service of a striving towards wholeness" (1959, p. 720).

In 1960, Hanscarl Leuner became a prominent figure in the field of low dose psychedelics. Leuner had been in analysis with Jungian analyst Gustav Schmaltz, which might explain his interest in symbolism, dreams and daydreams. Leuner developed a technique called Guided Affective Imagery, a daydream technique. After learning of the work of Sandison, he started to use low doses of psychedelics to further regression and catharsis. This in turn intensified and deepened therapeutically useful images (Leuner, 1983, p. 177). According to Leuner, "the correct dosage is one that evokes the desired psychodynamic material but at the same time allows part of the patient's reflective and observing ego to remain intact so that he will not be flooded with a glut of experiences" (1983, p. 178). His experience of combining low dose psychedelics with his daydream technique suggests that the technique of active imagination as suggested by Jung might also benefit from low dose psychedelics.

Practical Issues

From studies in the 1950s and 1960s it can be concluded that the use of low dose psychedelics has benefits for the psychotherapeutic process, including psychoanalytic orientated therapies. As stressed by Michael Fordham and Marion Curtner, it is important not to solely rely on the psychedelic substance as an agent for therapeutic progress. As became clear in the early days of psychedelic assisted psychotherapy, the relationship between the patient and therapist is more important for the effectiveness of the treatment. The psychedelic substance is used solely to assist in the analytic process. More recent research confirms this. For instance, Thal et al. found that the therapeutic benefits of substance-assisted treatments rely on the combination of psychological effects of the substance, "the shared interpersonal experience between client and therapist, the mindset of the client and the therapist, and successful psychotherapeutic integration of the experience" (Thal et al., 2011).

Contraindications for the use of low dose psychedelics should be considered and, when in doubt, a medical specialist should be consulted.

An analyst wanting to consider working with psychedelics should be aware of any physical health issues, such as heart conditions. Another important issue to consider is the use of psychopharmaceuticals, as psychedelics might interfere with the working of medication, or the medication might interfere with the working of the psychedelic substance.

Regarding the mental state of the patient, I have not been able to find studies identifying the contraindications for microdosing. Müller et al. (2020) even describe the successful treatment of a 39-year-old female patient suffering from severe, treatment-resistant depression and a complex personality disorder with a vulnerability for psychosis. The treatment was designed similarly to a microdose process, although over time they increased the doses from 50 to 200 micrograms LSD. This case study was described from a psychopharmaceutical viewpoint, which still leaves questions regarding the use of microdosing assisted analysis with patients suffering from severe psychopathology. From a Jungian viewpoint, the use of psychedelics should be supportive for psychological growth. Following this principle, the regressive tendencies initiated by microdosing will not support the development in every patient. During periods of analysis, when the main emphasis is on supportive work assisting a weak ego structure, furthering the regressive tendency could be counterproductive. Using psychedelics in low doses in this group of patients might lead to increased vulnerability to stress, an inability to integrate with higher danger of acting out, and in severe cases paranoid fear or a fear of disintegration.

During the preparation phase, possible risks that could arise during a session should be discussed. Especially with a low dose of psychedelics, the analyst might tend to consider the patient to be fully conscious and not perceptible to slight changes in ego functioning. Even being under the influence of a low dose, the patient may find himself in a vulnerable position. It is imperative that the analyst is sensitive to the mental state of the patient. The analyst will need to be empathic toward the patient and aware of the increased sensitivity to acting out, transference issues, and suggestibility (Carhart-Harris et al., 2015). As with full dose guided experience, the limits of behavior should be made clear with special attention for touching and violence.

Understanding the condition of being under the influence of a psychedelic could be addressed by the analyst having his own microdose experience. The problem that might arise from this is that the analyst might start to compare his or her own experiences with those of the patient. Apart from the different substances used and the differences in dose-body weight ratio and mental state, there are many factors—known and unknown—that influence the experience. Furthermore, the substances *activate* experiences rather than *produce* them, so every experience is an activation of the individual's unconscious.

Conclusion

The question addressed in this chapter concerns the implementation of microdosing in clinical practice. The topic has been approached from two applications: first, the use of low dose psychedelics and the indirect effect on analysis; and second, the use of microdosing in direct relation to the analytical hour. Although the full mechanism responsible for psychological changes is not fully understood and many issues still need to thoroughly be researched, it appears that microdosing—both indirectly and directly related to the analytic hour—could be well suited to support the psychodynamics during Jungian analysis. As research to date indicates that the effects of microdosing are overall positive, we should be encouraged to study this phenomenon more thoroughly and gain experience in the application of low dose psychedelics in analysis.

When a patient initiates microdosing as a way of self-medicating and to influence everyday functioning, there are indications that this could also support the analytic process. Three factors are important to consider. First, the intention for microdosing should be in service of psychological growth and not predominately relate to gratifying ego desires like the improvement of performance. Second, in comparison to patients using a medium or full dose, the microdoser will have to be more attentive to the inner process as unconscious material will not force itself upon ego. To make full use of microdosing, the patient would be advised to take time to attend to the inner world through periods of reflection and contemplation, meditation, daydreaming, or active imagination, and find ways to creatively express the unfolding content. Third, the gains from psychedelic use increase when the patient and analyst spend time on the integration process.

When used in direct relationship to the analytic hour, an effective microdose of psychedelics will support the patient to be more perceptive to unconscious material, more prone to opening up about painful, guilt or shame laden issues and more engaged in the analytic relationship. In this way, the substance will support an encounter with personal wounds, allowing for easier access to those parts of the psyche that are often difficult to approach. Therefore, psychedelic substances in low doses can augment and deepen the analytic work. Low dose psychedelics have benefits over the use of medium and full doses, which makes it worthwhile to consider as collaborator for analysis. The fact that there is a continuation of ego control without major perceptual distortions makes the experience less anxiety-provoking and intrusive for the patient, while still allowing for an increased openness to the unconscious. There does not have to be a major distinction between the normal therapeutic situation compared to the sessions in which the patient is under the influence, whereby this makes the experience less disruptive and unsettling for both the patient and the analyst. Furthermore, there is little or no need for expensive clinical oversight as is typical for medium and full dose experiences. Microdosing allows for a certain efficacy and immediacy that is different from the use of other doses. This means that the psychodynamics appear more favorable for the integration process.

As research remains in its early stages, the benefits and disadvantages of microdosing still require thorough grounding in both empirical as well as experience-based studies. For now, both research and subjective experiences suggest that even a small dose of psychedelics can be a useful collaborator to analysis.

References

Abramson, H.A. (1956). Lysergic Acid Diethylamide (LSD-25): XIX. As an adjunct to brief psychotherapy, with special reference to ego enhancement, *The Journal of Psychology*, *41*, 199-229.

Anderson T., Petranker R., Rosenbaum D., Weissman C.R., Dinh-Williams L-A, Hui K., Hapke E. & Farb N.A.S. (2019). Microdosing psychedelics: personality, mental health, and creativity differences in microdosers. *Psychopharmacology*, *236*, 731-740.

Bornemann, J. (2020). The viability of microdosing psychedelics as a strategy to enhance Cognition and well-being - An early review. *Journal of Psychoactive Drugs*, *52*(4), 300-308.

Cameron L.P., Nazarian A. & Olson D.E. (2020). Psychedelic micro-dosing: Prevalence and subjective effects, *Journal of Psychoactive Drugs*, *52*(2), 113-122.

Carhart-Harris, R.L., Kaelen, M., Whalley, M.G. et al. (2015). LSD en-hances suggestibility in healthy volunteers. *Psychopharmacology*, *232*, 785-794.

Carhart-Harris, R.L., Erritzoe, D., Haijen, E., and Watts, R. (2017). Psychedelics and connectedness. *Psychopharmacology*, *235*(2), 547-550.

Cavanna, F., Muller, S., de la Fuente, L.A. et al. (2022). Microdosing with psilocybin mushrooms: a double-blind placebo-controlled study. *Transational Psychiatry*, *12*(1), 1-11.

Chordorow, J. (Ed.) (1997). *Jung on Active Imagination*. Princeton University Press.

Curtner, M. (1959). Analytic work with LSD-25. *Psychiatric Quarterly*, *33*(4), 715-757.

Fadiman, J. (2011). *The Psychedelic explorer's guide: Safe, therapeutic, and sacred journeys*. Park Street Press.

Fadiman, J. & Korb, S. (2019). Might microdosing psychedelics be safe and beneficial? An initial exploration. *Journal of Psychoactive Drugs, 51*(2), 118-122.

Fordham, M. (1963). Analytic observations on patients using hallucinogenic drugs. In R. Crocket, R. Sandison, & A. Walk (Eds.), *Hallucinogenic drugs and their psychotherapeutic use.* 125-130. C.C. Thomas.

Forstmann M., & Sagioglou C. (2017). Lifetime experience with (classic) psychedelics predicts pro-environmental behavior through an increase in nature relatedness. *Psychopharmacology, 31,* 975–988.

Frederking, W. (1955). Intoxicant drugs (Mescaline and Lysergic Acid Diethylamide) in psychotherapy. *The Journal of Nervous and Mental Disease, 121,* 262-266.

Gattuso J.J., Perkins D., Ruffell S., Lawrence A.J., Hoyer D., Jacobson L.H., Timmermann C., Castle D., Rossell SL., Downey L.A., Pagni B.A., Galvão-Coelho N.L., Nutt D., Sarris J. (2023). Default Mode Network Modulation by psychedelics: A systematic review. *International Journal Neuropsychopharmacology, 26*(3), 155-188.

Glatter, R. (2015, November 27). LSD Microdosing the new job-enhancer in Silicon Valley and beyond. *Forbes.* https://www.forbes.com/sites/robertglatter/2015/11/27/lsd-microdosing-the-new-job-enhancer-in-silicon-valley-and-beyond/?sh=736445b8188a (Last accessed 21-07-2023).

Griffiths R.R., Johnson M.W., Richards W.A., Richards B.D., McCann U., Jesse R. (2011). Psilocybin occasioned mystical-type experiences: Immediate and persisting dose-related effects. *Psychopharmacology, 218*(4), 649–665.

Hill, S.J. (2019). *Confrontation with the unconscious: Jungian depth psychology and psychedelic experience.* Aeon.

Horsley, J.S. (1943). *Narco-analysis.* Humphrey Milford.

Johnstad, P.G. (2018). Powerful substances in tiny amounts: An interview study of psychedelic microdosing. *Nordic Studies on Alcohol and Drugs, 35*(1), 39–51.

Kashdan T.B., and Rottenberg J. (2010). Psychological flexibility as a fundamental aspect of health. *Clin Psychol Rev.*, *30*(7), 865-78.

Kaertner L.S., Steinborn M.B., Kettner H., Spriggs M.J., Roseman L., Buchborn T., Balaet M., Timmermann C., Erritzoe D. & Carhart-Harris R.L. (2021). Positive expectations predict improved mental-health outcomes linked to psychedelic microdosing. *Scientific Reports*, *11*(1), 1941.

Karim, F. (2017, December 30). A drop of LSD is 'new brain booster.' *The Times*. https://www.thetimes.co.uk/article/a-drop-of-lsd-is-new-brain-booster-w2kbtw559 (Last Accessed 21-07-2023).

Kuypers, K.P.C. (2020). The therapeutic potential of microdosing psychedelics in depression. *Therapeutic Advances in Psychopharmacology, 10,* 1-15.

Lea, T., Amada N. & Jungaberle H. (2020a). Psychedelic Microdosing: A Subreddit Analysis, *Journal of Psychoactive Drugs*, *52(*2), 101-112.

Lea, T., Amada N., Jungaberle H., Schecke H. & Klein M. (2020b). Microdosing psychedelics: Motivations, subjective effects and harm reduction. *International Journal of Drug Policy*, *75*, p. 102600.

Leonard, A. (2015, November 20). How LSD Microdosing became the hot new business trip. *Rolling Stone*, https://www.rollingstone. com/culture/culture-news/how-lsd-microdosing-became-the-hot-new-business-trip-64961/ (Last Accessed 27 July, 2023).

Leuner, H. (1967). Basic functions involved in the psychotherapeutic effect of psychotomimetics. In Brill, H. (Ed.): *Neuro-Psycho-Pharmacology*. Excerpta Medica, (445-448).

Leuner, H. (1983). Psycholytic therapy: Hallucinogenics as an aid in psychodynamically oriented psychotherapy. In Grinspoon, L. and Bakalar, J.B. (Eds): *Psychedelic reflections*. Human Sciences Press, Inc. (177-192).

Millière R., Carhart-Harris R.L., Roseman L., Trautwein F.-M., and Berkovich-Ohana A. (2018). Psychedelics, beditation, and self-consciousness. *Frontiers in Psychology 9*, 1475.

Müller F., Mühlhauser M., Holze F., Lang U.E., Walter M., Liechti M.E. and Borgwardt S. (2020). Treatment of a complex personality disorder using repeated doses of LSD—A case report on significant improvements in the absence of acute drug effects. *Frontiers in Psychiatry, 11.*

Novac, A. & Blinder B.J. (2021). Free association in psychoanalysis and its links to neuroscience contributions. *Neuropsychoanalysis, 23*(2), 55-81.

Passie, T. (1997). *Psycholytic and psychedelic therapy research 1931-1995: A complete international bibliography.* Laurentius Publishers.

Passie, T. (2019). *The science of microdosing psychedelics.* Psychedelic Press.

Passie T., Guss J., & Krähenmann R. (2022). Lower-dose psycholytic therapy - A neglected approach. *Frontiers in Psychiatry, 13,* 1020505.

Polito, V., & Stevenson, R.J. (2019). A systematic study of microdosing psychedelics. *PloS one, 14*(2), e0211023.

Petranker, R., Kim, J., & Anderson, T. (2022). Microdosing as a response to the meaning crisis: A qualitative analysis. *Journal of Humanistic Psychology,* 2216782210750.

Prochazkova, L., Lippelt, D.P., Colzato, L.S. et al. (2018). Exploring the effect of microdosing psychedelics on creativity in an open-label natural setting. *Psychopharmacology, 235,* 3401–3413.

Rifkin, B.D., Maraver, M.J., & Colzato, L.S. (2020). Microdosing psychedelics as cognitive and emotional enhancers. *Psychology of Consciousness: Theory, Research, and Practice, 7*(3), 316-329.

Rootman J.M., Kryskow P., Harvey K., Stamets P., Santos-Brault E., Kuypers K.P.C., Polito V., Bourzat F. & Walsh, Z. (2021). Adults who microdose psychedelics report health related motivations and lower levels of anxiety and depression compared to non-microdosers. *Scientific Reports, 11*(1). 22479.

Rootman, J.M., Kiraga, M., Kryskow, P. et al. (2022). Psilocybin microdosers demonstrate greater observed improvements in mood and mental health at one month relative to non-microdosing controls. *Science Report, 12*(1), 11091.

Sandison, R.A., Spencer, A.M. and Whitelaw, J.D.A. (1954). The Therapeutic value of Lysergic Acid Diethylamide in mental illness. *The British Journal of Psychiatry, 100,* 491-507.

Sandison, R.A. (1954). Psychological aspects of the LSD treatment of the neuroses. *Journal of Mental Science, 100*(419), 508-515.

Schmid Y., Enzler F., Gasser P., Grouzmann E., Preller K. H., Vollenweider F.X., Brenneisen R., Müller F., Borgwardt S., Liechti M.E. (2015). Acute effects of lysergic acid diethylamide in healthy subjects. *Biological Psychiatry, 78*(8), 544-553.

Solon, O. (2016, August 24). Under pressure, Silicon Valley workers turn to LSD microdosing Silicon Valley workers are taking tiny hits of LSD before heading to work. But are they risking their health or optimising it? *Wired.* https://www.wired.co.uk/article/lsd-microdosing-drugs-silicon-valley (Last Accessed 21-07-2023).

Stolaroff, M. (2015) Do we still need psychedelics? In Allen Badiner (Ed.), *Zig Zag Zen: Buddhism and psychedelics.* Synergetic Press.

Swanson, L.R. (2018). Unifying theories of psychedelic drug effects. *Frontiers in Pharmacology. 9,* 172.

Szigeti, B., Kartner L., Blemings A., Rosas F., Feilding A., Nutt D.J., Carhart-Harris R.L., and Erritzoe D. (2021) Self-blinding citizen science to explore psychedelic microdosing. *eLife, 10.*

Thal, S.B., Bright, S.J., Sharbanee, J.M., Wenge, T., and Skeffington P.M. (2021). Current Perspective on the therapeutic preset for substance-assisted psychotherapy. *Frontiers of Psychology, 12,* 617224.

Van Dusen, W. (1961). LSD and the enlightment of Zen. *Psychologica, 4,* 11-16.

Vojtěchovský, M., Safratová, V., and Havránková, O. (1972). Effect of threshold doses of LSD on social interaction in healthy students. *Act Nerv Super (Praha), 14*(2), 115-6.

Yanakieva, S., Polychroni, N., Family, N. et al. (2019). The effects of microdose LSD on time perception: a randomised, double-blind, placebo-controlled trial. *Psychopharmacology, 236,* 1159-70.

The Self as the First Principle
for a Psychedelic Experience

Leslie Stein

The book, *Shivitti: A Vision* (Ka-Tzetnik, 1989), is the almost unbearable story of a holocaust survivor undergoing treatment with LSD. It records the very gradual reconstitution of the narrator's soul as the abject horrors are brought vividly back to consciousness by the expansive and loosening power of the psychedelic. It reveals that the healing that occurred over time required the psychiatrist to provide a framework, a container, for the patient to hold onto to be able to unearth his deepest core, the mystery of his being, in stark contrast to the evil that had completely pervaded his psyche. As the psychiatrist explained to him: "the LSD won't work by itself" (Ka-Tzetnick, 1989, p. 33): it needed that framework. The therapist had to establish and then maintain the intention behind their work together, and during and after each session take him further into the content by asking over and over, "What do you see?" Out of this approach, a profound message emerged from the patient: "I watch the elusive There, There that revealed There, so incomprehensible, the destination of the endlessly rolling ball of yarn. It's my insides that stare and track the motion of the ball" (Ka-Tzetnick, 1989, p. 105). In Jungian terms, this is an alteration that has occurred, as Eric Neumann explains, because "the ego cannot cling to its position in consciousness, but must expose itself to encounter with the non-ego" (Neumann, 1948/1969, p. 380).

Psychedelics, if examined through the lens of the Jungian concept of individuation, must engage the participant at the deep, non-ego level of the Self, the numinous center of psyche, the God within, that which symbolizes wholeness. It is that framework, built up around this first therapeutic principle of the Self that points to individuation through a lasting alteration of consciousness.

Psychedelic therapeutic research and theory emphasizes that there is no therapeutic benefit without a framework that is formed through the effect of the "context" (Martin & Sterzer, 2022) as well as "the consolidation of these during the subsequent period of integration" (Letheby, 2021, p. 143). The context: set and setting, is critical to the creation of a framework by establishing a purpose and meaning for the experience. This is expressed in the literature as the element which establishes a coherent prior intention that orients the experience toward change by offering meaning and value for the significance of what is to be observed, as well as a setting that instills a sense of safety to open to the experience (Watts & Luouma, 2020). Having a clear intention and purpose are therefore the primary considerations, so the fascinating phenomena that arise as myriad visual effects or through uplifting experiences are not considered to have the same effect on psychological change as that which is preceded by a prior, purposeful orientation and intention (Haijen et al., 2018; Carhart-Harris et al., 2018).

Unlike the single-focused Jungian framework based on the Self, psychedelic therapeutic research does not yet refine the nature of the context by indicating the importance of engaging with any particular level of psyche, nor does it offer a goal or principle that must be realized. It also does not explain the depth of engagement that must be achieved at the stages of establishing the set or upon integration after the experience ends. The framework for psychedelic use is accordingly amorphous, as it is not subject to any consistent theoretical bases. It has been said, accordingly: "It is not yet well-understood how the milieu of psilocybin administration and the accompanying psychological-support model facilitate therapeutic change in psychedelic forms of therapy" (Modlin et al., 2023).

The importance of the existence of a clear, unambiguous framework for any model of psychological change cannot be underestimated. The participant requires a conceptual structure to contain what is occurring during and after the experience. The same is true of a mystical experience and thus a framework is at the heart of every esoteric, spiritual, and religious tradition as a noetic infrastructure for the ego to accept the purposive outcome of the occurrence. These frameworks permeate the experience and therefore provide a coherent explanation for understanding and accepting what is otherwise overwhelming, so that, as Gershom Sholem explains: There is no such thing as a mystical experience *per se*; "there is only the mysticism of a particular religious system, Christian, Islamic, Jewish mysticism and so on" (1941, pp. 5-6).

In the absence of a coherent theory or model as to the nature of the framework, the claim for legitimacy of psychedelic therapy is then derived by inference derived from reported instances of the psychological effectiveness of the experience assessed by a myriad of subjective measures. Accordingly, that efficacy has been proposed, for example, from the results of the Mystical Experience Questionnaire, the Emotional Breakthrough Scale (Roseman et al., 2019) or the categorization of insights according to the Psychological Insight Scale (Peill et al., 2022). Extrapolation from these and other positive scales is then the theoretical basis for requiring an effective support model based on a framework for intention and orientation as the means to achieve these states.

A potential framework in psychedelic research is usually constructed by three imprecise possibilities. The first draws loosely on elements used in the successful impact of ancient cultural settings where psychedelics are ritualized, such as with ayahuasca. The second is the use of generalized techniques that strive to create a universal world view with a focus on internal imagery, achieving ecstatic states, and a relationship to an unseen world (Winkelman, 2021). The third is by equating a psychedelic experience as containing elements of a mystical experience.

These approaches, although often vague and lacking clarity, are needed in an attempt to make the recipient who is overwhelmed by the experience, receptive. A framework will not, however, necessarily lead to an alteration of consciousness, as it is not possible to determine the receptivity of a particular individual to a mystical (Stein, 2019, Chap 2) or psychedelic experience. There are indeed many other indicia that affect receptivity, such as the developmental background, particular complexes, cultural and religious beliefs, all of which interact with fear, dread, and a reluctance to make a permanent change of a long-held static ego position. What follows logically is that the stronger and more coherent the principle underlying the framework, the more likely is the possibility of an individual accepting and integrating the psychedelic experience.

The Self as the First Principle

The spiritual and religious traditions that propose a congruent, specific framework for reception of a numinous experience have been developed over centuries, and therefore have reached a level of refinement that provides a clear basis for acceptance of these experiences. They all proceed on a *first principle* that is the basis for their world view, ideologies, goals, and practices. Aside from cultural paradigms where psychedelics are part of the ancient esoteric and ritual teachings focused on shamanistic first principles, there appears to be no intact Western esoteric framework that can provide a first principle that can be employed for psychedelics. In our society, the world view we have of psychedelics is, by its history and recent arrival as a capable therapy, immature and loosely derived from occult practices, reported mystical experiences, and eclectic new age world views. New age and occult practices have uncertain and unreliable first principles: "To be sure, Western occultists modified and adjusted religious teachings to fit their own agendas, curriculums, and world-view, which is certainly a phenomenon that should be considered with a critical eye" (Cantú, 2020, pp. 109-110). This is a phenomenon understood by Jung who insisted on the presence of a psychological first principle upon which a framework can be formed.

The process of Jungian psychoanalysis that relies upon the continued revelation of the purposive nature of the unconscious and the centering function of the Self as its *spiritus rector*, provides an orientation responsible for a change of the conscious position over time. Its essence is that it creates a specific cohesive, ordered framework made patent by the ongoing process of experiential awareness of the analysand's relationship to the unconscious, and the Self, the gradual realization of that centering function within psyche. This framework is the scaffolding in Jungian psychoanalysis in dealing with all pathologies, and in the consideration of dreams, fantasies, projections, narratives, as well as working through numinous experiences.

In the forthcoming publication of *Protocols to Memories, Dreams, Reflections* (Jung & Jaffe, 1958), Aniela Jaffe relates two previously unpublished comments where Jung expresses his views in reference to mescaline. These views appear to suggest that Jung had experience with mescaline by raising it as a comparison to other experiences, but his actual use is not known. However, they point to the nature of that first principle that is appropriate as the basis for the mindset and later integration of the psychedelic experience:

> It was as if I had undertaken a mescaline experiment where I am inside it without being objective. I could register objectively only what I was experiencing. I had no concepts with which I could comprehend this. It was not a philosophy, but neither was it an intoxication. I had absolutely nothing I could compare it to. It was something into which I surrendered myself of my own freewill, and yet was trapped by it as if I had experimented on myself with a toxin. …
>
> I was concerned to find out whether these things have a meaning or whether they are actually meaningless. I was strongly influenced by how meaningful these things are even if I could then understand the meaning only a little. My "scientific" question was this: what happens when I switch off consciousness? I notice from dreams that something stood in the background to which I wanted to give a fair chance of emerging. One subjects oneself to the conditions required for it – as in a mescaline experiment – that are required for it to emerge. (Jung & Jaffe, 1958, pp. 380; 381)

The first part of the quote explains that for Jung, overwhelming experiences, as in a psychedelic experience, are not able to be observed *objectively*; that is, by the ego comprehending its meaning as it is occurring to permit it to have a lasting change in the conscious position. This is re-stating Jung's significant limitation of the presence of the ego here imposed upon the effectiveness of psychedelics. This occurs because, as he refers to in the second quote, their use results in a switching off of ego consciousness: the conscious, discriminating mind is not active or is substantially reduced. The absence of the evaluative mind, overwhelmed by the drug, is a barrier to understanding the purposiveness of the experience as it is occurring that is the key to an alteration of the conscious mind. Jung explains elsewhere: "Nowhere is the basic requirement so indispensable as in psychology that the observer should be adequate to his subject, in the sense of being able to see subjectively but also objectively" (Jung, CW 6, §10). This reflects his clear view, repeated in all his discourse, that the basis of any psychological change requires a conscious, alert mind that can observe with clarity and understand logically the nature of that which is presented to it in an experience.

It is apparent that psychedelics can make an individual more receptive to change by the entropic effect of relaxing higher-level brain functions (Carhartt-Harris & Friston, 2019). Even with greater receptivity, however, the establishment of an intention in the set and setting, even offering apparent links to a deep meaning or wider ideas of interconnectedness, may not continue during the experience when the ego is overwhelmed, as he suggests in the first quote. This is because, as Jung explains in another context when speaking of mescaline, it causes the lowering of the threshold of that critical waking consciousness that "renders perceptible the perpetual variants that are normally unconscious, but on the other hand making it impossible to integrate them into the general orientation of consciousness" (CW 3, § 569).

His answer to this conundrum lies in his remarks that he noticed in dreams that "something stood in the background to which I wanted to give a fair chance of emerging" and, as he expresses it, to which there is a need to surrender to that something for "it to emerge" (Jung & Jaffe, 1958, p. 381). That something, although not named, is Jung's first principle, that which stands behind a change in consciousness: in Jungian terms, the realization of the Self, the God within.

Taken together, the two quotes indicate that from Jung's viewpoint, a psychedelic experience will have the necessary impact on the position of the ego *if* the individual opens to the reality that there is something that is seeking to make itself known as the experience is unfolding. This understanding that there is this purposive, generative layer to psyche, has precedence over any experiencing of a sense of interconnectedness or other numinous insights, which lack the same potential for psychological change. This difference arises because, following his reasoning, the lack of objectivity during the experience elevates only the most profound insight, the emergence of the Self, that is making itself known and is critical to psychological change. If this is made the basis for the set and integration, there is a possibility that the importance and nature of the Self can be seen as the proper framework for what is occurring and has occurred. It is this that is most likely to broaden the conscious mind.

A vignette from a patient is useful to explain what may be counterintuitive from the psychedelic research literature: that the emphasis should be on the possibility of the Self seeking to manifest in the experience. A male patient, a musician, related this experience that occurred during a moderate dose (3 gram) psylocibin experience:

> *I was talking to my deceased partner as if she was there with me but what I realized was that there was a force in me that was presenting this to me, whatever it was, both for my sake to heal my trauma, but more importantly, it seemed, for its own sake by increasing my awareness and, I guess, collective awareness.*

This conveniently expresses the first principle of Jung that he first enunciated in these terms in 1917 in *The Red Book* to the effect that opening to the ideal of the Self, that something that emerges, will make the occurrence of the experience indelible:

> I would have to confess to this experience and recognize the God in it. No insight or objection is so strong that it could surpass the strength of this experience. And even if the god had revealed himself in a meaningless abomination, I could only avow that I have experienced the God in it. I even know that it is not too difficult to cite a theory that would sufficiently explain my experience and join it to the already known. I could furnish this theory myself and be satisfied in intellectual terns, and

yet this theory would be unable to remove even the smallest part of the knowledge that I have experienced the God. I recognize the God by the unshakeableness of the experience. (Jung, 2009, p. 338)

By this interpretation, a change will occur in psychedelic and numinous experiences by a realization of the directing role of a non-ego aspect of psyche that extends beyond the lesser role of the ego's fixed position. A psychedelic experience changes consciousness to the degree that such a truth is revealed in whatever way and *to what extent*. The truth manifests itself in various ways with different intensities as an experience of wholeness, unity, and interconnectedness, which are then understood as manifestations of the Self that arise from the unconscious.

These are complex concepts, refined by Jung over time, but they all rely upon the idea that psychological change occurs when the subjective experience includes an objective intimation of a purposeful inner component, so that the conscious mind will submit to and absorb it to foster an alteration of consciousness. It is that level of impact that is needed, Jung explains about his own experience, because it is that which "seized me and beyond all measure and steadily goes on working in me" (Jung, 2009, p. 338).

Lasting change requires a new world view that shifts the conscious position from outer directed causation to inner direction, or else any change is transitory. This inward direction requires, as Sri Aurobindo so beautifully explained, "purification and consecration" (Aurobindo, 1972, p. 904). In the case of psychedelics, as Jung points out in the second quote, purification and consecration occurs when it is an experience of the objective reality of that something seeking to emerge for the sake of itself. That relativizes the ego, softens it, and is most important for the *set* to allow the power of the mysterious numen to be realized.

The Self in the Set

Fundamental to Jung's opus is this first principle of psychological growth. It provides the ideal of the realization of a centering function in psyche, the Self, which actively seeks to resolve the conflict of opposites that are our lives. The Self appears, when recognized, as pre-existent to consciousness, and with agency. Accordingly, giving over to the guiding agency of the Self has the effect of providing a point of reference in the maelstrom of confusion that is the conscious mind. For Jung, the Self was not a mere theory or abstract goal, as he found confirmation of its existence in many traditions and religions, such as the *Atman* in Hinduism, the pre-existent aspect of the divine within us that therefore confers on the Self divine qualities and aligns with our religious instinct.

The importance of the recognition of an inner force that seeks to resolve conflict is not easily explained because, as Sri Aurobindo states, the something within, which he calls the psychic being, "…except where it is very much developed has only a small and partial, concealed and missed or diluted experience on the life of most men" (Aurobindo, 2014, p. 354). There are many layers of mind that must be traversed for that something to be realized as the essential psychological essence, the first principle. In his writings in *Aion,* Jung therefore refers to the Gnostic idea that there is a strong distinction between the higher man, synonymous with the "'spiritual, inner' man" (CW 9ii, § 360) who has found this Self, and the lower man, the latter by implication not connected at all with that "something," but existing "in the sublunary world of matter" (CW 9ii, § 368).

By this approach, the lower man, where we all mostly reside to a greater or lesser extent, must proceed by a series of psychological steps until there is realization of the purposive nature of the unconscious when an intimation of the Self is likely to arise. This sensing or intuition of the Self fosters the presentation of unity and interconnectedness in psyche. Thus, this first principle would solve the question of providing an uplifting framework for a support model for an induction to psychedelics and its integration. It goes beyond imprecise new age or generalized descriptions of what to expect in a forthcoming experience, providing the framework of the healing power of a revelation of that inner guide standing behind the occurrence.

This element of the mind objectively realizing the existence of the Self must be present to some extent in the psychedelic experience for it to have efficacy, according to Jung, as it is the thinking mind that must be powerfully influenced and made to understand that there is more in psyche. This is most effective if it offers the chance of the introduction of a new secret or ideal in the set that can then be verified in the experience; as the ancient *Rg Veda* requires: "secret words that speak their meaning to the seer" (IV. 3. 16). For a mystical experience as an analogy, the revelation must be received and understood within a prior spiritual or religious framework, as it is that which provides an orientation for it to change a mind when otherwise overwhelmed (Stein, 2019, Chap. 4).

The Induction into that Something

If a psychedelic experience suspends the conscious, thinking mind, as Jung suggests, it is because it has been overwhelmed by a fantastical array of images without understandable content. How then is it possible for a prior framework relying on the first principle to have any effect on such a mind?

Repeating what Jung states in the second quote, "I notice from dreams that something stood in the background to which I wanted to give a fair chance of emerging. One subjects oneself to the conditions required for it – as in a mescaline experiment – that are required for it to emerge." His intention is to give the Self a chance to emerge in the experience and to allow oneself to be the means for it to emerge. The preparedness for it to emerge is the framework that he provides in another section of the *Protocols to Memories, Dreams, Reflections* (Jung & Jaffe, 1958) becomes a *prior* "unconditional saying yes" to what will have "stepped forward from within" during the experience.

In referring to a toxin, Jung is referring to the suspension of the ego because it is being overwhelmed. It is necessary therefore that a door be kept open to the emergence of the Self when that opportunity arises. How this occurs is not obvious but requires a reference to different states in the experience. By analogy, in a mystical experience there are stages where there is a suspension of the ego, and others where there is conscious awareness of what is occurring (Stein, 2019, pp. 62-63). The first stage of a mystical experience is the cognitive awareness of being overwhelmed as it begins. At this stage, the conscious mind is active and can provide a hypothesis of what is occurring through the framework. Just prior to a peak experience where there is a complete suspension of the mind, there is a view formed of what is beginning to be revealed. Again, the framework is there to keep the mind focused on the first principle behind the occurrence. Then there is the peak experience that Jung is referring to where the mind stops and there is no framework. In a coming down from the experience, cognitive thought enters to make sense of what has occurred (Stein, 2019, pp. 68-71).

The peak experience for psychedelics where the conscious mind is not active, is similar to mystical experiences, although there is no research that has delineated the subjective experience of these stages in a psychedelic occurrence (Majic et al., 2015). Thus, it has been said: "Despite extensive quantitative characterisation, no papers so far have reported a qualitative description of the subjective experience of orally administered psilocybin in healthy volunteers..." (McCulloch et al., 2022). What is obvious is that there are indeed experiences of a staged process of ego-dissolution using psychedelics that, even excluding the short acting and dramatic impacts of 5-MeO-DMT, are the onset of non-dual experiences where the subject and object merge. Accordingly, intermittent conscious states are reported that highlight cognitive awareness and assessment of a sense of interconnectedness, blissful moods, ecstasy, and awareness of an alteration of time and space (McCulloch et al., 2022).

Varying fugue states of ego dissolution, interspersed with periods of cognitive evaluation are therefore the norm in a psychedelic experience, as reported with medium dose psilocybin that may last four to six hours (Passie et al., 2002). If, as with a relatively brief mystical experience that lasts a matter of minutes at most, there will be a range of cognitive analyses at different stages, this will apply as well to a psychedelic experience. If this proposition is correct, this is how Jung's suggestion of the awareness of the emergence to that inner something, the basis of the framework, can emerge and be the basis for psychological change.

In establishing this framework, it will not emerge by providing the participant with a quick narrative or theory, but rather from the well-developed understanding that the unconscious is purposive and that the Self contains the ultimate mystery of existence. How long this awareness takes to coalesce in order to form a strong framework using a psychoanalytic modality is uncertain and its outcome depends on many variables. It is unlikely that it will manifest after a few induction sessions.

However, if this is indeed the most viable framework, it allows for the possibility of the construction of a narrative so that the images that will be encountered can be seen as purposive and can give way to a breakthrough. This will provide a *possible,* but by no means conclusive framework for conditioning the mindset prior to a psychedelic experience to the first principle.

Setting and the Self

A ritualistic, spiritual, all-absorbing environment can, to some extent, bring on a gesture or sentiment of the first principle. An intimation of unity conveyed by the setting may allow a descent into psyche to deepen the inward direction, to bring an intimation of peace, and thus to reach the gate of that inner being. Can the first principle be conveyed by the setting and not just prior narrative explanations or subsequent interpretation?

In all Jung's writings, he emphasizes the necessity of change within a "container" by the creation of a "sacred space," what he calls a *temenos.* In psychedelic therapy, in similar terms, there is a "consecration" created by the setting (Cwik, 2010). A meta-analysis of psychedelic research as to setting suggests it will be most effective because of elements that are not traditional in psychoanalytic settings, such as the impacts of music, rituals, and physically comfortable surroundings, as well as undefined but highly relational therapist attributes (Golden et al., 2022), the latter not being unusual. A pleasant setting, social and tactile support, as well as safety measures, without specificity, are promoted as an aid in a positive psychedelic experience, although: "Generally, the studies above have suggested, assumed, or tried to assert that environmental sociocultural context can influence psychedelic experiences and outcomes. However, they did not provide empirical controls or rigorous testing of these hypotheses" (Golden et al., 2022, p. 58).

There are, nonetheless, many reports in psychedelic research of the importance of a spiritual, ritual setting as being most aligned with promoting self-insight and mystical type experiences (Perkins et al., 2021; Golden et al., 2022, p. 58). The reasoning is that the setting itself combines with the set to create a *congruent* context for the intention or orientation necessary for the possibility of change (Golden et al., 2022,

p. 59). What is highlighted often in the literature is the importance of empathic resonance where a psychedelic therapist or facilitator helps the individual to navigate the process because of the therapist's own psychedelic experiences, as well as physical proximity. This is explicated, as is relevant here, by Julia Kristeva as creating a contact with "Being that extends beyond me," as she refers to the first principle that arises from the "nonverbal experience of the referent in the interaction with the other" (1989, p. 67).

From a Jungian point of view, it is unclear whether an analyst *qua* analyst can provide this therapeutic setting for a psychedelic experience. To do so would shift the existing paradigm of the transference/ countertransference dimensions and its ethical considerations, discussed elsewhere in this book. However, in the name of the first principle, it is always a possibility to take part in the setting, assuming it is appropriate and ethical in the circumstances. It is warranted by our duty to provide meaning through the introduction of the Self as the first principle of change. Having introduced the Self as a framework, carrying awareness of it through in facilitating an experience may precipitate the highest possibility of change; as Jung expresses it in a 1940 lecture: "If I discover that I have been anticipated, it makes an enormous impression on me. The feeling of meaning or purposefulness is part of that, even if, as I said, we cannot precisely pinpoint what that meaning, the specific purpose, is" (Jung, 2023, p. 143).

Symbols of the Self and Integration

The fantastical array of the contents of a psychedelic experience do not necessarily provide symbols that can be interpreted. According to *Protocols of Memories, Dreams, Reflections* (Jung & Jaffe, 1958), Jung questions the worth in experiences where one is overwhelmed by the images and loses cognition. Jung refers to this in the quote and elsewhere (CW 3, § 548) as the equivalent of being overcome by a toxin. However, he states in the *Protocols* in reference to vague fantasies, what aspect may be relevant: "What my fantasies showed me was a matter of actualization of the inner man who appears under the symbol of the Anthropos," the latter being also called by him the "inner, spiritual man" (CW 9ii, § 360).

Understanding how to employ the Self for integration after a psychedelic experience can be derived from Jung's comments about fantasies. He asserts that they "possess no realizable worth," but they can be developed to alter consciousness if they can be worked on with the "constructive method" (CW 6, § 93). This method proposes that symbolization of any kind becomes relevant when the unconscious is manifesting "a goal or purpose, but characterizing its objective in symbolic language" (CW 6, § 702). Its elucidation using the constructive method is to bring in associations to enrich the symbolic product so "that it eventually attains a degree of clarity for conscious comprehension" (CW 6, § 705).

This means that the fantasies that are relevant in the seemingly random, bizarre images that occur in a psychedelic session, may contain symbols that are purposeful because they point to the development of the awareness of the inner, spiritual Self. If this is the case, these experiences will be particularly powerful for certain drugs, such as DMT, because the insights come with direct force, less cluttered by complexes so that a change of consciousness is highly likely.

> By and large, it seems to me that structurally they are less complex than the narratives of dreams. Overall, what makes ayahuasca visions impressive is their magnificence, grandeur, supernaturalness, and the psychological and spiritual impact they have on their viewers. Only a relatively small number of the visions in my corpus of data define multi-unit, complex narrational structures. (Shanon, 2003, p. 110)

That which is of sufficient power to overwhelm the ego, as arises in a mystical occurrence, is that which presents some symbolic or intuitive communication of a sense of peace, unity, and interconnectedness as the experience would not exist if not for the emergence of these higher intimations. Accordingly, any visual effects in a psychedelic experience that offer a deeper connection, even if remote, where there is a merging of subject and object, an interconnection with nature, or even another entity, may all be considered direct communications from the Self. These are the images that need to be integrated as they are of the highest order, as Jung explained about images of the Self in a seminar in 1940:

These symbols have always belonged to the images, or at least the attributes, of God. Their becoming conscious has always meant *gnosis*, that is, knowledge of God as the center of human soul life, of which we are already somehow aware; it already coincides with the image of God, and, furthermore the experience of such contents is usually regarded as an experience of God. Such a judgment is not arbitrary, but is naturally based on the numinous character of the experience. (Jung, 2014, pp. 102-103)

In a psychedelic experience, the images and symbols vary greatly depending on the drug, the dosage, as well as the set and setting. There are no agreed clinical or theoretical models as to how to integrate that experience and work with the images after the experience has occurred: "empirical work addressing the sources of integration therapy's impact remains limited" (Earleywine, et al., 2022). This is most likely because there is no line of sight between the principles underlying the set, setting and integration, and, as well, the visuals are so bizarre that they defy historical symbolization. The only possibility for integrating the psychedelic generated images is by a greater congruence with a pre-existent mindset oriented to change, and a setting that has supported that intention, thereby creating a consistent theme that can be assayed in the symbols that are available for integration.

The Reality of the Self for Psychedelics

The Self is the name of a placeholder for that force within us that seeks continued expression. It is called the Atman, the Holy Spirit, divine providence, the God within, God's will, what Ralph Waldo Emerson called the Over-Soul, or what Jorge Luis Borges referred to as the Aleph. It could simply be called evolution or, as neurobiology has found, a centering function in the brainstem (Alcaro et al., 2017). When this is realized, practically, it creates a balance between the conscious mind and Self as the initiator and the doer. This balance is the greatest psychological possibility. The first principle then that can be the consistent basis for the set, setting, and integration is that the Self is behind the experience for one to realize its existence. Accordingly, taking psychedelics is an instrument of the Self that seeks its own realization.

The Self can be exposed in as many ways as there are religious, spiritual, or ritualistic orientations. It is, to be useful for the set and the basis for integration of a psychedelic experience, that which is related to the inner spirit within one, the spirit in others and in nature and their interconnectedness. In Jung's taxonomy of individuation, he refers to the importance of realizing that the inner Self is in all things, bringing that higher sense of unity that is its goal (CW 9ii, § 410). Psychedelic research has not used this orientation directly, but concludes that, for example, DMT decenters the ego (reduction of selfhood), offers non-judgmental processing, cognitive flexibility, emotional regulation, and a new sense of oneself: a sense of connection and openness to experience (Perkins et al., 2023). These are all aspects of the Self, or the realization that there is an aspect of psyche that is seeking higher consciousness for us and itself.

The practice of psychoanalysis has a particular rhythm in which the purposefulness of the unconscious and a trust in that process emerges slowly over time. Although various non-traditional methods can be introduced, such as mindfulness meditation, psychoanalysis is always oriented, directly or indirectly, to the constructive, synthetic idea of working with what points to the Self. Breakthroughs are slow, as the process of the unconscious integrating material that has arrived into consciousness occurs at its own pace. The fundamental first principle that there is a center in one's being that seeks the revelation of the balance between conflicts caused by duality, and that is achieved by its realization, is the work of a lifetime. A mystical experience that offers a direct reception of the unity of all things is the reason that Jung calls them the "real therapy" (Jung, 1974, Vol 1, p. 377).

The conclusion can only be reached that psychedelic usage that is accompanied by a mindset oriented to that inner unity and that then provides symbols that suggest a potential to be integrated, is to be welcomed. The degree to which the analyst working with psychedelics steps outside a traditional role in which transference and counter-transference issues arise, is uncertain. However, that may be unnecessary if the analyst first creates the necessary mindset to any degree and is later available for integration.

References

Alcaro, A., Carta, S., & Panksepp, J. (2017). The affective core of the self: A neuro-archetypical perspective on the foundations of human (and animal) subjectivity. *Frontiers in Psychology, 8* (1424), 1-13.

Aurobindo, Sri (1972). Letters on Yoga – Part two and three. *Sri Aurobindo Birth Centenary Library.* Vol. 23.

Aurobindo, Sri (2014). Letters on Yoga – III: Experiences and realisations in the Integral Yoga. *The Complete Works of Sri Aurobindo.* Vol. 30. Sri Aurobindo Ashram Trust.

Cantù, K. (2020). Don't take any wooden nickels: Western esotericism, yoga, and the discourse of authenticity. In E. Asprim, & J. Strube (eds.). *New approaches to the study of esotericism.* Brill. (pp. 109-126).

Carhart-Harris, R.L., Roseman, L. Haijen, E., Erritzoe, D., Watts, R., Branchi, I. & Kaelen, M. (2018). Psychedelics and the essential importance of context. *Journal of Pharmacology, 33*(7).

Carhart-Harris, R.L., & Friston, K.J. (2019). REBUS and the anarchic brain: Toward a unified model of the brain action of psychedelics. *Pharmacological Reviews, 71*(3), 316–344.

Cwik, A.J. (2010). From frame through holding to container. In M. Stein (ed.). *Jungian Psychoanalysis: Working in the spirit of Carl Jung.* Open Court, Chapter 16.

Earleywhine, M, Low, F., Lau, C. & De Leo, J. (2022). Integration in psychedelic-assisted treatments: Recurring themes in current providers' definitions, challenges, and concerns. *Journal of Humanistic Psychology*, April 2.

Golden, T.L. Magsamen, S., Sandu, C.C., Lin, S., Roebuck, G.M. Shi, K.M., & Barrett, F.S. (2022). Effects of setting on psychedelic experiences, therapies, and outcomes: A rapid scoping review of the literature. In F.S. Barrett, K.H. Preller (Eds.). *Disruptive Psychopharmacology.* Springer. (35-70).

Haijen, E., Kaelen, M., Roseman, L., Timmermann, C. Kettner, H. Russ, S., Nuff, D., Daws. R.E., Hampshire, A.D.G., Lorenz, R., & Carhart-Harris, R.L. (2018). Predicting responses to psychedelics: A prospective study. *Frontiers of Pharmacology, 9,* 897.

Jung, C.G. (2014*). Dream interpretation ancient and modern: Notes from the seminar given in 1936-1941.* J. Peck, L. Jung, M.M. Grass, (Eds.). Philemon Series. Princeton University Press.

Jung, C.G. (2023*). Jung on Ignatius of Loyola's spiritual exercises: Lectures delivered at the ETH Zurich.* M. Liebscher (Ed.). C. Stephens (trans.). Volume 7. Philemon Series. Princeton University Press.

Jung, C.G., & Jaffe, A. (1958) *Protocols to memories, dreams, reflections.* (Forthcoming as S. Shamdasani, Ed. Philemon Series. Princeton University Press).

Kristeva, J. (1989). *Black Sun: Depression and melancholia.* Columbia University Press.

Letheby, C. (2021). Philosophy of Psychedelics. Oxford University Press.

McCulloch, D. E-Wen, Grzywacz, M.Z., Madsen, M.K., Jensen, P.S., Ozenne, B., Armand, S., Knudson, G.M., Fisher, P.M., & Stenbaek, D.S. (2022). Psilocybin-Induced mystical-type experiences are related to persisting positive effects: A quantitative and qualitative report. *Frontiers in Pharamacology, 13.*

Majić, T., Schmidt, T.T., & Gallinat, J. (2015). Peak experiences and the afterglow phenomenon: When and how do therapeutic effects of hallucinogens depend on psychedelic experiences? *Journal of Psychopharmacology, 29*(2), 241-253.

Martin, J.M., & Sterzer, P. (2022). How level is the 'cognitive playing field'? Context shapes alterations in self-conception during the psychedelic experience. *Philosophy and the Mind Sciences, 3.*

Modlin, N.L., Miller, T.M., Rucker, J.J., Kirlic, N., Lennard-Jones, M., Schlosser, D., & Aaronson, S.T. (2023). Optimizing outcomes in psilocybin therapy: Considerations in participant evaluation and preparation. *Journal of Affective Disorders, 326,* 18-25.

Passie, T., Seifert, J., Schneider, U., & Emrich, H.M. (2002). The pharmacology of psilocybin. *Addiction Biology, 7*(4), 357–364.

Peill, J., Trinci, K.E., Kettner, H., Mertens, L.J., Roseman, L, Timmerman, C., Rosas, F.E., Lyons, T., & Carhart-Harris, R.L. (2022). Validation of the psychological insight scale: A new scale to assess psychological insight following a psychedelic experience. *Journal of Pharmacology, 36*(1).

Perkins, D., Schubert, V., Simonová, H., Tófoli, L.F., Bouso, J.C., Horák, M, Galvão-Coelho, N.L., Sarris, J. (2021). Influence of context and setting on the mental health and wellbeing outcomes of Ayahuasca drinkers: results of a large international survey. *Frontiers of Pharmacology, 12,* 623979.

Perkins, D., Ruffell, S.G.D., Day, K., Rubiano, D.P., & Sarris, J. (2023). Psychotherapeutic and neurobiological processes associated with ayahuasca: A proposed model and implications for therapeutic use. *Frontiers of Neuroscience, 16.*

Roseman, L., Haijen, E., Idialu-Ikato, K., Kaelen, M., Watts, R. & Carhart-Harris, R. (2019). Emotional breakthrough and psychedelics: Validation of the emotional breakthrough inventory. *Journal of Pharmacology, 33*(9).

Shanon, B. (2003). *The antipodes of the mind: Charting the phenomenology of ayahuasca experiences*. Oxford University Press.

Stein, L. (2019). *Working with mystical experiences in psychoanalysis: Opening to the numinous.* Routledge.

Watts, R. & Luoma, J. (2020). The use of the psychological flexibility model to support assisted therapy. *Journal of Contextual Behavioural Science, 15,* 92-102.

Winkelman, M.J. (2021). The evolved psychology of set and setting: Influences regarding the roles of shamanism and ethnogenic ecopsychology. *Frontiers in Pharmacology, 12.*

The Setting

Jung's vas Hermeticum
Bion's Container-Contained

Renée Cunningham

Current literature on psychedelic treatment emphasizes that the experience of the *set and setting* strongly determines treatment outcome. The set and setting is defined as the inner and outer conditions involved in the preparation and execution of a psychedelic journey. The security of the environment and sense of wellbeing of the journeyer are essential considerations in undergoing a psychedelic experience (Leary, 1964). The importance of set and setting can be extended into the experience of analysis as well. The inner and outer conditions of the participants play an important role in the couple's capacity to traverse the inner world of the patient's trauma and, through analytic fielding of dreams, imagination, and intuition, rebuild the patient's capacity to self-contain, soothe, and connect with the outer world.

Psychedelic research shows that feelings and memories can be accessed and experienced again where trauma has foreclosed on one's capacity to feel. The upsurge of feelings, emotions, and experiences becomes material ripe for integration in post-psychedelic sessions. However, questions arise around the integrity of the individual's ego, the state of the transference, and the impact of bypassing important alchemical procedures in service of a direct experience of the self. A porous or rigidified ego may have difficulty integrating psychedelically induced material, because it has not been slowly acclimatized to the depths of the unconscious (Hill, 2013). This process is exceedingly delicate and needs the support and trust of an analyst whose capacity to be a container is solid and dependable and whose treatment plan contains specific protocols for containment before, during, and after treatment. The work of Carl Jung and Wilfred Bion can be helpful in the development of protocols for the use of psychedelics because both men have a comprehensive understanding of psychotic states and how to treat and contain them.

According to psychoanalyst Wilfred Bion, *container-contained* represents the unconscious, dynamic urge to seek and find meaning through object relations. This urge begins at birth with the "infant's searching and being found by the mother's breast" (Symington, p. 52). Accessing the unconscious often involves working in liminal states where the couple may dream the patient's life into being by utilizing dreams as a safe harbor for revisiting traumatic experience. Current research supports the notion that working in liminal states with dreams, imagination, and intuition is healing for trauma patients (Kraehenmann, 2017; Zang, 2013, 2015). In infancy, the baby experiences these states through reverie with the mother.

The essential query of this writing revolves around the integrity of a psychedelic psychoanalysis[1] when psychedelically induced images are introduced into the *temenos* from the outside as tincture. To what extent are psychedelics effective in repairing trauma when structurally introduced and maintained in a healthy container-contained environment, and finally, what role do psychedelics play in dreaming the patient's life into being where trauma has created an impasse in a patient's access to the unconscious? In exploring these questions, Jung's *vas Hermeticum* and Bion's container-contained will be explored and discussed while analyzing a psychedelically augmented psychoanalysis with a patient.

Jung's Self and Bion's O

Wilfred Bion and Carl Jung shared a primary interest in the cosmos of psychic life; its creative expression through intuition, dreaming, and imagination, all borne through the temenos of relationship. Jung and Bion both held an intense reverie with the transcendent realm, defined in terms of Jung's concept of the archetypal Self and Bion's idea of O, and their respective relationships to these ideas were important to each. In recent decades, contemporary psychoanalytic schools, particularly relational psychoanalysts such as James Grotstein, Michael Eigen, and Stephen

Mitchell, have been increasingly interested in the transpersonal aspects of the psyche. Here, Winborn (2017) cites Grotstein comparing Bion's and Jung's ideas of the transcendent:

> So I think that with Bion's notions of myths, of transcendence and transformations, and of prenatal, unborn selves, we are hearing someone who was very much influenced by Jung and/or working parallel to him without knowing it … Bion is also one of the very few people in the psychoanalytic field who respects religion, spirituality, the numinous, the ineffable. And that certainly is Jung. (Grotstein in Culbert-Koehn, 1997, p. 16)

Indeed, the cohesion in the depth psychology schools seems to point to an emergent interest in the transpersonal realm of the psyche. Repeatedly, Bion and Jung springboarded into the depths of their understanding of the psyche through the door of the infinite and ineffable Self and O. Essentially, Bion and Jung's ideas of the transcendent refer to a life of meaning beyond the boundaries of an ego-defined life. Throughout his writings, Jung emphasizes that an individual's singular urge is not to get to know one's own ego, but instead, to have a relationship with the divine. Indeed, the urge of the Self is transcendence. When the Self announces its presence through an archetypal experience, it can induce tremendous alterations in the personality and the ego's sense of omnipotence. Jung (1959) states,

> I usually describe the supraordinate personality as the 'self,' thus making a sharp distinction between the ego, which, as is well known, extends only as far as the conscious mind, and the whole of the personality, which includes the unconscious as well as the conscious components. The ego is thus related to the self as part to whole. To that extent the self is supraordinate. Moreover, the self is felt empirically not as a subject but as object. (CW 9i, § 315)

Bion, like Jung, also expounds upon the transcendent aspect of the psyche through his idea of O. Similar to Jung's archetypal Self, O lives in each individual, yet also intersects with a cosmic O. Bion emphasized that O in the consulting room exists within and between each individual (Stephens, 2020); the in-between is a subjectively held experience similar to Jung's archetypal field emerging between and within the analytic couple. Jungian analyst Barbara Stephens Sullivan states:

> The domain of O has been explored by philosophers and mystics under titles like the absolute, ultimate reality or ultimate truth, the ground of being, God or the Godhead. O is the world of Plato's ideal forms, Kant's things-in-themselves, Bion's pre-conceptions, Klein's inborn phantasies and Jung's archetypes. (2020, p. 38)

Like Jung's archetypes, we can sense Bion's O through our feelings (Sullivan, 2020). He refers to emotional and psychological experience as Knowledge (K). Bion emphasizes the idea of experience, or K, and the importance of surrendering preconceived notions in analysis as much as possible to experience O in its truest form (Bion, 1970). It is a highly creative, mysterious process. Here, Stephens expounds upon "domain K":

> The 'domain K' is that aspect of the universe of one's life experience that one can hope to get to know by interacting with it in an open and receptive frame of mind. Here, Bion (1970) is emphasizing that he is not talking about book learning, which will never reveal O. We sense O by sinking into our experience and letting it absorb us until we can intuit the intangible fundamental reality that is making itself known through our lived experience. This will not lead us to know O. What we can hope for is a sense of the leading edge of O as it evolves into material existence. (2020, p. 40)

An increase in K is similar to a newfound awareness that occurs when the ego is defeated by the Self, introducing one to the transcendent aspect of psyche. Depth psychology, psychedelics, religion, and theology all support the desired contact between the human being and the transcendent.

Jung's vas Hermeticum

In Jungian analysis the analyst's office becomes a container, or the alchemical *vas Hermeticum* (the grail cup) which provides the necessary reverie for the soul-making experience being created by the participants. Depth psychotherapy is a form of spiritual communion, a religious culture shaped by the two individuals participating in the ritualistic act of creation. The paradigmatic experience of psychotherapy culls the unnecessary, revealing a universal truth of Self, located at the core of one's being and becoming. In his book, *Dionysus: Myth and Cult,* Walter Otto discusses the concept of analysis, and its power to emotionally and psychologically transform. As a system or variety of worship, analysis, "as a totality belongs to the monumental *creations* of the human spirit" (Otto, 1965, p. 18).

Jung's work on alchemy focused on the act of creation or the revelation of the inner deity through one's devotion to self-awareness. The image of the *vas Hermeticum* is one of a glass container representing the subjective experience created within an individual when encountering the Other. Jung believed that two people hold the mysteries of the universe within the infinite number of experiences that can be made from the union of their psyche. Jung states,

> For two personalities to meet is like mixing two chemical substances: if there is any combination at all both are transformed. In any effective psychological treatment, the doctor is bound to influence the patient; but this influence can only take place if the patient has a reciprocal influence on the doctor. You can exert no influence if you are not susceptible to influence. (CW 16, §163)

The transformation takes place within the unconscious attraction in similarities and differences held deep within the couple's unconscious world. This *participation mystique,* a term initially coined by Lévy-Bruhl (1926) drives the couple, urging them to newer landscapes of development within each other and themselves. Indeed, the unconscious base matter of the psyche, or *prima materia,* becomes enlivened through the *participation mystique,* leading to an unconscious attraction. The couple begins their mutual developmental life through projection (transference) and projective identification (countertransference). This phenomenon, the projection of inner contents onto and into the other, becomes a critical change agent.

The burgeoning field of psychedelic psychoanalysis is designed to augment treatment with a substance that weakens the ego's calcified defenses, thereby introducing the patient to aspects of the Self that exist beyond the ego's impaired field of vision—but within the ego's reach to experience something new. It will be through (Levy-Bruhl, 1910) the fertilization of the relationship that the death states may transmute into a living substance, germinating into a language and image the analytic couple can understand. Within the *vas Hermeticum,* the dismembered parts of the soul relegated to the storehouse of the unconscious may be called back through the relationship with the other, and through *re-membered* suffering, the soul may stand a chance for resurrection. Otto explains the mystery:

> The creative phenomenon must be its witnessed. And its testimony has only one meaning: that the human mind cannot become creative by itself, even under the most favorable circumstances, but that it needs to be touched and inspired by a wonderful Otherness; that the efficacy of this Otherness forms the most important part of the total creative process, no matter how gifted men are thought to be. (1965, p. 26)

The act of creation is born through the imaginal world and the liminal spaces of the psyche that burst through the gates of relationship in imagery and feeling. In trauma, the dream world is impaired, and the dreamer struggles to access solutions that feeling provides, such as the critical capacity for self-reflection. Through dream work, untenable feelings may be approached and metabolized through active imagination. Psychedelic psychoanalysis is designed to augment this process. But Jung disagreed with the use of psychedelics due to the unpredictable and wily nature of the unconscious, and the forces let loose on the ego in a confrontation with the Self: "Generally speaking, the ego is a hard-and-fast complex which, because tied to consciousness and its continuity, cannot easily be altered, and should not be altered unless one wants to bring on pathological disturbances" (CW 8, § 430). Here, Jung warns against disturbances in the ego's capacity to integrate unconscious content. The inner other's emergence then, whether induced through psychedelics or cultivated through the analytic relationship, bears consideration. Bion's theory of container-contained offers another prism of exploration into psychic development through the augmentation by psychedelics.

Bion's Container-Contained

Wilfred Bion emerged from the Kleinian school of psychoanalytic thought. His psychoanalyst was Melanie Klein; his foundational thinking stems from that experience. For Bion, the relationship between mother and infant asserts a primary influence on the child's becoming and an equally destructive erosion in the integrity of the personality when early experiences are foreclosed by trauma and/or maternal deprivation. Bion emphasizes the patient's experience of themselves in the analyst's presence (Bion, 1983). More importantly, Bion's work focuses on the healing potential of the analytic bond. Grotstein explains:

> He aimed to acquaint man with the awesomeness and wonder, rather than the dread, of the effable Otherness within and beyond him and to lead him to respect the truths that constantly evolve from it. Bion's analytic stance is to encourage man to allow himself to become incarnate by his ineffable, infinite reservoir of cosmic being. (2007, p. 52)

Jungian analyst Barbara Stephens Sullivan states,

Bion's theory is revolutionary. It focuses on the ways
the individual fails to *have* his emotional experiences
rather than the ways the person defends against knowing
about them. This theory describes a hypothetical inner
'apparatus' that we must have in order to handle emotional
life, an apparatus that develops throughout the life cycle,
hopefully towards increasing levels of robustness, but
never attains perfect reliability. (2010, p. 68)

The inner apparatus Sullivan refers to sits at the core of Bion's
theory. It is the foundational psychic capacity to hold and contain raw,
inchoate psychic material and transmute this energy through relationship
into a living experience informed by feeling and image. Stephens aptly
describes this apparatus as the 'α (alpha) function:

Raw sensations of life, saturated with unformed
protoemotional energies, assault us at every moment. At
first, these are neuronal impulses traveling to the brain.
How does the mind turn this raw data into something
thinkable and feelable? Bion (1962) calls this fundamental
process 'α (alpha) function,' and I would suggest that it
accomplishes a task that all higher mammals (and perhaps
other creatures, too) must accomplish. (2010, p. 68)

To appreciate the subtle and powerful complexities of Bion's
descriptions of the alpha function and container-contained, it is important
to comprehend the role of the alpha function and its relationship to alpha
elements, β (beta) elements and the contact barrier.

Psychoanalysts Joan and Neville Symington describe psychological development as an unconscious phenomenon whereby outer
and inner experiences find each other and through their union, experience
is born. "The mating of container and contained is how mental growth
occurs at every stage of development" (2004, p. 53). The container
simulates the mother and her ability to physically, emotionally, and

psychologically attend to her baby's needs (contained), and through reverie (holding and containing) or her alpha function, she can dream her infant's becoming (Grotstein, 2007). The potent image here is of the infant's locating and latching onto the mother's breast (Symington, 1996). The reverie that was once defined by an in utero cosmos becomes in the outer world a psychic container born from mother's eyes, arms, skin, and prosody of voice. In reverie, whether it is between outer and inner or through image to experience, the union is a dynamic process of seeking and finding, culling and sorting, as relational sparks begin enlivening the archetypal experience of being.

Reverie is central to the integrity of the alpha function and the maternal capacity for transmuting proto-sensorial and proto-emotional (beta elements) states into alpha elements (emotions) or dream (waking and sleeping) material and psychic nutrients for symbolization. "The primitive matrix from which thoughts develop, the processed and unthought data, are named beta elements" (Symington, 1996, p. 39). Psychic landscapes begin taking shape as beta elements are transmuted. According to Stephens, "Bion's hypothetical alpha function turns beta elements into alpha elements: integrated atoms of sensory emotional experience that have been symbolized and taken in as parts of the person's developing self. These elements can be stored and used by the psyche in any of the psychological activities (like thinking[2], feeling, dreaming, or remembering) that constitute emotional work" (2020, p. 71).

The alpha function can be witnessed in the mother's reverie and ability to psychologically and emotionally hold the frustrating, untenable, negative bits cathected from the infant's overwhelmed psyche. In reverie, a calming, soothing experience indicates that beta elements have penetrated the contact barrier. The image utilized by Bion to express the contact barrier is the nervous system's synapse (Bion, 1962; Lopez-Corvo, 2003; Symington, 1996). Both beta and alpha elements come in contact with this barrier as energy is transmuted. The form of the transmutation (conversion to alpha) depends on the integrity of the alpha function, a reflection of the mother's capacity to contain the infant's inchoate states:

> The contact-barrier is supposed to be located amid the
> conscious and the unconscious, demarking their contact as

well as separation between each other and discrimintating outside from inside realities. It will perform as a kind of permeable membrane whose nature will depend, on how the supply of α-elements is established, and on how they relate with each other. (Lopez-Corvo, 2003, p. 69)

According to Symington: "It is while this membrane is being produced that there is an ongoing correlation of conscious and unconscious elements which, after abstraction, results in comprehension of the emotional experience. It also allows for storage in memory and for repression" (Symington, 1996, p. 65).

Containment provides an environment for the conversion of beta to alpha elements as some psychic bits make their way through the barrier and others fall away. The baby's experience of the mother's containing alpha function provides an environment for the baby who can, through the shaping of a healthy contact barrier, begin breaking ground into the relational world. In essence, the mother's alpha function "absorbs, defuses, transduces, detoxifies—that is 'dreams'—her infant's projections" (Grotstein, 2007, p. 45). It is within the container-contained experience that the relationship with the other emerges and later produces in the infant the ultimate capacity for self-containment and symbolization.

Symington states that the container-contained is an internal-external experience: "The container is *internal*, whereas, holding or the holding environment is external or in the transitional stage between internal and external; the container is non-sensuous, but the holding environment is predominantly sensuous; the container together with the contained is active" (1996, p. 58). Grotstein supplements Bion's idea of the container-contained by considering the internal model (self) that the infant is born with, which becomes activated by the maternal reverie: "While I certainly believe that Bion is correct in his conception (of the container-contained)…I posit that the infant is born with rudimentary [inherited] α-function with which it is prepared to generate pre-lexical communications and to receive prosodic lexical communications from mother" (2007, p. 45). Grotstein echoes Jungian analyst Michael Fordham's model of the Self: that the infant is not born *tabula rasa* but that the Self is born incarnate and unfolds through an ego/Self paradigmatic phenomenological relationship (Fordham, 1956; 1973).

Through the ego's states of de-integration, integration, or disintegration the archetypal world is activated and mediated by the mother. Her capacity to contain the infant's falling apart and re-integrating greatly effects the buoyancy of the baby's developing ego (Fordham, 1973). The mother's emotional acuity informs her level of faith, the strength of her alpha function and her relationship to O. According to Bion, "faith is a state of mind that is receptive to O, the source of what we call reality" (Sullivan, 2020, p. 44). Faith is critical to the couple's navigation of the unknown, for it directly impacts the couple's dreaming and becoming together. The mother's alpha function, in waking and dreaming states continues to process alpha elements, organizing sense impressions. "These elements as they proliferate, may cohere, agglomerate, get sequentially ordered to give the appearance of the narrative, get logically or even geometrically ordered" (Bion, 1962, p. 17). Resonances of the alchemical process of *coniunctio* can be detected here as archetypal patterns constellate and shape the mother/infant relationship, the Self's expression organizing the couple's cosmos.

Psychedelics and the Container-Contained

To discuss Bion's concept of container-contained and the effectiveness of psychedelic psychoanalysis, I will utilize the article entitled *Psychedelic Psychoanalysis: Transformations of the Self,* by psychoanalyst Megan Rundel[3]. Rundel describes a ketamine-supplemented psychoanalysis with a patient named Ari, who she treated for approximately four years. At the age of ten, Ari had suffered the loss of his father, and had very few childhood memories prior to his father's death. Consequently, he had developed dissociative defenses to cope with a childhood of impending death. His mother was equally opaque in the analysis, her ghostly presence palpable. Rundel states: "Ari's mom hovers around the analysis like a phantom, almost as absent as the father. He doesn't remember much about her, good or bad: no comfort, no punishment, no contact…She didn't seem depressed or afflicted; just remote. Ari was on his own…" (2022, p. 471).

Ari was ensnared in the archetypal experience of the dead mother. Any movement towards life was met with a dread of being engulfed by the other. To expose himself to the negative or the unknown was risky at best. His dissociative defenses contributed to the mutual state of emptiness (within the couple), filling the analytic container with dread, shifting Ari's experience of O from awe-inspiring and numinous to an awful dread of the other. Rundel iterates: "Transformations in O can feel turbulent and anxiety-producing, as anchors in normal narrative security and identity are threatened. Bion spoke of "an intense catastrophic emotional explosion, O" (Bion, 1965) that brought about a radical shift in one's sense of knowability and separateness" (Rundel, 2022, p. 476).

Ari's descent into the underworld occurred before his ego could handle such a trauma. Without maternal mediation, archetypal forces engulf the ego leaving it incapable of coping. Splitting ensues, fragmentation and dissociation result and self-integration is thwarted. Rundel describes an ongoing transference-countertransference experience:

> ...[W]e couldn't find life or feeling between us. His relational trauma had locked him in an emotional dissociation that felt impossible to enter. I grappled with questions about how to work with the impasse. For months and years, we tolerated it, spoke to the felt sense of it, and linked it to the absence of both parents. I could feel despair settling in for both of us. (Rundel, 2022, p. 471)

The reported lack of feeling between the couple points to an impairment in the container-contained. The health of the container-contained can be compromised when the container is highly taxed in its capacity to contain psychic content, or when the container is "so rigid that it compresses the contents, rendering them static or even depriving them of their qualities" (Symington, 1996, p. 53). Indeed, Ari's parents had impaired Ari's alpha function. Such an impairment causes a disruption in the "translating of sense impressions or beta-elements into more sophisticated elements, useful in the process of thinking, or creating alpha elements" (Lopez-Corvo, 2003, p. 263). In such circumstances a screen of beta elements is constructed between conscious and unconscious (Lopez-Corvo, 2003). reflecting not just a reversal of (α) function, but "is responsible for a state of confusion similar to dreams, as well as massive projections of beta elements" (p. 203). Indeed, one indication of this occurrence can be experienced in the therapist through projective identification, such as when Rundel describes states of apathy and frustration at not being able to make contact with Ari. She is caught in the throes of Ari's parental interjects "that arrive in the internal world either due to parental projective identification interjected into the self, or to trauma from the real that violates the self, or both" (Bollas, 1999, p. 94).

The stuckness experienced in the field also indicates that the dreaming states accessible in reverie are lacking, making the forging of being through dreaming difficult at best. Here, Bion describes the disconnect Rundel might be experiencing in the transference/countertransference:

> Instead of sense impressions being changed into alpha elements for use in dream thoughts and unconscious waking thinking, the development of the contact barrier is replaced by its destruction. This is effected by the reversal of the alpha function so that the contact barrier and the dream thoughts and unconscious waking thinking, which are the texture of the contact-barrier are turned into alpha elements, divested of all characteristics that separate them from beta-elements and are then projected thus forming the beta screen. (1962, p. 25)

In Jungian terms, the couple exists in *participation mystique,* a state of unconscious identification. Ari has descended into the alchemical state of *nigredo*. In the *nigredo,* nothing is moving; it is the beginning of the alchemical procedure defined by Jung as the "chaos, the *massa confusa,* an inextricable interweaving of the soul with the body, which together formed a dark unity" (CW 14, § 696). It is only through the peeling back of projections that the soul can begin to be freed. According to Jung, "projections can be withdrawn only when they come within the possible scope of consciousness" (CW 14, § 697). However, in a container-contained environment defined by maternal deprivation, consciousness may not come for some time because the soul has yet to be born. The self-egg is still very much in incubation. It will be through renewed feeling states that the unfolding of the self begins.

Rundel and Ari eventually decided on ketamine therapy. They hoped it would help to loosen the grip of the archetypal dead parents, allowing for something new to emerge. Rundel's treatment plan prescribed several pre-ketamine sessions followed by a few low dose sessions "in which we both got a feel for the ketamine and how we could best form a relationship with it in service of his healing" (Rundel, 2022, p. 472). The low dose consults were followed by four high dose sessions, as well as sessions in between for integration of the material. Rundel was present during all of the sessions.

Rundel reports on the results of the initial sessions: "The low-dose sessions were remarkable in themselves; Ari was able to perceive more subtle aspects of his experience than he ordinarily could, and he developed an awareness that there was 'something missing' inside. He could feel the presence of an absence" (Rundel, p. 472). His capacity to notice the subtleties of his absent mother, while becoming aware of an inside emptiness, indicates that Ari has made contact not only with his shadow, but the feelings that are linking up to an existential trauma that must be grieved. New relational ground is being broken as the archetypal experience of the dead mother is emerging in the field. The container-contained, or Rundel's capacity to hold and feed Ari's projective contents allows for a shared intimate experience to take shape, this intimacy providing the *prima materia*, or base matter for dreaming, while giving a name to the previously unknowable and dreaded other. For the couple, this dreaming is critical in repairing the lost reverie with the mother and delivering Ari's world into technicolor.

Ari states that in his first experience, he encounters hospitable and inhospitable life forms, and at one point, gets petrified as he comes upon his father's grave. Critically, Ari does not flee but instead decides to stay and face his fears:

I decided to just stay there and see what happened. Nothing happened, it felt dark and stagnant, oppressive and claustrophobic, and I wanted to find a way out. I found a kind of escape hatch above me, which relieved me, but I realized that I needed to stay a while longer. Then spirits gathered around me in a circle, and I knew they were ancestors...Their presence was comforting. They were there to support me and offer me guidance. (Rundel, p. 475)

Ari's ability to sit with anxiety indicates a shift in his capacity to hold the unknown, an essential discipline in psychological health. His holding and containing of fear during a regressive condition indicate an increase in trust in self and other, serving as a metaphor for a bridging between the ego and the Self. This capacity is supported by neuroscience and the effects of psychedelics on emotions, and in Ari's case, on his relationship to fear (Matte Blanco, 1998a, 1998b; Hill, 2013; Krahenmann, 2017; Rundel, 2022; Strassman, 2001).

Recent research with animals indicates that the use of psychedelics may play a large role in elimination of conditioned fear memories (Krahenmann, 2017; Zhang, 2013; 2015). Not only do psychedelics "enhance associate learning and memory consolidation...it is conceivable that psychedelics might facilitate conditioned fear extinction if the conditioned fear memory is retrieved (e.g., via exposure to the relevant stimuli), and if the psychedelic-experience during and after this fear exposure is modified and re-consolidated by positive, self-protective information within a trustful interpersonal context" (Krahenmann, 2017, p. 1035). Ari's psychedelic encounter with his father, along with the presence of Rundel in a contained, trusting environment confirms the current research. The increase in feeling and trust, and the decrease in fear, allows for a dreaming of Ari's new world. Since dreaming for Bion includes the processing of conscious and unconscious states, the psychedelic sessions serve as dream material for integration.

Ari is liminally altered in a state in which dreams become a mediating safe harbor, where he can tolerate the unknown while allowing the analyst/mother to provide a reverie he has been deprived of in his trauma. In integration sessions, the experience serves as dream material for psychic integration. Psychedelic experience as dream material is affirmed by neuroscientist Rainier Kraehenmann: "Given that both dreams and psychedelics acutely induce characteristic changes in subjective experience, one may hypothesize that therapeutic effects of psychedelics in psychiatric patients may be mediated by the dreamlike experiences of the patients during psychedelic treatment" (2017, p. 1032).

In Jungian psychology, dream work is critical to overall health, and neuroscience affirms this notion. Dreams can revitalize and restore imagination and creativity, encourage self-understanding, and restore feelings once numbed by trauma. According to Kraehenmann: … [D]reaming has the cognitive advantage of facilitating creative insight— the forming of associative elements into new image-based combinations which lead to greater understanding and are useful to solve a problem. This notion is further supported by some data which support the idea that dreaming cognition can be superior to waking cognition in tasks which require cognitive flexibility, formation of new associations, or insight into hidden abstract rules (2017, p. 1034). Indeed, "The broad overlap between dreaming and psychedelic states supports the notion that psychedelics acutely induce dreamlike subjective experiences which may have long-term beneficial effects on psychosocial functioning" (Kraehenmann, p. 1038).

As the ketamine sessions unfolded, Ari could make contact with an existential state of loneliness he carried around in and outside of therapy. Rundel states:

> Ari became intensely aware of his own painful loneliness and tracked it through his daily life, in interactions with friends, coworkers, and especially his mother and sister, and in his somatic sensations. At first this feeling was overwhelming to him; it was frightening, and he worried that he would be forever exiled to solitary confinement. He felt intense energy and pain in his heart and belly, areas where he had always been numb. (2022, p. 476)

Early trauma can impair the infant's capacity to self-soothe, creating a rupture in the psyche-soma relationship. For Ari, the psyche-soma ruptures would play a significant role in his psychedelic journeying and his ability to feel emotions moving through his body, a significant ailment in the dead mother archetype. According to Rundel:

> He felt a quickening of feeling around his heart that was spacious but often painful, a literal experience of heartbreak...for Ari, the change emerged from a previously sealed off world of the death, which also contained his affects and meanings. Each journey took him back to the underworld; he felt a mixture of fear, grief, and expansion with greater depth of emotion that we had accessed in prior work. (2022, p. 477)

Ari's suffering begins to feed the dreams of the life to come. Through his relationship with Rundel, several areas of psyche soma repair are witnessed. Ari's capacity to face his fears and work with his loneliness indicates an increase in what Bion calls *Negative Capability*, the capacity to suffer uncertainty, doubt, ambiguity, and frustration. The *negredo* activates the deep sadness which is finally released up and through the body.

Ari's ego has undergone a *solutio*, the shadow integration allowing for a new appreciation of things. Neuroscientist Lawrence Fishman affirms the neurological and psychoanalytic benefits of ego dissolution from psychedelics: "This process coincides neurobiologically and psychodynamically deactivating defense mechanisms which mitigate the threat of losing the loved object. It also enables the dreamlike imagery, symbols, and metaphor of the primary process, a regression to earlier ways of relating to objects, and feelings of love and connectivity" (2019, p. 53). Rundel also began integrating aspects of her own shadow as she openly admits to finally feeling pent up anger at Ari for his lengthy withholding of affection for her. It is here that an increase of K occurs as the couple begin circumambulating the whole human relationship. The bouyancy of the container-contained reflects the couple's capacity to navigate these truthful, relational waters.

These robust affective states reflect a restoration of Ari's alpha function. Equally, Rundel's alpha function provides a substantial container-contained experience for Ari, as he responded with deep feelings of grief. The *solutio* of grief closed the chasm of the distance between the couple, opening a wellspring of deep feelings previously capped off from trauma. According to Rundel:

> When psychedelic agents are used in a safe, therapeutic setting, the opportunity arises in which to experience a range of effects in a safe and reliable container, so that they can be defended against less and a greater range of emotions can become available This can allow for the repair of old wounds. (2022, p. 478)

Integration sessions are essential in post-psychedelic experiences. The consults serve as metaphors for the great mother and the container-contained where images, feelings, and memories of the psychedelic experience become food for lucid dream work. As dreams are the royal road to the unconscious, "psychedelic states are a true royal road to the unconscious: dreamlike thoughts in which affectively charged, symbolic contents of the primary proces are experienced during wakeful consciousness (Masters and Houston, 1966, p. 235). Utilized as one reality psychedelic states and dreams shape a landscape of psyche which can be plummed for symbolic material, strengthening the causeway between the ego an the self. "It is plausible to assume that the lucid dreaming mindset may enhance core processes of psychotherapy such as self-understanding and psychological insight, and may therefore facilitate psychological change—a prerequisite of symptom reduction and behavioural adaptation" (Kraehenmann, 2017, p. 1038).

Finally, psychedelic therapeutic augmentation sublimates the ego to Self through the transpersonal experience of visits from ancestors. "Through the ketamine work he consulted that circle of ancestors he contacted in his first journey for guidance, and they helped him to share his feeling of isolation with others, including me, which brought them together" (Rundel, 2022, p. 476). The ancestors provide faith and experience of the ineffable O through contact with the archetypal Self. This is a remarkable example of the states of betwixt and between (liminality) that can provide a safe passage for Ari's going on being, finding meaning in his life, and the dreaming of his future.

Rundel's work with Ari is a poignant example of how psychedelic implementation in psychoanalysis can enrich a patient's life, creating an adaptive bridge to overall wellbeing; however, there were also challenges that emerged in conjunction with the Covid-19 pandemic. Enforced separation of pandemic lockdown gave rise to Ari's emotional distancing. During the electronic sessions, Rundel states that Ari experienced "my voice as remote, tiny, flat, vanishing. He was again all alone, sealed off, and even I couldn't reach him" (2022, p. 480). A deep period of mourning ensued, but with an important caveat: Ari could feel and sit in the suffering, which was different than before. Indeed, Rundel reports that she no longer feels invisible to Ari, even though they still "oscillate between times of connection and painful disconnection" (Rundel, 2022, p. 480).

Rundel's work with Ari is impressive, and if the results are long-term, she provides a solid case for the implementation of psychedelics. The unearthing of image and feeling through the ketamine provided rich dream material which restored his faith in the other, while also introducing him to his greater potential. However, it is useful to question the short circuited ascent of Ari from the *negredo* through the use of psychedelics. While sitting in the stuckness held a particular agony for Rundel, it may be important for the patient to hold the stuckness until their ego is ready to transition from the *negredo* on its own. What cost does the ego pay when its organic seeking and finding of the Self is bypassed through the use of medicine? Developing a relationship between the ego and Self is essential to overall health and is a skill set which unfolds over time in the analytic work. Active imagination and dreaming provide the road map. But what might happen when the map is forced by psychedelics instead of arriving organically within the temenos of the work? The answer may lie in the bouyancy of the ego. Michael Fordham believed that the difficulty lies not in whether psychedelic images engage one, or whether one can engage the images in active imagination, but whether one's ego "relates actively to unconscious material that initially emerged without conscious intention or participation, that is a valid integrative process" (Hill, 2013, p. 150).

The capacity to attend to and participate in the unconscious material is an indicator of a healthy ego capable of withstanding the intensity of the engagement of the psychedelic experience (Fordham, 1956). Moreover, the ego that can engage in the unconscious material can access the liminal states required for bridging to the self and dreaming themselves into being. Indeed, Rundel's container, along with Ari's preparedness and symbolic capacity, as well as his attitude towards the engagement of psychedelics, played an important role in the progress made.

The health of one's ego, trust in the analyst and the analytic process, and the capacity to hold suffering fulfills many of the requirements for psychedelic augmentation. Indeed, the bouyancy of the ego sits at the center of one's capacity to withstand the unconscious realm and its tendency to overwhelm the ego during developmental storms. Ongoing research indicates that: chronic instability in character structure; regressive, entrenched negative transferences; and narcissistically inflexible or dependent ego structures are more apt to identify with the darker side of the Self, making psychedelic augmentation dangerous for some patients. It is within the throes of archetypal possession that adaptation is thwarted and psychosis threatens to consume the ego. It will be up to the analyst to determine with great refinement whether the patient's ego is functioning in relationship to the Self, or if the ego is unable to manage the forces of the archetypal world.

References

Bion, W. (1962). *Learning from experience*. Jason Aronson, Inc.

Bion, W. (1965). *Transformations: Change from learning to growth*. Karnac Books.

Bion, W. (1970). *Attention & Interpretation, in Seven Servants Four Works by Wilfred Bion*. Jason & Aronson, Inc.

Bollas, C. (1999). Dead mother, dead child. In G. Kohon (Ed.), *The dead mother: The work of Andre Green*. (pp. 87-108). Routledge.

Culbert-Koehn, J. (1997). Between Bion and Jung: A talk with James Grotstein. *The San Francisco Jung Institute Library Journal, 15*(4) 15-32.

Fischmann, L. (2019). Seeing without self: Discovering new meaning with psychedelic-assisted psychotherpy. *Neuropsychoanalysis, 21*(2), 53-78.

Fordham, M. (1956). Active imagination and imaginative activity. *Journal of Analytical Psychology, 1*(2), 207-208.

Fordham, M. (1973). *Analytical Psychology: A modern science* (pp. 12-38). Karnac Books.

Grotstein, J.S. (2007). *A beam of darkness Wilfred Bion's legacy to psychoanalysis*. Karnac Books.

Hill, S.J. (2013). *Confrontation with the unconscious: Jungian depth psychology and psychedelic experience*. Aeon Books.

Houston, R.E.L.; Masters, J. (1966). *The varieties of psychedelic experience*, Fourth Printing. Holt, Rinehart & Winston.

Kraehenmann, R. (2017). Dreams and psychedelics: Neuropheno-menological comparison and therapeutic implications. *Current Neuropharmacology, 15*, 1032-1042.

Levy-Bruhl, L. (1910). *Les Functions Mentales don Les Societies inferieures,* translated (1926) from French as *How Natives Think*. (No publisher listed).

Lopez-Corvo, R.E. (2003). *The dictionary of the work of W.R. Bion.* Routledge.

Otto, W.F. (1965). *Dionysus.* Indiana University Press.

Rick Strassman, M. (2001). *DMT: The spirit molecule.* Park Street Press.

Rundel, M. (2022). Psychedelic Psychoanalysis: Transformations of the Self. *Psychoanalytic Dialogues, 32*(5), 469-483.

Sullivan, B.S. (2020). *The mystery of analytical work.* Routledge.

Symington, J.A. (1996). *The clinical thinking of Wilfred Bion.* Routledge.

Leary, T., Metzer, R., Alpert, R. (1964). *The psychedelic experience: A manual based on the Tibetan Book of the Dead.* University Books.

Winborn, M. (2017). Bion and Jung: Intersecting vertices. In R. S. Brown (Ed.), *Re-Encountering Jung Analytical Psychology and contemporary psychoanalysis* (pp. 85-111). Routledge.

Zang, G.S. (2015). The role of serotonisn 5-HT2 receptors in memory and cognition. *Front Pharmacology, 6,* 225.

Zhang, A.C. (2013). Stimulation of serotonin 2A receptors facilitates consolidation and extinction of fear memory in C57BL/6J mice. *Neuropharmacology, 64,* 403-413.

Endnotes

[1] Psychedelic Psychoanalysis is a coin termed by psychoanalyst Megan Rundel (2022).
[2] For Bion, thinking was not just the cognitive capacity to process thought, it also included feeling.
[3] I have not treated Rundel's patient, and therefore, it would be inappropriate to analyze him. The skeletal information is utilized to discuss, define and explore the ramifications of psychedelic augmentation in treatment, as well as to imagine what might be happening within the unconscious world of patient. It is with great respect that I appreciate the contributions Rundel's work has made in the pioneering field of psychedelic psychoanalysis.

The Range of the Jungian Frame

John R White

Recent findings in empirical research concerning the potential therapeutic value of psychedelics have led to widespread optimism and considerable interest in the development of psychedelic assisted therapy. In turn, this situation has demanded the development of new ways of imagining psychotherapy in general, and psychoanalysis in particular, so the core values remain intact while introducing psychedelics, which is not a traditional dimension of these disciplines. Running parallel to the aforementioned optimism is a more cautious approach among some mental health professionals, in part born of the concern that classical forms of psychotherapy must change in nature with the introduction of psychedelics, since such practices admit into what was traditionally *talk therapy* something alien to it.

In the following chapter, I consider one aspect of this general problem: the therapeutic environment—or what has become known generally as the *therapeutic frame*—in which psychoanalytic psychotherapy occurs. The therapeutic frame is the system of conditions which make sound psychoanalytic psychotherapy possible, but which conditions often become areas of concern within the therapeutic process. One of the achievements of psychoanalytic research in the past fifty years is that it has recognized the significant role the therapeutic frame can play in therapeutic process, as well as its sometimes looming presence in the unconscious material of patients. The introduction of psychedelics into therapy, or even the willingness to see patients using psychedelics on their own, can pose potential conflicts with the traditional concept of the therapeutic frame.

In the following, I will consider three things. First, I will offer a general description of the therapeutic frame, based primarily on the work of Freudian analyst Robert Langs. Second, I will suggest that that the frame is at times posed in too unyielding a form, one which perhaps confuses the principle of the frame with some definite description of the frame. Finally, I will offer some reflections on changes in the therapeutic frame if psychedelics become considered part of the therapeutic process, and what rationale there might be for such changes.

The Therapeutic Frame

The idea that the practice of psychoanalytic psychotherapy has or should have a specific and clearly delineated therapeutic framework, one which (1) sets conditions mutually acceptable to therapist and patient and that are conducive to sound therapy and (2) is acknowledged and adhered to by both therapist and patient, is nothing new in psychoanalytic traditions. It has been observed since the time of Sigmund Freud that if certain conditions associated with, but in some sense external to, the therapeutic process are not properly set and observed, it can have negative effects on the therapeutic process itself. Consequently, a Jungian psychoanalyst or in fact any analytically oriented therapist is responsible not only for the elements of the therapeutic process but is also obliged to keep the therapeutic process secure from such potentially inhibiting or interrupting circumstances associated with the conditions of therapy. Some decades into the psychoanalytic movement, the recognition of the set of such factors by psychoanalytic practitioners acquired the technical name *therapeutic frame* or simply *the frame*.

The importance of the therapeutic frame came especially into focus in the 1970s and 1980s, largely due to the work of Freudian psychoanalyst, Robert Langs. Langs himself recognized that he neither initiated the idea of the frame nor was the first to recognize its value, tracing his own conception of the frame in principle back to Freud, but textually back to the work of Margaret Little (Langs, 1979; Langs, 1982). Langs's unusually forceful emphasis on the importance of the frame, however, underlines an aspect of psychoanalysis and psychoanalytic psychotherapy that can sometimes be missed or ignored, virtually always to the detriment of both the patient and the therapeutic process. Frequently, therapists will consider therapy to consist only in the lived relationship between therapist and patient, e.g., verbal and other types of communication as well as the interventions on the part of the therapist. Langs's emphasis on the frame was in part a reaction against this view, highlighting that there are often psychologically significant factors emerging in therapy that have less to do with the specifics of the therapeutic relationship and more to do with the reaction of patient or therapist to the general conditions of therapy and the unconscious meanings which they may or may not possess.

The notion of the frame is relatively easy to define, though its elements might be debated (and will be debated below). The therapeutic frame consists of all the factors and conditions necessary to make either therapy in general or successful therapy in particular possible, yet which are not themselves internal to the therapeutic process. For example, setting the fee for therapy is a condition of therapy but is not necessarily internal to a given therapeutic process. Though a condition of therapy, the price of therapy often has further therapeutic and particularly unconscious meaning for both our patients and ourselves, especially in capitalist societies where money often acts not only as economic means of survival but also as symbolic surrogate for significant life values and self-esteem. Consequently, though the setting of the fee is certainly a condition of therapy, the latter may also enter the process at some point, often unconsciously, demonstrating symbolically that the frame is no mere *physical* condition of therapy but is also a *psychologically* important one. Similarly, leaving our patient in as much anonymity as possible is a condition perhaps not of therapy but certainly of sound therapy, and thus is an element of the frame. Indeed, such anonymity often does not come up in therapy at all, in part because it is assumed from the outset. However, if there is a breach in anonymity unexpected by the patient, the therapist will often see just how psychologically important that condition is, by the intense affect this situation arouses.

In Langs's final book on technique (2004), written in the last decade of his long publishing career, he delineated fourteen different factors which he believed belonged to the ideal frame, including the character of one's office (e.g., that it is soundproof and used only by one person), privacy, confidentiality, no note-taking or production of other materials which could be seen by third parties, relative anonymity of the therapist, absence of physical contact, agreed and consistent time, offering of neutral interventions, and others. While Langs did not assume that one could always have an ideal frame, especially in the age of managed care which requires the possibility of third-party access, he did think that one should consistently strive for that ideal.

Underlying Principles

While the above might be sufficient for *describing* the therapeutic frame, it does not penetrate to the deeper issues of *principle* which initiated the concept of the frame in the first place. Stepping back for a moment to look at those principles can help us understand the importance of the therapeutic frame, especially in the case of patients using psychedelics.

Though Langs always considered himself a "classical [Freudian] psychoanalyst," his ideas, especially later in his career, are often closer to Jung than to Freud (White, 2023). I oversimplify here to illustrate a point: whereas Freud tended to see unconscious processes as a product of repression and other conscious defenses and thus always in need of integration by consciousness, Langs and Jung both recognized at least a limited autonomy to aspects of the unconscious psyche (Langs, 2004; Frey-Rohn, 1990). And though Langs's and Jung's theories of the unconscious psyche are quite different, the correlations between these theories in one central area indicate the importance of the frame.

For both Langs and Jung, the sector of the psyche termed *unconscious* is not comprised exclusively of repressed or denied contents or other distorted products of ego defenses, but also includes a center of valid and valuable perception. For Jung, this aspect of the unconscious psyche is symbolized in a number of ways. The most obvious such symbol is the Self, an ideal of balance and wholeness which often communicates itself through unconscious processes and especially dreams. It is also symbolized in Jung's adherence to the soul's teleology, an impulse toward development, expansion, balance, and wholeness internal to the psyche and to psychic experience (Jung, 1948). Furthermore, one of Jung's two concepts of adaptation expresses this power of perception on the part of the unconscious psyche, in that adaptive issues indicate where developments toward expansion and wholeness are demanded of the patient (White, 2023). In other words, written into the nature of the psyche, by Jung's account, are not only denied and repressed contents but also a system of psychic impulses, all of which are designed to aid and instigate movement toward individuation, directed by the Self. An essential part of Jungian psychoanalysis consists in reading from the patient's material where these deeper, impersonal impulses toward individuation might be at work, interpreting to the patient the fundamental truth about their individuation that these communications express (Winborn, 2019; Dieckmann, 1991; White, 2023).

Langs, in contrast, did not have an explicitly teleological conception of the psyche, something which I suggest leads him to underestimate the importance of some of his insights (White, 2023). At the same time, it should be noted that Langs was an avid empiricist, tending to eschew more speculative forms theory about the psyche until the last fifteen years or so of his career when he could no longer avoid such theorizing (Langs, 2004; Langs, 2004a). Langs's own clinical experience throughout his years as a psychoanalyst confirmed the idea that there is more to the unconscious than repressed and denied contents. More than perhaps any other psychoanalyst (Gill, 1984), Langs's conception of clinical work consists largely in listening for derivative communications in sessions, in order to recognize what unconscious contents needed to be brought to consciousness. Through this approach to clinical listening, Langs found that the unconscious derivatives were not as a rule distorted communications, as Freud's theory of contents born of defenses would suggest. Langs instead found these to be typically valid (even if partial) perceptions of reality and the psychological directions in which the patient needed development. Listening for such derivative communications became the primary locus of Langs's analytic style (Langs, 1982; 2004), not because they were distorted but because they contained the insight into what the patient needed.

In his later work, Langs referred to this aspect of the unconscious psyche as a *wisdom system*. He contrasted that unconscious wisdom system with those unconscious contents born of repression or denial by calling the former the *deep* unconscious (Langs, 2004; 2004a). The deep unconscious mind, for Langs, not only validly perceives aspects of the individual psyche and its adaptive relationship to the world but even includes its own ethical system—something which, Langs suggested, is often a cause of ethical conundrums since it is an ethical system somewhat different from our conscious ethics (Langs, 2004; 2004a). But the deep unconscious is, in any case, a source of wisdom and insight and nothing like a cauldron of repressed, denied, or distorted contents. In this respect, though Langs has no correlating concept to Jung's Self in his theory, he evidently experienced the same phenomenon clinically. What is essential in this comparison between Jung and Langs: both considered aspects of the unconscious relatively autonomous from the conscious mind, and both assumed that a substantial part of analytic listening and formulating interventions consisted in understanding the unconscious psyche's point of view on the material given by the patient, precisely because it was *not* distorted.

Though descriptions of the frame, such as that given above, often focus on the negative consequences that occur if one does keep the frame, it must be understood that there is a more central and definitively more positive issue of principle at stake than a set of problems that might occur if the frame is not honored. The conception of the therapeutic frame is neither a mere cautionary tale of actions to be avoided nor is it an end in itself to be kept inviolate because *those are the rules*. The point of the frame is to be at the service of the therapeutic relationship by setting conditions which *encourage worthwhile unconscious communications*, so that the work of analysis can proceed as smoothly and richly as possible.

How does the frame aid this work? By highlighting certain general factors which condition therapy and which are likely places of unconscious meaning and unconscious distress—not only on the part of the patient, I should add, but also on the part of the analyst. Put more succinctly, we can say that most of the factors associated with the frame are such that they tend to invite unconscious acting out on the part of patient, therapist, or both. The importance of the frame, and the primary reason Langs offers a somewhat rigid picture of the frame, is to inhibit those tendencies of acting out, thereby positively encouraging a therapeutic field which *symbolizes* the unconscious processes and correlating distress, rather than *literalizing* the distress by unconscious acting out (Langs, 1982; 2004; Goodheart, 1980).

The importance of these principles which ground the frame should not be lost on us, for at least two reasons. First, the relative value of the therapeutic frame has everything to do with it being a context for talk therapy; it was definitely not designed to be a frame for therapy which was not fundamentally talk therapy or which introduced a factor which falls outside of the mutually adaptive relationship of patient and analyst, such as psychedelics. While one might wonder whether this point also applies to non-psychedelic drugs like SSRIs, the parallel is by no means exact because the latter do not aim at dramatically different sorts of conscious experiences than can count as normal, which are both endemic to psychedelics and a substantial reason why psychedelics might be used clinically. Consequently, if there is a parallel here, it is not one relevant to our concerns.

Second, it does not follow that no dimension of the frame is valuable for working with people using psychedelics therapeutically. I will suggest, to the contrary, that the frame of therapy must be modified to the extent that one aims to work with patients using psychedelics, but that some elements of that frame remain the same. Thus, in our attempts to formulate the frame, we must keep in mind the principle articulated above, namely, that we modify the frame only to the extent that such modification will likely lead to richer unconscious communication, in part through inhibiting likely forms of acting out.

Psychedelics and the Frame

In the following, I will not attempt to give a strict definition of the frame, either in general or in the specific case which includes psychedelic use, but simply offer reflections on how to understand the frame when we are working with patients using psychedelics. This is in part because the relationship between therapy and psychedelic use and how to work with the latter is a still developing issue, and it would be premature to set out anything too definitive. I will also be assuming that the therapeutic ideals we are working with are basically Jungian, e.g., aiming for a richer and more positive relationship to one's unconscious life, expanded adaptive potential due to typological development and making complexes more conscious, wholeness, spiritual openness (e.g., to archetypal experiences), and other standard Jungian goals of treatment.

My reflections are divided into three subsections, the first a question about the existing literature, the second an imagined case where a Jungian analyst is a part of a psychedelic assisted psychotherapy process with their own patient, and the third an imagined case where an analytic patient is using psychedelics on their own. While these do not cover all possible situations where psychoanalytic psychotherapy and psychedelics might cross paths, they should be sufficient for understanding something of how the frame might validly be altered due to the presence of psychedelics within the process.

Recent Research

The outburst of recent research on psychedelics has produced a good deal of optimism about their therapeutic use, and rightly so. Reviews of empirical literature have consistently shown that, in clinical settings which include prior screening of patients regarding their existing mental health and also include clear and followed protocols concerning dosage, the use of MDMA and of classical psychedelics is safe and can be conducive to symptom reduction for psychological conditions ranging over PTSD, end-of-life anxiety and depression, and moderate to severe depression (Garcia-Romeu & Richards, 2018; Barber & Aaronson, 2022). Despite some lingering popular views of psychedelics which characteristically overrate their potential adverse effects (Bender & Hellerstein, 2022), current practices in clinical trials suggest that adverse effects are not due to psychedelics themselves but to improper dosage (as is the case with virtually all forms of drug) and/or inadequate settings (Schlag et al., 2018).

Nonetheless, there are reasons still to be cautious with the use of psychedelics. Though the research around psychedelics is promising, the amount of research is still relatively sparse, due in the USA largely to the difficulties of researching Schedule 1 drugs. Indeed, according to one calculation, "post-1991 published psychedelic literature consists of only fourteen clinical trials, reporting on 315 patients" (Bender & Hellerstein, 2022: 1927), too small an *n* from which to draw definitive conclusions about either safety or clinical usefulness. Furthermore, the research itself has been on highly screened populations and in highly supervised environments, which may tell us very little about how to work with one of our analytic patients using psychedelics on their own. This sparsity of literature is no minor point and demands that we be realistic about what we actually know and do not know about psychedelics.

While this point might seem extrinsic to our discussion of the frame, it is central to our discussion for a number of reasons. First, it is important to keep in mind that psychedelics are in part characterized by the significant shift in consciousness they produce. Ideally, one would hope that the use of psychedelics would accelerate a positive therapeutic process, and the clinical studies mentioned suggest they could do just that. Generally, psychedelics, when taken according to current protocols, seem to decouple patterns of thought and feeling, allowing for some release from old patterns while also encouraging re-integration afterwards (Garcia-Romeu & Richards, 2018; Carhart-Harris et al., 2017). Nonetheless, the relative sparsity of research should be kept in mind. For example, whatever value psychedelics have for resolving mental health issues, the literature does not at all support that they cure these conditions (Bender & Hellerstein, 2022) and we do not yet know, due to the sparsity of literature, what other factors still need to be accounted for when working with patients using psychedelics. In the case of the use of an agent which can have such a large impact on conscious functioning, knowing the range, but also the limits, of the literature is itself an inherent part of the frame, without which the conditions of aiding the patient in this regard are not met.

Second, and following on the previous point, as with most empirical literature concerning mental health issues, the highly positive results are measured by symptom relief. While we naturally want our patients to feel better in some unspecified sense, the relief of symptoms is not always—and usually not—the primary goal of Jungian psychoanalysis. On the contrary, symptoms are often an important portal into unconscious processes, and the process of individuation often includes periods of anxiety and depression that are simply part of the process, which we may not be able to work through if non-analytic practices short circuit that process. Do psychedelics cut that process short? The literature suggests they do not, due to the decoupling mentioned above and the ease of integration of previously unconscious material after the use of psychedelics. However, the literature, though promising, is generally not focusing on the goal of Jungian psychoanalysis, individuation, and thus it is not entirely clear what that literature indicates specifically with respect to analytic process.

Third, as we have seen above, both Jung and Langs in their respective ways affirmed unconscious perception, i.e., that unconscious psychic experience is not purely immanent to the person but transcends the psyche by having points of view not only on the inner psychic reality of the person but also, for example, on the adaptive struggles a person has with the outer world. Furthermore, classical analytic concepts such as projective identification as well as Jung's understanding of the collective unconscious show that it is possible for there to be what we might call unconscious contagion, whereby one experiences in oneself what is actually a content of someone else's psyche (White, 2023). It is in part because of this fact that Langs considered what he termed *neutral* interventions a part of the frame: they are neutral in the sense of being disinterested or, in other words, not trying to persuade or move a patient, but rather offering interpretations which leave the patient in their own autonomy to accept or reject.

Retaining this neutral stance is more important with regard to patients on psychedelics because an individual's state of mind and expectations (*expectancy effects*) greatly affect the experience, including the expectations of others, all the more so due to the intensity of the subjective experiences (Garcia-Romeu & Richards, 2018). Consequently, whatever one thinks of the burgeoning literature on the therapeutic use of psychedelics, it is important that some stance of neutrality is retained in the actual interaction with a patient considering their use, lest one's positive or negative feelings about it also influence the patient's experience. This point also highlights that some of the most researched aspects of psychedelic treatment, the so-called set and setting, are also themselves additional parts of the frame when working with patients on psychedelics. These are at least far less important aspects of the frame with typical talk therapy.

Imagining the Frame in Psychedelic-assisted Therapy

As noted above, the therapeutic frame in its classical form was designed for talk therapy, where the primarily verbal communication between patient and therapist is understood to be the means of healing. Introducing something from outside that range of experience into therapy for the purpose of healing, such as psychedelics, with the substantial change they bring to conscious experience and the "marked changes in perception, emotion, ego function, and thought" (Cohen, 1967), cannot but require some modification of the frame. While Langs considered a firm therapeutic frame to be a more or less an inviolable condition of sound analytic therapy and further considered all the elements of the frame he outlined to be constitutive of the frame, forbidding any essential changes to it, he does not seem to have envisioned a kind of psychedelic assisted therapy as it is envisioned today (though it is. interesting to note that Langs's earliest publications in the late 1960s were in LSD research).

The current design of psychedelic assisted therapy might give us a way to imagine a process that is in one sense outside typical psychoanalytic psychotherapy and its characteristic frame but also at the service of such therapy. While there are certain variations in clinical style, psychedelic assisted psychotherapy is generally divided into three stages: preparation, dosing, and integration. The preparation stage includes meeting with a psychiatrist, who performs an evaluation of the patient for psychedelic psychotherapy and who works with the patient to reduce existing medications. This stage also includes three preparatory therapy sessions, typically with a lead therapist and a co-therapist, which include describing the potential range of experiences under the influence of psychedelics, issues associated with set and setting, and potential ways of navigating challenges that might occur during dosing. During this phase, there is often an emphasis on trusting the process and letting go, so that the patient has as positive an experience as possible, keeping in mind the expectancy effects mentioned above. After the dosing session, there is a further set of meetings with a psychiatrist for post-dosing evaluation, safety assessments, and the like, as well as three more therapy sessions to aid integration of the insights attained (Garcia-Romeu & Richards, 2018; Barber & Aaronson, 2022).

Now there is little doubt that the process I have just described is incoherent with the classical therapeutic frame as articulated within analytic traditions. For example, the elements of relative privacy of the patient are set aside for a process including a number of mental health and medical professionals. Furthermore, the therapy sessions prior to dosing are not specifically analytic in orientation, i.e., they do not thematize unconscious processes, but focus on conscious expectations, biological and psychological possibilities under the influence of psychedelics, as well as directives such as taking a stance of letting go. Certainly, were we to judge this process according to the standard psychoanalytic understanding of the frame, there are so many frame violations here that anything like sound psychotherapy would not be possible. But, of course, the point is that we cannot judge the frame in this case by that standard understanding because this is not talk therapy, but something different.

If we recall the point that the frame is not an end itself but rather something formulated to aid in unconscious communications by inhibiting acting out, it should be clear that the above description actually does conform to the *principle* of the frame, given the nature of psychedelic assisted therapy, even though it does not conform to the specific *form* the frame takes in talk psychotherapy and psychoanalysis. These procedures were formulated so the patient could have the maximal positive psychedelic experience, which must include psychiatric evaluation, understanding the uniquely intense experiences associated with the use of psychedelics, and recognizing dangers associated with this process. Furthermore, the above process emphasizes not only the psychedelic experience but the integration of those experiences, by including post-dosage work with both psychiatrists and therapists. The existing literature suggests that these maximal psychedelic experiences include "phenomenological experiences that...reframe and reorient...the strongly held beliefs which underly [sic] their mental illness" (Barber & Aaronson, 2018, p. 585) as well as "sensory-aesthetic, psychodynamic-autobiographical, cognitive-intellectual, symbolic-archetypal, challenging, and mystical experiences" (Garcia-Romeu & Richards, 2018, 11)—each of which suggests the presence of newly available unconscious material, ripe for interpretation and integration.

It is easy to imagine a situation where a Jungian analyst is a lead therapist in such a process and, potentially, even working with their own patient—though admittedly the principles of such an interaction might still have to be worked through. For example, given the differing processes, would this be experienced by the patient more as a continuation of analytic work or would it be experienced more as a kind of dual relationship? In any case, what should be clear is that, to the extent that the above process is in fact dedicated to the goal of enriching the patient's relationship to their unconscious and at the service of unconscious communication, though incoherent with the letter of therapeutic frame, it is in fact coherent with its spirit. Once the difference between the demands of the frame for psychoanalysis and the demands of the frame for psychedelic assisted therapy are understood, and assuming both patient and analyst recognize that the psychedelic experience should be oriented toward the same goal as their analysis—enriching the relationship to important, unconscious processes by limiting acting out—psychedelic assisted therapy could be used as an auxiliary to Jungian psychoanalysis and work to its benefit.

The kinds of experiences which are reportedly the outcome of the clinical use of psychedelics, such as those listed above, suggest that there is in fact a need for Jungian analysts to be involved in this growing field. This is so because the majority of such experiences appear to render unconscious processes, in both the classical Freudian and the classical Jungian senses, more available for interpretation and integration. What Grof says about LSD, that it "is seen as a catalyst that activates the unconscious processes in a rather unspecific way" (2008, p. 32) seems generally to apply to psychedelics and requires that they be interpreted and integrated by therapists with both an aptitude and a training conducive to working with patients' unconscious processes. Who better than Jungians to work in such a field?

Working with Patients using Psychedelics on their own

A recent survey estimated that there are 32 million lifetime users of psychedelics in the USA alone, though psychedelics are heavily controlled and regulated substances, not only in the USA but throughout the world (Krebs & Johanson, 2013; Pilecki et al., 2021). Some psychedelic substances are inherent to spiritual traditions which have become widely popular beyond their original borders and, furthermore, word has gotten round that psychedelics may have a therapeutic use. Given these factors, it is unlikely that any Jungian analyst working in the Western world will fail to have at least one patient who is actively using psychedelics.

Now this situation poses definite problems for therapists. On the one hand, many patients use psychedelics with the idea that they bring therapeutic benefits. On the other hand, many therapists have resisted involving themselves in psychedelic assisted therapy, due to the fact that all forms of psychedelics other than ketamine (in the USA) were illegal until recently, though the latter is changing in some states and municipalities. The situation of a patient using illegal drugs can certainly pose ethical and legal issues but can also pose problems associated with the therapeutic frame. For example, an analyst might be uncomfortable discovering that a long-term patient has been using psychedelics, due to their being illegal or due to feeling that by working with the patient they be seen as implicitly condoning their use of illegal psychedelics. The analyst may in fact be unsure whether to continue with the patient or refer them out. Or again, a relatively well-informed analyst might understand that the use of psychedelics under controlled clinical settings is certainly safe but have no way to know or to monitor a patient using them on their own or with friends or at a concert, where it can be significantly less safe to use them. In this case, definite frame issues could arise, especially if the patient is not using psychedelics prudently, because something outside of the therapeutic process can inhibit or derail aspects of the therapeutic process and because the analyst might not find it easy to retain the relatively neutral stance mentioned above when it comes to interventions, for fear of being implicated in the patient's psychedelic use.

One possible response to a situation like this is to use what is termed a *harm reduction approach*. On this model, once one knows a patient is using psychedelics, one focuses a part of therapy on assuring that the patient is using in a way that reduces the risk of harm.

> Harm reduction assumes that it is better to provide space
> for clients to be honest about their substance use with
> a therapist who is nonjudgmental and has their best

interests in mind, rather than establishing a situation in which clients need to either terminate therapy or hide their use or lack of commitment to abstinence to avoid judgment or treatment rejection. (Pilecki et al., 2021, p. 4)

In essence, what a harm reduction approach encourages is that a therapist do what the preparatory sessions in the controlled clinical sessions described in the previous section do: point out the risks of using psychedelics (especially outside of controlled clinical sessions), and encourage the patient to do what is in their best interests to limit the likelihood of any actual harm.

An analyst in this situation might, for example, help the patient clarify the reasons for psychedelic use and suggest alternative ways to achieve such goals or educate the patient at least by pointing to certain resources whereby the patient can educate themselves. An analyst would naturally want to encourage a patient on psychedelics to pose medical questions to medical providers, also underlining thereby that the analyst is no substitute for a medical professional in this regard (unless the analyst happens to be a psychiatrist or medical doctor). The analyst can also help the patient with plans of action in case support is needed. Further, one can in principle help the patient to benefit therapeutically by urging them to educate themselves on how best to use psychedelics without likely negative side effects (Pilecki et al., 2021).

It should be emphasized that using a harm reduction approach is by no means without risks for the analyst, ranging over accusations of ethics violations, criminal prosecution, or potential litigation, simply due to the currently heated atmosphere around the use of psychedelics. But providing the analyst neither gives access to psychedelics nor coordinates with underground guides, is consistent in stating that they do not facilitate access to controlled or illegal drugs, obtain adequate training in psychedelics, and understand the strengths and weaknesses of psychedelics, they also reduce their own risks a good deal (Pilecki et al., 2021).

Does this approach in any way violate the ideal therapeutic frame? Only insofar as one is, as in the previous example of controlled clinical trial, focusing not on unconscious processes and their interpretation, but on substantive conscious-level emphases on safety, gaining information, and giving advice, all of which, as a rule, are not considered ideal analytic interventions. However, if one goes beyond harm reduction, as suggested above, and, through psychoeducation, aids the patient to understand not only how to use psychedelics safely but also how best to use them for experiences conducive to unconscious communication and individuation, here too one has perhaps violated the letter of the frame, but retained its spirit. Indeed, treated in this way, the emphasis on harm reduction and the use of psychedelics for enriched relationship to the unconscious is virtually the same as what I termed the principle of the frame: to improve unconscious communications by limited acting out, in this case limiting the kinds of acting out that an imprudent use of psychedelics might bring.

Conclusion

What I have offered here is far from a comprehensive statement of the frame and its function in the case of patients using psychedelics. But that of course was not my goal. My primary goal was to underline two considerations: (1) that the concrete nature of the therapeutic frame in psychoanalysis will necessarily be somewhat different from the nature of a therapeutic frame where psychedelics are involved, either in strict clinical settings or outside them; (2) the fundamental question is not whether the frame in these two cases is the same, but whether the principle underlying the frame, i.e., limiting unconscious acting out in the service of an improved connection to the unconscious and richer unconscious communications, is what determines the nature of the frame in either case. So long as one keeps that principle in mind in designing the frame, such alterations can be clinically justified.

References

Barber, G. & Aaronson, S. (2022). *Current Psychiatry Reports, 24,* 583-590.

Bender, D. & Hellerstein, D.J. (2022). Assessing the risk–benefit profile of classical psychedelics: A clinical review of second-wave psychedelic research. *Psychopharmacology, 239,* 1907-1932.

Carhart-Harris R.L. et al. (2017) Psilocybin for treatment-resistant depression: fMRI-measured brain mechanisms. *Scientific Reports* 7(1):13187.

Cohen, S. (1967). Psychotomimetic agents. *Annual Review of Pharmacology, 7*(1), 301-318.

Dieckmann H. (1991). *Methods in analytical psychology: An introduction.* Chiron Publications.

Frey-Rohn, L. (1990). *From Freud to Jung. A comparative study of the psychology of the unconscious.* Shambhala.

Garcia-Romeu, A. & Richards, W.A. (2018). Current perspectives on psychedelic therapy: use of serotonergic hallucinogens in clinical interventions. *International Review of Psychiatry, 4*(4), 291-316.

Gill, M. (1984). Robert Langs on technique. A critique. In J. Raney, (Ed.) *Listening and Interpretating. The challenge of the work of Robert Langs.* New York: Aronson.

Goodheart, W. (1980). Theory of analytic interaction. *San Francisco Library Jung Institute Journal, 1,* 2-39.

Grof S. (2008). *LSD psychotherapy* (4th ed.). Multidisciplinary Association for Psychedelic Studies.

Krebs, T.S. and Johansen, P.Ø. (2013). Over 30 million psychedelic users in the United States. F1000Research, 2:98.

Langs, R. (1979). *The therapeutic environment.* New York: Jason Aronson.

-    (1982). *Psychotherapy. A basic text.* Jason Aronson.

-    (2004). *Fundamentals of adaptive counseling and psycho-therapy.* Jason Aronson.

-    (2004a). Death anxiety and the emotion-processing mind. *Psychoanalytic Psychology, 21*(1), 31-53.

Pilecki, B. et al. (2021). Ethical and legal issues in psychedelic harm reduction and integration therapy. *Harm Reduction Journal, 18,* 40.

Schlag, A. et al. Adverse effects of psychedelics: From anecdotes and misinformation to systematic science. *Journal of Psychopharmacology, 36*(3) 258–272.

White J.R. (2023). *Adaptation and psychotherapy. Langs and analytical psychology.* Rowman & Littlefield.

Winborn M. (2019). *Interpretation in Jungian analysis. Art and technique.* Routledge.

Integration
in Practice

The Sacred Journey

James A. Fidelibus

"A profound sense of the sacred."

This was the unhesitant response offered by a relatively new analysand when I asked him to describe what was distinctive about his exploration into psychedelic experience. I was specifically wondering how images encountered under the influence of psychedelics might differ from those he encountered in dreams. The difference, he said, was that in the psychedelic experience he felt the presence of a sacred "center of love" that undergirded its eight-hour duration and contextualized all that occurred therein. It formed a loving sense of oneness—an empathy with all that exists—that moved him deeply. He wept, to the extent he knew, for hours.

Gabriel is a young psychiatrist beginning his last year of residency. He has a history of anxiety including episodes of depression and the use and intermittent abuse of drugs and alcohol. The son of a physician-father whom he respects and loves, his acceptance into medical school succeeded as an interest in becoming an effective healer of the psyche began to awaken in him. During his medical training, Gabe underwent more than two years of Freudian analysis—an experience that he found transformative in its own right. He had tried psychedelics recreationally in earlier years and, coming to recognize their therapeutic potential, arranged to have a psychedelic experience in the supportive company of a physician-friend who could serve as an effective guide. Having made important connections with Jung's psychology, when residency training brought him to the university town in which I practice, in conjunction with his psychedelic experiment, he sought out a Jungian analyst for the work of integration.

Gabe saw a connection between the therapeutic use of psychedelics and Jungian psychology that is generally acknowledged. While Jung himself had cautioned against the use of psychedelics in working with the unconscious, field investigators have tended to recognize in psychedelic experience something akin to a "confrontation with the unconscious" that Jung described in *The Red Book* (Harris, 2021). Leading psychedelic researcher Stanislav Groff regards Jung's mythopoetic approach to the psyche as important grounding for the most advanced "transpersonal" stage of psychedelic psychotherapy (2008, p. 227). For his part, Jung was concerned that the use of mescaline, the psychedelic substance familiar to him at the time, would risk acute psychosis by overwhelming the psyche with collective images (Hill, 2019, p. 47). His concerns are worth heeding as there are indeed contraindications and risks to consider. Andrew Huberman (2021), for example, considers psychedelic intervention to be contraindicated if the patient is under the age of 25, has a personal or family history of psychosis, or has been taking antidepressant medications at any time in the previous 30 days. There is also care to be taken with regard to the choice of setting, training of support guides, attitude or intent in approaching the experience, and dosage. All this notwithstanding, however, given their affinity, there can be little doubt as to the relevance and inevitable impact of Jungian thought and practice on the currently reemerging field of psychedelic therapeutics.

A distinctive of the contribution of Jung's psychology is its prospective orientation. There is a movement-toward-novelty that occurs with the integration of archetypal meanings in the development of individual identity. This prompts a reconfiguration of the individual's relationship to the collective as the living repository of culture and tradition. It involves, as Jung put it, "the development of the psychological individual as a being distinct from the general, collective psychology," which, at the same time, "must lead to more intense and broader collective relationships and not to isolation" (CW 6, § 757-758). Such a move takes courage as it can be initially confusing, at times subtle, at other times pronounced, and even occasionally harrowing. Disorientation and risk to one's persona can elicit anxious avoidance or depressive withdrawal that may further complicate the clinical picture.

From a Jungian standpoint, however, baseline symptoms are not simply signs of illness but represent unique individual potentials that yearn to be lived. They are the *prima materia* of personal transformation. Dreams, particularly when understood archetypally, and active imagination are the innovations of classical Jungian praxis that help patients find their unique path and muster *the courage to be*. So, the question that I posed to Gabe at the beginning of our work, in addition to being prompted by genuine intrigue, also betrayed a partial skepticism. Granting, for the sake of argument, that adverse effects could be avoided, what, if anything, would psychedelics add to the adequacy of analytic practice?

"The courage to be," a phrase borrowed from the existentialist theologian Paul Tillich, is used here advisedly. Courage, for Tillich, implies a decision in the face of anxiety and doubt (1952, p. 176). Here is where a therapeutically regulated use of psychedelics may be helpful, and perhaps powerfully so. While a decision for *the courage to be* is implied in all analytic endeavor, it has one's back-to-the-wall, so to speak, once psychedelics are administered. Under the influence of psychedelics, the ego must decide here and now whether or not it will submit itself to what it cannot know. Particularly at higher dosages of psilocybin, there is a decision to either resist or to go with an undefined experience. "I was quite scared," one participant admitted in approaching his psylocibin session:

> I had read a lot of things about "ego death." I almost accepted I was going to die in a way, it was that scary. I felt I was being brave, I had no idea about what was going to happen to me, if I would come out in one piece, where it would take me, how terrifying it would be. I'd read some terrifying experiences, and you are just jumping off. (Watts, 2017, p. 549)

Will the ego decide to cooperate with its own relativization in the face of this larger, incomprehensible reality or not? An affirmative answer requires an embodied decision calling for participation of the total person in an experience that the ego can neither contain nor control. When the uncertainty, fear, and doubt this involves is met with positive resolve, it constitutes, as the theologian would have it, an act of faith.

Making this choice opened Gabe to the core experience of his psychedelic journey. It was an encounter with the *mysterium tremendum et fascinans* (Otto, 1923) in which he sensed losing himself in a merger with *all-that-is*. While this is not necessarily the experience of every psychedelic explorer, in Gabe's case, as in many, it opened up an alternate and numinous realm which can properly be called *mystical*. He entered an existential state of awe as he found himself in the presence of, and one with, what he later identified as the *ground of Being*. He felt embraced by a loving presence that connected him with all that exists and produced in him a profound sense of compassion for all of creation. It was an experience that initially consumed him and then sustained a background presence that supportively held him through the duration of what had become a sacred journey. Now, a year-and-a-half later, it has not entirely left.

The choice point that immediately preceded this experience presented itself as an erotically charged image of four colorfully clad, dancing Latino women. In contrast to the breakdown in subject-object distinctions that had occurred during the state of merger, there was yet a separate sense of *I* when the dancing women at first appeared. Gabe's experience of the dancing women caught him by surprise. The image was unexpected and was very much felt to be *other*. It was an affectively complex image which, while feeling alien, simultaneously drew him in. It presented a choice point that we both understood in Jungian terms as the seductive lure of the anima into the great unknown of the unconscious.

After having encountered the dancing women, then being drawn into the aforesaid state of merger, Gabe next moved into a third phase of the experience, a biographical phase, that was introduced by the appearance of a trickster. This was an unnerving jester figure in its proverbial three-pointed Harlequin cap, seeming both clever and sinister, that brought Gabe to a scene from his childhood. He found himself alone in a bathroom sitting on a potty looking abandoned and confused. Throughout the psychedelic experience, Gabe wore a blindfold and headphones, with ethereal music as background. As the encounter with the traumatized child was unfolding, he instinctively verbalized the experience to his guide. Gabe then heard his guide speak the words, *"Inhabit him."* Gabe entered the child and became one with him. He found himself merged into a real-time experience of sitting on a potty as a young child feeling abandoned, scared, and ashamed.

The child then, in the fourth phase of the journey, morphed into a Native American brave which Gabe and I both understood in Jungian terms as a symbol of the Self. He was lifted by a sense of wholeness that emerged within him. This was an embodied experience in which chthonic-spiritual, earthy-transcendent dichotomies fell away. The experience affirmed his strength and gave him the reassurance that he was okay. Following the psychedelic session, Gabe's identification with this image came back to him on regular occasions and in ways that moderated formerly impulsive or angry reactions.

A Jungian analyst would readily see the four-part organizing framework of Gabe's psychedelic journey as a quaternity, regarded by Jung, of course, to be symbolic of wholeness. Throughout this four-phase journey, Gabe's level of consciousness seemed to fluctuate. A centered orientation that preserved some level of subject-object distinction appeared to trade off with a state-of-merger. This centering was evident in the experience of the dancing women as well as in the experience of the trickster as they were both felt to be *other*. There was a consequent sense of both attraction and repulsion felt toward both these images. In all apprehension, Gabe made a decision to move toward them, a choice that took him into a realm of experience that he could not have anticipated.

The memory of childhood trauma that presented itself was not new. Gabe had recalled the potty-training incident in his former psychoanalytic work. The surfacing of this memory at that time brought a strong emotional response that prompted him to query his parents about what had happened. He learned from his father that there had indeed been concern about developmental delay with regard to potty training. Behavioral techniques were apparently employed to remedy the problem. So, suppositories were inserted by his father, something Gabe found painful, and Gabe was left in a bathroom, unresponded to, isolated and alone, until he succeeded in producing the desired result.

Following the surfacing of this memory in his psychoanalytic treatment, Gabe noticed that his general sense of anxiety had lessened. This was an important outcome given his long-term struggle with anxiety. Later, however, under the influence of psychedelics, Gabe entered the experience again but in a way that was substantially more vivid and direct. With the assistance of psychedelics, Gabe was able to tolerate a reliving of the trauma, not a mere recalling of it, that permitted a fuller processing of the traumatic affects and, in turn, promoted their gradual integration through analytic work. In his book on trauma, Bessel Van der Kolk makes the important point in several places that healing involves the ability to tolerate what were formerly overwhelming affects associated with the original trauma. Among the ways that a capacity for tolerance can be enhanced, he considers the potential use of psychedelics, specifically mentioning MDMA (2014, pp. 223-224). It was psylocibin, instead, that had this kind of effect for Gabe.

From a Jungian perspective, however, developing the capacity to tolerate traumatic affects somewhat understates the work. Individuation requires not only a growing tolerance for difficult affects, but also involves their connection to inner psychic structures or part-personalities that Jung called complexes. Complexes, in Jungian theory, have an archetypal core which carries a feeling tone associated with a group of often suppressed memories and their related conscious fantasies. As suppressed, when the affective energy of a complex heightens, it can temporarily overtake mind and body, autonomously discharging in ways which are quite independent from ego control. "Complexes interfere with the intentions of the will," Jung writes, and they "behave like independent beings" (CW 8, § 253). A large part of the analytic process is integrating these inner parts by developing a more conscious relationship to them.

Grof discovered something similar in his work with psychedelics. COEXs or "condensed experience systems," as he calls them, are "a specific constellation of memories (and associated fantasies) from different life periods of the individual...accompanied by a strong emotional charge." They can "function relatively autonomously," selectively influencing "the subject's perception of himself or herself and of the world, his or her feelings and thoughts, and even somatic processes" (2008, p. 68).

Gabe's experience of his father may be described in terms of COEX or complex formation. His father imago was one of an all-knowing, almost God-like authority, who set the parameters within which Gabe was expected to succeed. Gabe was the inheritor of an intergenerational family tradition in which the men became physicians. This expectation was carried forward by Gabe's father, and the pressure Gabe felt for compliance seemed to trigger a reactivation of suppressed complex-related affects that had surrounded potty-training during early childhood.

Gabe's childhood trauma had involved an abrupt and confusing switch in which a loving and responsive father had suddenly turned tyrant and, to a degree, seemed willing to induce conformity through the infliction of pain. With the pressure he felt to enter medical school, old parental expectations for conformity seemed to resurface. Now, as an adult, the expectations for conformity triggered a passive rebellion. A lack of motivation sabotaged his ability to satisfy admission requirements and resulted in a rejection of his application to medical school. But the failure also shook loose a determination. It ignited a competitively motivated need to prove himself in which he redoubled his efforts and worked hard to pass the qualifying exams. This time it worked; he succeeded in being admitted. Gradually, however, the drive Gabe felt to prove himself yielded to a growing aspiration to become an effective healer of the psyche. It was as though the rebellion he initially felt was a precursor to this new development. The conformity-rebellion polarity in response to parental expectation was transcended as a new vision for his future took hold. We mused that while his father's job as an anesthesiologist was to put people to sleep, Gabe's attraction to psychiatry was, figuratively speaking, to wake people up. Making this distinction was a humored way of recognizing the shift toward an individuated value, which at the same time was not a complete rejection of the collective one. Gabe didn't like everything about medical school. Indeed, medical school itself carried its own collectivized expectations which could at times be triggering and evoke complicated, dissonant affects. Nevertheless, with an initially fragile yet increasingly individuated sense of purpose, Gabe's motivation for admission and ultimate success in medical school was sustained.

The time of Gabe's entry into medical school, however, signifi-cantly preceded the time of his psychedelic experience. One wonders, then, how any possible case could be made for the psychedelic journey to have impacted events that preceded it. The time difference, however, may actually help to put the utility of psychedelics in perspective. Grof describes LSD, psilocybin, and mescaline, what he calls the "classical psychedelics," as "nonspecific catalysts and amplifiers of the psyche" (2008, p. 11). They "do not have any specific pharmacological effects," meaning that they do not induce experience by their chemical action on the brain. Rather, "they increase the energetic niveau in the psyche and the body which leads to manifestation of otherwise latent psychological processes" (2008, p. 11). In other words, it is a dynamic inherent to the psyche itself that produces the healing experience—one that is catalyzed by psychedelics, not created by them.

What was catalyzed in the third phase of Gabe's psychedelic journey was a direct experience of past trauma that allowed it to be fully entered and processed in a way that it had never been. It was a centered experience, although seemingly not centered on the ego typified as the center of consciousness. Rather, it became situated in a larger and broader, perhaps transcendent reality, that gave it new meaning. This meaning included its transitional nature as it served to move Gabe from the confusion and shame of childhood trauma into the strength and confidence symbolized by the Native American brave. The injury, as it were, was the precursor of a novel development. This development was a newfound experience of inner strength. It was, to be sure, an existing potential of Gabe's inner psychic reality that, with the assistance of psychedelics, became an actual experience that could be integrated in our work together. With access to this part of himself, as the process of analysis unfolded, there was a new context for revisiting the traumatic past in a way that permitted integration of what had previously remained fragmentary and devoid of meaning. Psychedelic experience, while by no means the only way, may be a particularly potent way of facilitating this kind of retroactive healing. Old experiences can be reinterpreted and re-narrated in the light of a new personal vision that opens up the flow of healing energy.

But something began to bother me when a couple of the dreams Gabe reported strongly suggested the presence of an inner struggle with the feminine. In the initial phase of his psychedelic journey, when Gabe first described encountering the dancing Latino women, we regarded the figures as the contrasexual anima—the gateway to the unconscious in the male psyche—and moved on. Gabe had moved through the image of the dancing women in his psychedelic journey quite easily—perhaps too easily. Did the use of psychedelics permit him to bypass a struggle that then showed up in his dreams?

Gabe dreamt that he was at a gathering in which he met a young woman who, in life, had been a platonic friend during his college days. In the dream she showed an erotic interest in Gabe and wanted to be with him physically. The public setting, however, made Gabe feel uncomfortable. But the young woman did not want privacy; she wanted to kiss him, even in public—something from which Gabe recoiled. In the next dream, Gabe found his car stuck in a deep pit inside the Roman Coliseum. There he saw a young woman, a perfect-looking, glowing blonde. Her home was also at the bottom of the Coliseum where he found her in a golden bathtub. She invited him to join her. As he was drawn to do so, the young woman's boyfriend entered the scene and Gabe became immobilized with guilt. Both dreams suggested difficulty connecting to the feminine. The former depicts the difficulty in relation to the persona where the public setting evokes resistance to an erotic connection. The latter relates to archaic, perhaps ancestral shadow material. Gabe was immobilized as awkwardness and a shadowy sense of guilt stepped between him and his erotic interests. In both cases, the path toward integration was blocked.

Significantly, these two dreams form a unit that was bookended by two additional dreams that gave them context. The immediately preceding dream had Gabe at a wedding in which the wedding party, of which he was a part, was split-off, located in a balcony above a larger group of people gathered in the common space below. This splitting seemed to take on the more specific sense of splitting-from-the-feminine in the two dreams that followed. Then, in the concluding dream, Gabe found himself in a desolate, lifeless boarder zone between Ukraine and Russia where a catastrophic nuclear explosion left only a single structure standing: a tower that was emitting smoke. Sensing danger, Gabe hopped a train for the airport only to find all flights cancelled. An exorbitant fare precluded the train as a further option for escape.

A detailed consideration of the dreams aside, their sequence shows a progression of meaning. The splitting evident in the first dream might be explicated by the two dreams that follow as a dissociation from feminine energy due to persona and shadow resistances. The final dream, with its imagery of a bombed-out, barren field, carries a sense of desolation and imminent danger as well as an urge to escape but with no escape being possible. It seems that this final dream in the sequence was cornering Gabe into facing something he found threatening.

I well recall the session in which we worked on the last of these four dreams. It was unsettling for both of us. We grappled with the dream imagery in a way that failed to satisfy the desire for a coherent understanding. As time ran out, we were left hanging. I ended the session feeling anxious and disoriented telling Gabe that we would pick up the discussion next time. When the next time arrived, Gabe showed up angry. Who did Jung think he was to be dabbling in the unconscious? Before the end of the hour, however, we both recognized that Gabe was diverting anger toward Jung that he mostly felt toward me. He was tortured by what had come up for him in the intervening time and questioned if I knew what I was doing.

In the evening following the prior session, a new and disturbing childhood memory had broken into awareness in which Gabe and a friend had been plucking the feathers out of a caged bird as it was crouching away from them to protect itself. Seeing this, the friend's mother looked horrified—a reaction that registered poignantly with Gabe. Now as a budding psychiatrist, looking back, Gabe thought that he would likely have diagnosed this kind of behavior in someone else as psychopathic. But this was not someone else, it was him! Shaken by the memory, he tossed and turned sleeplessly that night for what seemed like hours. Then yet another memory hit him in which, as a child in daycare, he had pulled the diaper out of the pants of a young autistic girl—as though he was acting out anger related to his own presumed developmental delay in projection. These combined recollections brought up shadow material that was almost too intense for Gabe to face. I thoughtlessly tried to reassure him that he was not a psychopath. Then, recognizing my reaction as an enactment of the primitive rescuer in me (Schore, 2012, p. 159), I attempted to reenter the experience with Gabe more reflectively.

We picked up on the smoking tower in Gabe's last dream, the analogous towering figure in his life, of course, being his physician-father. Gabe associated the image of the smoking tower in his dream to a similar tower-image in Tolkein's *Lord of the Rings*. The connection was painful. Was his father to be associated with the resident evil of the tower's Dark Lord Sauron? Gabe loves his father dearly, so the implication that his father was in any way evil was intolerable to him. Yet, the best of men are not without their own shadow sides, and the dream could reasonably be taken to suggest that this was an element within his father's character with which Gabe needed to square. Beyond this, however, the tower stood as the sole structure remaining in a bombed-out field—the image of a field under more typical circumstances being associated with life and fecundity.

Gabe had formed a sense of connection to his father that was lacking in relation to his mother. While he both loved and felt love from his mother, he also experienced her as an unstable emotional presence. Her labile emotional displays, which could run the gamut from tears to flying-off-the-handle, often left Gabe confused. He wondered, at times, how his father managed to stand steady amidst the chaos surrounding him. The mother-son relationship also lacked softness and warmth. In ways, it was not the fertile field in which emotionally secure attachments could grow and flourish. So, while Gabe could identify with his father, his mother complex involved an inner distrust of his own psychic makeup. Through the experience of his mother, Gabe had unconsciously become dissociated from the qualities he perceived in her that defined the feminine within him. Taken prospectively, the seductive dream images were inviting Gabe to form a new connection to these inner parts.

As of this writing, recovering and affirming these parts of himself is the direction of Gabe's ongoing analysis. In the process it has become apparent that Gabe's difficulty relating to himself has something to do with his familial past. His maternal grandfather had cheated on his grandmother, which created an emotionally damaging childhood environment for his mother. Was this something he inherited? An indiscretion had occurred under the influence of alcohol in Gabe's dating days—something that at the time deeply hurt the woman he was dating and about whom he genuinely cared. He was tortured wondering about who else he might have hurt, without recollection, while under the influence. Recognizing in this the evidence of a conscience and a genuine caring, and as he began to see his mother's erratic behavior in light of her own early life wounding, he found forgiveness for his mother as well as himself. Some of the inner feminine was reclaimed.

Our relationship itself, with its transference and counter-transference dynamics, has folded into the process of healing. As we entered what I consider the crisis in our relationship with Gabe questioning my competence, being the same age as Gabe's father and recognizing a version of the father-figure I likely represented, I was able to receive a criticism from Gabe in a way that he had probably not previously experienced, at least not with his actual father. As we reflected on it together, how could he not feel doubts and mistrust toward me given the sensitive and difficult issues we were moving into? At times, one needs to test the bridge one is walking across to have the courage to take the next step. A mutual reaffirmation has since contributed to a deepening of trust and warmth in our relationship, and it seems likely that, to the extent we have been able to work through transference-countertransference enactments, a deconstruction of the infallible father in the context of our relationship has served to further Gabe's healing.

The overall claim being made here, however, is that Gabe's ability to move into and through his work with the complex material and relational dynamics just described pivoted on an experience of the numinous that was catalyzed by the use of psilocybin. His encounter with the numinous provided a new context within which he could reframe the emotional wounds of his childhood and put them in a new perspective. With numinous experience, "The sense of enlargement of life may be so uplifting," writes William James,

> ...that personal motives and inhibitions, commonly omnipotent, become too insignificant for notice, and new reaches of patience and fortitude open out. Fears and anxieties go, and blissful equanimity takes their place. Come heaven, come hell, it makes no difference now! (1991, p. 217)

With a broadened and deepened awareness of his connection to what he identified as the *ground of Being*, all the particular events and experiences of life, including the shortcomings of his parents, as well as his own, were viewed in a new light. Gabe saw his parents, along with the rest of humanity, in their frailty and began to account for the ways that he had been hurt by them with respect to their own wounding in life. Particularly in reference to his mother, Gabe discovered his heart shifting toward an acceptance that prompted forgiveness as a new narrative began to form around the possible ways in which she herself may have been emotionally damaged. Gabe also moved toward reconciliation with himself, accepting a part of him that he feared was unstable, impulsive, or even psychopathic. He felt an inward prompting to say to himself, *I can love this part too.*

But a question remains: in mystical experience, psychedelic or otherwise, who or what does the experiencing? It would seem not to be the ego. According to Jung, the ego is to be understood as, "the complex factor to which all conscious contents are related" since "no content can be conscious unless it is represented to a subject" (CW 9ii, § 1). But what about mystical experiences in which there is not a separable subject, but subject-and-object are merged as one? Who or what then does the experiencing?

The Christian mystic Meister Eckhardt wrote of a reconciliation of opposites by discovering God within the dynamism of his soul (CW 6, § 418). Finding his soul was also Jung's preoccupation in *The Red Book* (2009, p. 127). Escaping precise definition, Jungian analyst Donald Kalsched sees the soul as "a certain essential something that links us through love to the divine, to each other, and to the exquisite beauties of the natural and cultural world" (2013, p. 10). This emphasis on linkages or interrelatedness, including that to the divine, leans toward the view of mathematician-philosopher Alfred North Whitehead. As represented by interdisciplinary researcher Matthew Segall, Whitehead views "soul" as the "correspondence between the World-Soul and the varying grades of finite souls, including humans, that affirms the co-creative role of every organism no matter how seemingly insignificant...." It is nothing static, but "the process of erotic evocation of intensities...whereby egoistic aims are sublimated by their inclusion in a greater whole, a 'Supreme

Adventure'" (Segall, 2021, p. 157-158). Soul, accordingly, is part of all existing entities, and all are united to a cosmic or World-Soul. There is no subject-object distinction in this kind of experience but an interrelated oneness with *all-that-is*.

Such experience exceeds the capacities of the ego but does not exclude it. In an analogized if not literal sense, a human being may be thought of as a "walking wave function" (Wendt, 2015, p. 37), that is, as existing in a field of potentialities whose actualization involves something like quantum indeterminacy. As, in quantum mechanics, an act of observation participates in the collapse from wave into particle, so the role of the observing ego contributes to what is brought into the actuality of conscious experience out of a pleroma of potentialities. This relativized role of the ego is cultivated in the work of integrative psychotherapy. In the wake of a psychedelic experience, the ego reenters its role as center of consciousness relativized to a larger reality. Emeritus professor of philosophy and psychedelic explorer Christopher Bache comments that, "The more successfully we have integrated our psychedelic experiences into our conscious awareness [i.e., ego consciousness], the 'closer' and more familiar our shamanic self [or, perhaps, soul] will feel to our ordinary sense of self" (2019, pp. 314-315).

For Gabe, the experience of the numinous assisted by psilocybin provided an opening through which he was able to move through his traumatization as a child into strength. As the ego regained its center in the days, weeks, and months following, he noticed a less competitive mindset, greater compassion, a sense of forgiveness, and a numinous oneness with other beings, whether plant, animal, insect, or human. Not all struggles, of course, are over. Rather, the ego seems to be in ongoing connection to a larger, transcendent reality.

One might legitimately ask if Gabe's experience of healing could have happened without the assistance of psychedelics. The answer, it seems to me, can only be in the affirmative. Did the assistance of psychedelics, however, add something—perhaps something powerful—in turning a potentiality into a realized actuality? This also would be difficult to deny. An experience of the numinous may be a birthright that materialist values have stolen from us. While there are many paths that can be taken to the numinous, the use of psychedelics is one path that may be available to those of us who are not, and may never be, among the spiritual masters.

In 1945, Jung wrote to a colleague that,

> ...[T]he main interest of my work is not concerned with the treatment of neuroses but rather with the approach to the numinous. ...the fact is that the approach to the numinous is the real therapy and inasmuch as you attain to the numinous experiences you are released from the curse of pathology. (1973, p. 377)

What may account for the sustenance of this optimized ego-Self relation is that, according to philosopher of mind Peter Sjostedt-Hughes, psychedelic experiences "have a tendency to shift metaphysical beliefs" (2023, p. 6). The ego then becomes oriented to an ultimate reality in a way that helps to preserve what was encountered in the psychedelic journey. This tendency, in the philosopher's opinion, "...implicitly suggests that more focus needs to be placed on metaphysics in psychedelic-assisted psychotherapy" (Sjostedt-Hughes, 2023, p. 6).

There indeed was a metaphysical shift in Gabe's worldview through the course of his integrative work. When I first mentioned Whitehead to Gabe, as is the case for too many, the name was unfamiliar. Gabe had previously felt drawn to the new atheism popularized through the books of Sam Harris. Synchronistically, however, as we wrestled with some of Whitehead's metaphysical concepts, including a concept of God, Gabe shifted out of his initial skepticism when he independently began reading *The Matter with Things,* the neuroscience trilogy written by psychiatrist-philosopher Iain McGilcrist, where references to Whitehead occur 149 times. It was in particular the panpsychist implications of Whitehead's thought that was helpful to Gabe.

What is panpsychism? Psychedelic experience is often reported to be more vivid and real than the experiences of normal consciousness. This despite the fact that seemingly bizarre things can happen: trees may breathe, for example, or plants speak. If the classical psychedelics are not the creators but the catalysts of experience, then the experiences they catalyze may not merely be hallucinatory but amplifications of a reality beyond the capacity of normal sensate ability. In psychedelic experience, in other words, there seems to be access to the deep interiority of things. This kind of experience can be accounted for in Whitehead's panpsychist perspective in which soul is a part of every self-organizing entity (Moore, 2023). This is not a radical idealism in which all experience can ultimately be reduced to mental states. It is grounded in a realism by which mental and physical poles become co-constituents of all self-organizing entities: from the electron to the molecule, to the cell, and to their nexus in plants, animals, and humans, with God as the ultimate actuality. While human consciousness is in a relatively sophisticated place along this continuum, consciousness, at least in some primitive form, reaches all the way down to the simplest and most basic entities. In some basic sense, then, even an electron is sentient.

Jung and Wolfgang Pauli were onto a version of this in proposing what they called the "psychoid": a fundamental level of reality in which mental and physical poles are indistinguishable. Jung writes,

> Since psyche and matter are contained in one and the same world, and moreover are in continuous contact with one another and ultimately rest on irrepresentable, transcendental factors, it is not only possible but fairly probable, even, that psyche and matter are two different aspects of one and the same thing. (CW 8, § 418)

In place of Jung's reference to "thing," a Whiteheadian view would substitute the word *process*. Process, in Whitehead's system, is the ultimate metaphysic of nature. It is not a substance, not a type of monism, but a *concrescence* or a growing-together of the interrelatedness of all entities which derive physicality from their objective, intergenerational past, and mentality from the potentialities of an indeterminate future. Both are co-constituents of each and every occasion of actuality no matter how simple or complex. This constitutes the *unus mundus* of which Jung spoke and with which we merge in numinous experience. Numinosity, or merger with the sacred, is the merger of consciousness, itself a process, with a universal process in which we, along with all entities, are one.

Jung was often on the defense and at times in denial when it came to the metaphysical implications of his work. Yet, there is evidence that *experiential metaphysics*, as part of a psychedelic assisted approach, contributes to positive therapeutic outcomes. "Experiential metaphysics" refers to experiences such as:

> Transcendence of Time and Space (loss of usual sense of time or of space), Positive Mood (joy, love, peace, or blessedness), Sense of Sacredness, Unity (Internal and External), Transiency of Unity, Objectivity, or Reality (insights into being and existence in general). (Sjostedt-Hughes, 2023, p. 12)

Relating his experience to Whitehead's notion of panpsychism provided Gabe with a mental framework that affirmed the reality of his mystical experience. Gabe lost time in an encounter with the *ground of Being* which overwhelmed him with a sense of love for the universe and all in it. It was a profoundly sacred experience in which he was one with *all-that-is*. To him, it was no delusion. "We're all really in this together," he told me, "plants, animals, insects, humans—we're all one." It is an experience he now returns to on a daily basis for grounding, and from which he continues to draw inspiration and meaning.

References

Bache, C.M. (2019). *LSD and the mind of the universe: Diamonds from heaven.* Park Street Press.

Grof, S. (2008). *LSD psychotherapy.* Santa Cruz CA: Multidisciplinary Association for Psychedelic Studies.

Harris, J. (2021). Psychedelic-assisted psychotherapy and Carl Jung's Red Book. *JAMA Psychiatry, 78*(8), 815.

Hill, S. (2019). *Confrontation with the unconscious: Jungian depth psychology and psychedelic experience.* Aeon Books.

Huberman, A. (Host). (2021-present). *How psilocybin can rewire our brain, its therapeutic benefits and its risks.* [Huberman Lab]. Apple Podcasts. https://podcasts.apple.com/us/podcast/how-psilocybin-can-rewire-our-brain-its-therapeutic/id1545953110?i=1000612139039 (Last accessed 23 May, 2023).

James, W. (1991). *The varieties of religious experience.* Triumph. (Original work published 1902).

Jung, C.G. (1973). *C.G. Jung letters, Vol. 1.* (Selected and edited by G. Adler and A. Jaffé). Princeton University Press.

Kalsched, D. (2013). *Trauma and the soul.* Routledge.

Moore, J. (Host). (2023 Jan.-present). *Matthew Segall, Ph.D.–Whitehead, process philosophy, and ecology.* [Psychedelics Today]. Apple Podcasts. https://psychedelicstoday.com/2018/04/10/matthew-segall-whitehead/ (Last accessed 8 July, 2023).

Otto, R. (1923). *The idea of the holy.* Oxford University Press.

Schore, A. (2012). *The science and art of psychotherapy.* W. W. Norton & Co.

Segall, M.D. (2021). *Physics of the world-soul: Whitehead's adventure in cosmology.* SacraSage Press.

Sjostedt-Hughes, P. (2023). On the need for metaphysics in psychedelic therapy and research. *Frontiers in Psychology, 14*:1128589.

Tillich, P. (1952). *The courage to be.* Yale University Press.

Van der Kolk, B. (2014). *The body keeps the score.* Viking Penguin.

Watts, R., Day, C., Krzanowski, J., Nutt, D., Carhart-Harris, R. (2017). Patients accounts of increased connectedness and acceptance after psilocybin for treatment-resistant depression. *Journal of Humanistic Psychology, 57*(5), 520-564.

Wendt, A. (2015). *Quantum mind and social science: Unifying physical and social ontology.* Cambridge University Press.

Active Imagination in Psychedelic-Assisted Psychotherapy: Building Bridges to the Self

Felicia Matto-Shepard

So long as religion is only faith and outward form, and the religious function is not experienced in our own souls, nothing of any importance can happen ... The man who does not know this from his own experience may be a most learned theologian, but he has no idea of religion. ...

(Jung, CW 12, §13)

Analytical psychology embraces paradox, the uncanny, and the numinous. Seeking contact with this mysterious reality is often necessary, even instinctual, on the path of individuation. This chapter considers how psychedelic assisted psychotherapy can support this process by opening portals of connection between the known and unconscious, between the rational and irrational realities, between inner defenses and the original wound. When paired with active imagination and supported by a skillful guide who is "not afraid to tread the darkest paths of neurotic fantasy" (Healy, 2017 p. 21), psychedelic assisted therapies can potentially help seekers build a bridge between worlds where aspects from the unconscious can be engaged, metabolized, and integrated—with the risk of being overwhelmed by a torrent of unconscious material reduced.

Many people are interested in psychedelic assisted therapies for the media-hyped silver bullet effect that promises to cure their ills. But almost as often, I find a patient's interest is born of a religious attitude—a longing to bind themselves to something greater, to experience something that is perceived as real but not fully known, just as the ego reaches for the Self: *I want to know my true, essential self. I want to see God. I want to connect to the universal web of life.* Behind common presenting issues such as depression, relational conflicts, and trauma, I witness an almost universal longing to know one belongs to something larger than oneself. Many never identify this as a desire for *the spiritual*, but they speak of a yearning to know their life has a deeper meaning or is part of something more than this manifest reality. Helen Marlo contextualizes this longing when she writes, "The instinct to seek the numinous is basic to humanity and should be considered natural" (2022, p. 47).

Patients are not the only ones interested in the spiritual nature of psychedelics. Evidence-based psychedelic researchers are demonstrating a respect for the spiritual psyche. Science and spirituality intersect, even collaborate, in the realm of psychedelic assisted psychotherapy. Johns Hopkins University studies the use of psilocybin to treat end-of-life anxiety. Outcomes demonstrate a correlation between having mystical-type experiences and successful treatment outcomes (Griffiths et al., 2011). Relatedly, the Multidisciplinary Association for Psychedelic Studies (MAPS), which conducts research in the use of MDMA to treat PTSD and other mental health issues, directs study participants toward a concept they call "inner healing intelligence," which is not unlike soul (Carlin, 2021, p. 151). It is a subjective experience of inner knowing, beyond the therapist's expertise, beyond the patient's ordinary cognition, identity, or self-knowledge. Patients are directed to listen *internally* for this guidance as it comes from the depths of the psyche. In these ways, spiritual experiences and the religious attitude are recognized as intrinsic to psychological healing. Like Jung, who persevered to prove the reality of the unconscious and its numinosity, many psychedelic researchers aim to demonstrate that a spiritual attitude and subjective numinous experiences are healing (Griffiths et al., 2011).

I trained in analytical psychology because it is one of the few psychologies that recognizes a real and autonomous psyche that extends beyond the personal conscious and unconscious. Engaging with this wide field is considered essential to psychoanalysis and individuation. As Jung wrote, "The approach to the numinous is the real therapy and in as much as you attain to the numinous experience you are released from the curse of pathology" (1973, p. 377). Similarly, psychedelic substances have been used for thousands of years in religious and spiritual healing. Today analytical psychology can play a vital role in the Western medicalized psychedelic movement by supporting the spiritual longing that seems embedded within it. I propose that, specifically, Jung's active imagination is a practice par excellence that can be used both during a psychedelic assisted psychotherapy session, as well as in the integrative process following. Active imagination connects ego awareness and the latent unmanifest self, where the veil is thin and an experience of the mystery can foster the path of individuation (Raff, 2000, p. 9). Additionally, I will demonstrate how I am expanding on the practice of active imagination by utilizing my experience in non-ordinary psychedelic states to collaborate with others within an active imagination.

Jung and Psychedelics

Jung frequently referenced the spiritual and autonomous nature of the psyche but wrote very little about the use of psychedelics. The few comments he made were cautionary. In the 1950s when Western researchers were experimenting with the potential healing uses of psychedelic medicine, he expressed concern that people would be flooded by unconscious material without knowing how to maintain a foot in the conscious ego, which he considered critical for psychological stability.

> I am profoundly mistrustful of the "pure gifts of the Gods." [psychedelics] … If you are too unconscious it is a great relief to know a bit of the collective unconscious. But it soon becomes dangerous to know more, because one does not learn at the same time how to balance it through a conscious equivalent. … (Jung, 1976, p. 173)

Jung's own confrontation with the unconscious gave him a first-hand experience of the immense disorganizing power of unbidden archetypal energies. Unfamiliar and terrifying images broke through from the unconscious and flooded his ego with emotion-filled symbolic material. He feared he was plummeting into psychosis like his patients

(Jung, 1977, pp. 233-244). Relatedly, early observations of subjects under the influence of LSD suggested that it might simulate a psychotic state.

Jung, out of sheer necessity, was doing his own experimentation navigating the wild realms of the unconscious, sans psychedelics. Two learnings from this period are relevant to this discussion. First, he discovered that one needs help when encountering the depths. "Go thus into the depths, but do not do this alone; two or more is greater security since the depths are full of murder" (Jung, 2009, p. 244). Toni Wolff was Jung's guide and support as he opened himself to this deluge of archetypal energies (Healy, 2017, p. 116).

Second, Jung and Wolff developed a method for engaging the upwelling forces: Jung anchored himself in his conscious ego reality, then, quieting his thoughts and surrendering his rational mind, he willingly opened himself to the uprising material. Dynamic images, strange thoughts, moods, and emotions came through the ego-Self axis. He observed and then intentionally engaged with these forces from the depths. With Wolff's reassuring presence, he held the tension between his ordinary rational mind and the information coming through the irrational activity of interacting with images and inner figures. He learned "how to balance" the forces of personal and collective unconscious "through a conscious equivalent," namely, active imagination. Jung kept a foot in his conscious moral ego while interacting with what came through the portal from the unknown.

Afterward, Wolff and Jung discussed and explored the material in an integrative process. Inadvertently, they had discovered a technique that can and is being used to navigate the material that comes through the portal of a psychedelic opening. Today, many psychedelic therapy training programs promote this type of active engagement with the images, feelings, and memories that arise during a medicine session, and they recognize the value of continuing this active imagination practice in the post-session integrative process. After looking at the commonalities between Jung's theory and psychedelic assisted psychotherapy, I will demonstrate how active imagination can be used during both stages of psychedelic therapy.

A Context for the Potential of Psychedelics in Psychoanalysis

It is a bit paradoxical that Jung was opposed to psychedelic use, yet his psychological theory shares similar concepts for healing and development which recognizes the importance of: building a bridge between ordinary consciousness and non-ordinary states; grounding in the ego while intentionally engaging that which hovers at the edges of the unconscious; and actively making meaning of that material through a conscious moral stance to weave these learnings into everyday life. Analytical psychology is built on the knowledge that a living relationship between conscious and unconscious is the path toward wholeness and individuation. *How* one develops such a relationship must be carefully considered. For some, such as Jung himself, the membrane between the material and spiritual plane is naturally highly permeable. Dreamwork, psychoanalysis, and active imagination are effective methods for reaching the depths. For others, the membrane is denser, defenses are more entrenched, and the personal unconscious and imaginal realms are further from reach. Psychedelic medicines, approached with adequate preparation, a clear mindset and within an intentional setting, have the potential to thin the veils, allowing the seeker to build a bridge to deeper aspects of soul and beyond. According to Clark in his recent paper weaving scientific research and analytical psychology, psychedelics have been described as "psycho-integrators" that facilitate integration between ancient subcortical brain systems underpinning unconscious cognitive process and our more recently evolved cortical systems associated with ego consciousness (Winkelman 2007; 2010). Significantly, Jung's concept of individuation essentially involves the integration of consciousness and the unconscious, resulting in the achievement of a state of inner wholeness—a process that is believed to be effectively facilitated by psychedelics (Hill, 2013, pp. 34–35) (2021, pg. 9).

Different than Dreaming

Analytical psychology utilizes dreamwork and active imagination as a window into unconscious complexes, shadow material, and potential pathways of growth. So why risk the use of psychedelics to create such openings? In a study of the similarities and differences between dreams and psychedelic experiences, Rainer Krähenmann concluded, "The broad overlap between dreaming and psychedelic states supports the notion that psychedelics acutely induce dreamlike subjective experiences which may have long-term beneficial effects on psychosocial functioning and well-being" (2017, p. 1038). He demonstrated that there is an overlap of dream and psychedelic states, but he also highlighted important differences between the two. Within ordinary nocturnal dreaming, the ego has neither agency nor metacognitive-processing abilities. The dreamer cannot make conscious choices nor reflect from their ego awareness. Much of the psychological benefit from dreaming is derived when the dreamer wakes, consciously contemplates the dream, and makes meaning of the symbolic material. "The ego needs to be fully awake, aware and capable of holding its position while interacting with the unconscious image" (Raff, 2000, p. 18). This cannot be accomplished during a dream.

Differently, during a psychedelic session, the seeker is in a unique mind state where they might witness their inner unfolding like a dream and *simultaneously* have access to associative reasoning, creative problem solving, and the use of metaphor and symbolic thinking. They possess access to a "clarity of consciousness and meta-cognitive abilities" (Krähenmann, 2017, p. 1037). Insight, linking, and meaning making are more possible. Both psychedelic medicine and nocturnal dreaming open portals between inner defenses and the original wound, between the familiar and the bizarre, between rational and irrational realities. Yet in a psychedelic state, the default mode network (Carhart-Harris et al., 2014) is softened while the ego gains new ways of perceiving and engaging beyond the limitations of language, sensory perception, and linear organization. Rigid narratives can be actively disentangled and dissolved, making way for wholly new ways of thinking. In these rich and creative states, the seeker might intentionally dialogue with an unfamiliar figure and gain non-ordinary knowledge or willingly join with a non-human life force and become infused with its capacities.

Case Example

In a medicine session, a figure appears next to Rose. Rose perceives her as a solid form, yet of another place, as if this figure has taken on this body in order to make herself visible. The figure sits quietly wearing a blanket as a shawl. She emanates potency, certainty, and quiet wisdom. Rose chooses to engage with her, inquiring into her reason for coming. In response, the figure invites Rose to walk around the physical landscape with her. She shows Rose the living reality within the plants around them. Rose is able to see inside the leaves where the cells pulsate and dance with life force. Each plant has its own rhythm, purpose, and teaching. In this state, Rose does not question the reality of what she is shown but approaches the situation with curiosity. She receives the transmission of each plant—one teaches about death, another about music, and another about cross-species collaboration. Post session, all these themes continue to emanate numinosity to Rose. New avenues of inquiry open through ongoing reflection and integration.

Active Imagination

If we accept that there is a place for psychedelics in depth psychology, we must consider how to navigate their use in a wise manner. This requires a thoughtful conversation with many voices, one of the reasons for this collection of essays. My contribution to this conversation explores how active imagination might offer an ego-stabilizing technique when psychedelic assisted psychotherapy is offered within a therapeutic setting by a knowledgeable and trusted therapist with a patient who has a clear intention and mindset. Today, I cautiously incorporate psychedelic assisted therapy into some of my practice and active imagination plays an important role in the work. I teach many patients to use active imagination as part of their ongoing analysis so they are accustomed to engaging figures, moods, and landscapes that appear in the imaginal field. This has been additive both within the psychedelic assisted psychotherapy session and during the ongoing integrative phase in the weeks, months, and years following a medicine session.

The Challenge of Active Imagination

Active imagination can be used to inquire into a mysterious mood, dilemma, dream, and so on. The technique itself is rather simple: quiet the thoughts, hold an inquiry in mind, and open to what arises in the body, mind's eye, intuition, or reverie. Suspend judgment, but maintain your ground. Engage what arises through techniques such as dialogue, writing, movement, and painting, and then contemplate the experience until it reveals meaning that can be woven into daily life. (For a full discussion of the active imagination process, see Raff, 2000, pp. 32–38).

Despite its seeming simplicity, this technique challenges many people because they doubt the reality of the psyche and suspect they are just making things up. According to Raff, in active imagination, "The ego's task is not an easy one, for it must preserve its integrity while not being too rigid or dogmatic" (2000, p. 21). The ego must practice "flexible strength" and listen to the unconscious while bringing honesty and integrity to the encounter, Raff continued: "The ego must not simply engage in an intellectual conversation with the unconscious, but must try to bring as much real affect to the discussion as it can" (2000, pp. 21–22); and then "the ego scrupulously observes the manifestations of the self and harmonizes itself with them" (2000, p. 3). Thus a dynamic relationship between ego and the latent self is fostered (Raff, 2000, p. 7). Imaginal dialogue, automatic writing, painting, dancing and more can be used in this harmonization process.

I have found that the flexibility, creativity, and metacognitive quality of a psychedelic mind state is especially conducive to this inner dialogue. Using a psychedelic medicine, the limitations of the rational linear mind soften. The seeker has access to the symbolic, to new modes of reasoning and channels of creativity. The imaginal is subjectively experienced as real. Jung and Wolff's commitment to navigating the treacherous depths provided me with a model and a tool for navigating psychedelic experiences.

Case Example II

A woman uses active imagination during a psychedelic session. Late in a session, she encounters an indescribable pulsing entity that shifts form like a cloud. It communicates an urgency without words. Having practiced active imagination, she turns her attention and curiosity toward the entity and silently inquires as to its purpose. It speaks through color and emotional transmission. She listens without the limitations of rationality as it urges her to pay attention to the dangers of "divisiveness and polarization." It shows her the profound suffering that such behaviors are causing humanity and the natural world. It seems to propel immense emotion into and through her, so that she feels and understands what is at stake. With effort, she stays grounded within herself and receives its messages. She then asks if the entity has guidance for her. It shows her certain people in her life and again warns of the danger of divisiveness, emphasizing the possibility for collaboration. After the medicine session, she continues using active imagination in the form of painting and authentic movement to explore this encounter. She becomes increasingly aware of her own shadowy divisive behavior and sees it more acutely in the collective. She continues to integrate this experience as layers of learning unfold.

Collaborative Active Imagination

Building on the practice of active imagination, I have discovered that I am sometimes able to join my patient in their imaginal field and together we co-imagine. This type of *collaborative active imagination* is woven into the roots of analytical psychology: In 1914, during the period that Jung and Wolff were intensely involved in the confrontation with the unconscious, they stumbled into a kind of "co-imagining." They were in Ravenna, Italy, exploring the Baptistery when they came upon "shimmering Byzantine mosaics on the wall" and they "discussed the images at length, marveling at their vibrant colors, and analyzing their symbolic meaning" (Healy, 2017, pp. 124-125). Later they discovered that these mosaics had been destroyed centuries before and no longer existed in physical form. The two, in fact, had experienced a shared vision of something outside of time and space and they interacted with each other within that field. They shared in a kind of co-imagining. Today, my experience as a psychoanalyst and my subjective research using psychedelic medicines teaches me how to intentionally navigate in such a shared field.

First, as a Jungian analyst, I recognize that an analytic duo is always interacting consciously and unconsciously within a psychic field together. The two submerge into the watery depths of the psyche where they impact, influence, and resonate with each other. Wordlessly, the patient's unconscious transmits images into the mind of the analyst, the analyst's unconscious transmits to the patient, back and forth, in a shared field of resonance. Psychoanalysts learn to trust their reverie as communications from the shared field and use it to shape their interventions during an analytic hour. This is especially applicable in a psychedelic assisted therapy session where psychic boundaries soften and the rules of *me* versus *you* and consensus reality don't apply as much.

In addition to my analytic training and experience, I have been experimenting with colleagues and peers to subjectively learn more about skillfully engaging others in a psychedelically enhanced shared field. I have gathered experiences that inform me about when to sit in silence and focus on my reverie as well as when to engage verbally and, importantly, *how* to engage verbally with someone in such an amplified and perceptive state. In these study groups, we explore non-ordinary ways of communicating within a psychedelically enhanced shared field. We then compare our subjective experiences, post session. These studies have led me to new ways of working with my patients during psychedelic psychotherapy sessions.

In one peer psychedelic experiment, all participants consumed the psychedelic and then focused attention on one person who attempted to transmit their present moment experience through word, sound, or movement. The group members opened their multi-perceptual awareness and followed one participant into their visual, sensational, and emotional landscape. With the expanded perceptivity that psychedelics can offer, the participants developed a capacity to transmit intentionally their inner experiences and co-experience dimensions, which were previously unknown to the other.

In one experiment, five of us sat in a circle and someone sang in a language I don't know. At first, I perceived movements like color waves, emanating from the singer. I closed my eyes, and I saw a long geometric passageway. I walked through it and then a door opened to a completely unfamiliar architecture that pulsed with the sacred. I opened my eyes and looked at the singer who nods at me, confirming that I have entered the landscape from which this song emerges. I got there by feeling and intuiting my way into the landscape the other was already in. I have discovered that when an unfamiliar field arises in my inner vision during such an experiment, I am likely entering into a field that is further from my personal psyche and moving closer to the field of another.

In another experiment with a peer group of experienced psychedelic practitioners, I was pondering themes of inheritance and personal destiny and found myself in a midnight blue starscape. It emanated ancestry and belonging. At some point I purposefully shifted my attention to another group member, wondering about our individual destinies and how they intersect. I focused my attention and intention on connecting with her in the field, and waited as my visual landscape transformed. Through one eye, I continued to see the midnight blue starscape that seems of my personal lineage. But through the other eye, a transformation occured, and I saw a black grid between me and the blue starscape. I noted this without understanding it. Then I shifted my attention to another group member. This time, the blue starscape developed bright clear light, illuminating the edge of my visual field. I mentally noted this.

After the session and during the reflection process, I shared my experiment and observation. The first participant confirmed that what I perceived was accurate—she was "taking down structures" (the black grid) during the session and she considers this part of her life's work, to see beyond the cultural constructs. The other participant described that he was immersed in the brilliance of pure radiant love, which he perceived as pure light. From this and other similar experiments, I hypothesize that within a psychedelic state, we can hone our attention and intentionally share perceptions, information, and images in non-ordinary yet real ways. I am exploring how this might be possible when just one person, namely the patient, takes the medicine and the other attempts to join them in a shared field.

Shared Active Imagination in Practice

In high dose psychedelic assisted psychotherapy, as the patient's inner process unfolds, the therapist must sit as a witnessing presence for long periods of silence or strong undifferentiated affect. The primary activity occurs between the patient and their *inner healing intelligence*. The patient might speak aloud but often does not require nor desire a verbal response. Other times, they seek reassurance or guidance or want more engagement with the therapist. Here, the usual dialogue and pace of a psychotherapy session would be intrusive and overwhelming to someone in a highly permeable psychedelic state. The therapist's own knowledge of and subjective experience of such states, in addition to their training and experience as a depth therapist, can help them discern a response. Later in the session when the effect of the medicine is tapering off, or in a low dose psycholytic session, verbal engagement with the therapist is more likely to be desired and beneficial (Passie et al., 2022). As a general rule, the more altered the patient's consciousness, the less the therapist says out loud. The approach is like that of the medial who knows more subtle—and less verbal—ways of working within the deep unconscious: "According to Wolff, the *medial* leads those who are compelled to enter into non-ordinary realities, and, in doing so, she initiates them into a deeper understanding of the psyche" (Healy, 2017, p. 144).

By combining active imagination with my findings from the peer experimentations described previously, I have developed a manner of working verbally during collaborative, or shared, active imagination. I have used this approach—always with a degree of caution—in low dose psycholytic sessions, and in the latter part of high-dose medicine sessions when the patient is more cognitively organized. Prior to the psychedelic assisted therapy sessions, these patients have developed some facility with active imagination as part of their ongoing analysis. As ongoing patients in my practice, their inner landscapes are familiar to me, and a strong relational resonance has been established long before adding psychedelic-assisted sessions.

In order to engage in collaborative active imagination during a psychedelic assisted psychotherapy session, the patient is in a state where they are able to narrate their inner unfolding. As the patient speaks aloud, I (without the aid of psychedelic medicine) quiet my own thoughts, open my imagination, and extend my inner awareness toward the patient's inner field. I listen to their words, images, and feeling tone, and then watch for a resonance within my own associations, body sensations, visual imagery, emotional field, and thoughts. This is not so different from what I do when engaging my reverie in a typical analytic session. But here, I am additionally informed by my subjective psychedelic research. Once I see, sense, or feel a resonance, I hold it in mind and wait for the image to make the next move, just as in a typical active imagination. If the image evolves of its own accord within my mind's eye, I tell the patient what I am seeing in as few words as possible. One of three responses generally occurs:

1. The patient shows no response, in which case I return to silence and follow the patient;

2. The patient responds with confusion or struggles to make my words fit. In this case, I assume I am out of resonance and suggest they drop my words and return to their interior.

3. The patient then sees/perceives what I describe and they engage it with interest. In this case, we continue to co-imagine, sharing what we perceive and following where the image takes us.

I have found that when the field is strong between the two of us, the image deepens and enlivens from our joint attention, allowing it to reveal itself more fully, offering its message and medicine.

Case Example III

Maya is a woman in a current analysis with me. About two-thirds of the way through a high-dose psychedelic psychotherapy session, we engage in collaborative active imagination. Maya's eyes are closed and her expression is pained. She says that at the base of her being, her "roots are bitter and rotten, contaminating everything." She despairs, "How can I grow if my roots are rotten?" She is both seeing the tree and she is the tree.

I recognize this rottenness as a complex that is strongly woven into Maya's identity. The image sparks my imagination. "Stay with the rotten," I encourage and close my eyes to see if I can join her. A little overeager to help her transform this complex, I jump in prematurely from outside the resonance and suggest that she bring in some fire to dry up the rot. She takes my offer, but "it doesn't work" and she feels a familiar pervasive disappointment. "I'm stuck." Realizing my lack of attunement, I pull my energy back and still my thoughts. I open my inner awareness and perceptivity to the rotting, bitter roots. In time, I sense the soggy decaying tree base and suspect I am now closer to Maya's field.

I wait here, and let Maya or the image take the next step. Maya says she is tired of relying on her own strength to override this lack of sturdy foundation. In my mind's eye, the soggy tree base morphs into a giant healthy redwood tree with a burned-out hollow at the base. (Perhaps this is related to the fire I had suggested a few minutes earlier?) The tree is growing despite the wounding it has endured. I tell Maya what I see, and she slowly senses it, too. Now her torso/trunk rises. We continue in this way, speaking what we notice. The image seems to participate and reveal more until we both perceive the wholeness of the tree and its place within the forest—the burn scar, solid trunk, and the high view all co-exist. My mind's eye is high up, looking at the vastness of the forest when Maya speaks more of a vulnerable aloneness and overdeveloped self-sufficiency. Now in my mind's eye, the high forest view shifts to the underlayer of redwood forest, an entangled system of mutually supporting root systems. It comes strong and unbidden, so I describe this. Maya picks this up and begins naming people and resources in her life that help sustain her. Her energy increases as she notes the ways she is not alone, that she is, in fact, supported by others.

In the post-medicine session, Maya continues to work with this image of roots and shared resources. She discovers a mycelial web, a mass of interdependent filaments, which is both a physical reality and a living symbol, an entity that Maya can reach and touch when she needs to remember that everything is not up to her. Similarly, she has been more able to access the high view of the forest in moments when her *bitter and rotten* complex is activated. There is more distance between the activated wound (the burn scar) and the actual here and now issue, resulting in increased psychological flexibility.

Art Making as Active Imagination During Integration Stage

So far, I have emphasized the psychedelic assisted therapy session itself. Now I will turn to the post-medicine integrative stage where there is tremendous potential for the use of active imagination. This integration phase, which can last for weeks, months, or years, is approached in vastly inconsistent ways. Some approaches emphasize physical care such as rest and food. Others suggest time in nature or rituals to honor and continue the work that started in the medicine session. There are peer-led integration groups, and there are clinicians who offer psychedelic integration psychotherapy.

I am particularly interested in what happens when the integration includes a creative combination of active imagination and process art. Process art emphasizes the inner exploration of the artmaker, with the aesthetics of the artwork a secondary consideration. It allows space for the unconscious to insert itself in ways that are simultaneously "inventive and unreasonable" (Wilson, 1998, p. 31). In this form of active imagination, the seeker moves slowly with paints, colors, clay, collage, or other materials, while listening at the edge of awareness for whispers from the other side. Subtle associations, disturbances, impulses, and insights appear in the imaginal field between the seeker and the mystery and are added to the artwork. A wordless dialogue takes place as the seeker cycles between conscious self-expression and surrendering the creative process to an autonomous other.

I have found that this process, which I call *alchemical art,* is an ideal way to re-engage, explore, and metabolize a psychedelic therapy session. Process art is a middle language living between the seeker's actual subjective experience and the challenge of putting a non-ordinary experience into the confines of words and narrative. Alchemical art is a visual and kinesthetic conversation that is akin to aspects of the psychedelic experience itself. The language centers can remain quiet while symbolic thinking is stirred. When this process is taken up in the weeks and months following a medicine session, the flexibility and creativity of the medicine state can still be accessed. Color, shape, texture, and image bring what had been an indescribable subjective experience into an external manifestation. As the artwork makes its way into physical form, it becomes a visible expression of something that was deeply experienced, while simultaneously mirroring and affirming the reality of the inner world. Or it might take on an autonomous quality and *speak* to the maker. Process art allows time for inquiry and contemplation, whereas expressing the internal in words too quickly can risk reifying a still emerging experience. This is art making as active imagination.

When working with groups in psychedelic art integration classes, I offer help if someone becomes frustrated or confused by their inner conversation or if they hit a roadblock in the art making. At this point, paradoxically, it can be helpful to shift to language to open up the creative flow. If I sense they need privacy or a more introverted approach, I might suggest they write in a free format using words, phrases, or stream of consciousness. Ideally, they write directly on the art piece so that this part of the active imagination is woven into the piece. Other times, I engage the participant in a more extroverted way, inviting them into verbal dialogue. I ask questions: What are they stuck in? What *is* working and what is *not*? What do they hear in their inner commentary? Are they having any associations? Body sensations? What do they see when they look at the page?

An interesting thing often happens. Just as speaking a dream aloud can help the dreamer hear something they hadn't noticed before, speaking about the art process can illuminate the inner dilemma and free up the creative flow. They hear a metaphor in something that had been concrete. For example, someone says, "The whole painting is too chaotic." I ask, "Does this have any relevance to your inquiry? Is this a familiar place?" Most often, they laugh with surprised recognition. "Yes, I resist the messiness of chaos." "The wildness scares me." "I am never allowed to be messy." Now, the creative flow re-opens and a conversation with chaos might ensue.

Case Example IV

In an alchemical art psychedelic integration workshop, Gabriella is working with layers of paint and collage. Deep into the art making, she appears flustered as she moves two collage pieces around the page—both pictures of infants with bright round faces—placing them together, then apart, then removing one, then adding it back. After some time, I approach Gabriella to ask if she'd like help. She thinks out loud, "There are these two babies. I think it's too many. One baby is fine, but both? It's too many. But I *want* both!"

Then she hears herself say "I don't want them to be alone." Her eyes widen as she makes connections to her recent learning about herself as a solo person in the world who has needed lots of time for her individual work. New perspectives have been emerging in her psychedelic sessions indicating that it is time for her to be less solo, to collaborate with others more, and to offer herself and her ideas more publicly. By speaking this out loud to another (rather than being alone with it in her thoughts), she hears herself and sees herself again for the first time. Even in this moment, in a parallel process, Gabriella finds herself more fully through dialogue with another.

Conclusions and Further Considerations

There are significant clinical and ethical considerations when entering into the deep imaginal realms with another. Given the limited scope of this chapter, I have neither identified nor discussed many critical factors. As the role of psychedelics in analytic psychology unfolds, I imagine a collaborative and thoughtful inquiry within the greater community will ensue. For now, I will offer a few ideas for future consideration.

I could argue that depth therapists already interact with patients in the dark of the psyche and are thus prepared for this work. But the unpredictability of the unconscious and the hyper-perceptivity of a psychedelic state require new and grave consideration. The psyche is autonomous, and unbidden chaos may be unleashed once the portal is open. We must keep in mind that within an amplified state, an otherwise small lack of attunement could lead to a relational rupture between patient and therapist. We must also consider the impact of the analyst's personal psyche, filled with complexes and biases, and how this might be amplified within the patient's extremely permeable psychedelic state of mind. Relatedly, the analyst consciously and unconsciously seeds the field with imagery that will likely influence the tone and content of a given session. How do we as clinicians best prepare ourselves for such sensitive work? What kind of training, supervision and consultation should be required? I believe it is imperative that the analyst has firsthand experience with psychedelic medicines. Additionally, a personal practice of active imagination, a refined ability to attune within non-ordinary states, extensive knowledge of psychedelic medicines, capacity for extended focus, and genuine humility are all required.

And then we must consider the patient. Who is a good candidate for psychedelic assisted psychotherapy and what conditions can be effectively treated? There is an international explosion of psychedelic research exploring the use of medicines such as MDMA, psilocybin, ketamine, LSD, ibogaine, ayahuasca and DMT to treat conditions such as PTSD, depression, suicidality, anxiety, eating disorders, obsessive-compulsive disorder, substance abuse disorders, autism and more. The findings of such research will help clinicians create best practices as these medicines become approved for clinical use.

Meanwhile, psychoanalytic communities are taking on other important questions: How and when might a psychedelic assisted session be introduced in an existing analysis? How is the frame of analysis maintained and altered? What might be the co-transferential impact? How do we navigate the projections onto psychedelic medicine itself?

These are important considerations, but my hope is that analytical psychology can also bring its relationship to the spiritual psyche into the psychedelic-assisted therapy conversation. Our respect for the autonomous nature of the psyche can offer a unique and relevant viewpoint. May we bring a full and considered voice to the psychedelic assisted therapy table while maintaining humility and reverence for not knowing.

References

Clark, G. (2021). Carl Jung and the psychedelic brain: An evolutionary model of analytical psychology informed by psychedelic neuroscience. *International Journal of Jungian Studies 14*(2), 97-126.

Carhart-Harris, R.L., Leech, R., Hellyer, P.J., Shanahan, M., Feilding, A., Tagliazucchi, E., Chialvo, D.R., & Nutt, D. (2014). The entropic brain: A theory of conscious states informed by neuroimaging research with psychedelic drugs. *Frontiers in Human Neuroscience, 8,* Article 20.

Carlin, S. (2021). Cultivating inner healing intelligence through MDMA-assisted psychotherapy. In T. Read & M. Papaspyrou, Eds. *Psychedelics and psychotherapy: The healing potential of expanded states* (pp. 151–162). Park Street Press.

Griffiths, R.R., Johnson, M.W., Richards, W.A., Richards, B.D., McCann, U., & Jesse, R. (2011). Psilocybin occasioned mystical-type experiences: immediate and persisting dose-related effects. *Psychopharmacology, 218*(4), 649-65.

Healy, N.S. (2017). *Toni Wolff and C.G. Jung: A collaboration.* Tiberius Press.

Jung, C.G. (1973). *Letters of C.G. Jung, Vol 1, 1906-1950* (Gerhard Adler & Aniela Jaffé, Eds.). Princeton University Press.

Jung, C.G. (1976). *Letters of C.G. Jung: Vol 2, 1951-1961* (Gerhard Adler & Aniela Jaffé, Eds.). Princeton University Press.

Jung, C.G. (1977). *C.G. Jung speaking* (W. McGuire & R. F. C. Hull, Eds.). Princeton University Press.

Krähenmann, R. (2017). Dreams and psychedelics: Neurophenomenological comparison and therapeutic implications. *Current Neuropharmacology, 15*(7), 1032-1042.

Marlo, H. (2022). Experiencing the spiritual psyche: Reflections on synchronicity-informed psychotherapy. *Jung Journal: Culture & Psyche, 16*(4), 44-69.

Passie, T., Guss, J., & Krähenmann, R. (2022). Lower-dose psycholytic therapy—a neglected approach. *Frontiers in Psychiatry, 13,* 1020505.

Raff, J. (2000). *Jung and the alchemical imagination.* Nicolas-Hays.

Wilson, J.M. (1998). Art-making behavior: What and how arts education is central to learning. *Art Education Policy Review, 99*(6), 26-33.

Sharing in the Field: The Art of Working Energetically with Psychedelics

Susan Williams

Not I, not I, but the wind that blows through me!
A fine wind is blowing the new direction of Time.
If only I let it bear me, carry me, if only it carry me! ...

What is the knocking?
What is the knocking at the door in the night?
It is somebody wants to do us harm.

No, no, it is the three strange angels.
Admit them, admit them.

D. H. Lawrence, *Song of a Man*
Who Has Come Through (1994, p. 195)

Beginnings

This chapter is an outgrowth of a *strange*, yet transformative exploration of what psychedelic plants and medicines are trying to communicate. Is something trying to break through? *Admit them, admit them.*

The art of working energetically with psychedelic medicines is my attempt at co-dreaming with the plants, allies, entities; with each other; and with the wider community to honor the dream-like nature of reality. Can we work collaboratively in the field as an energetic mycelium network? Just as this vast, dazzling hyphal system in a forest allows the sharing of nutrients between trees and plants, there may be an energetic equivalent in the field between human and non-human beings. How do we share our gifts and identify our shadows and complexes that may block the flow within and between us? I will explore these questions through a clinical case that demanded an expanded orientation toward wholeness and meaning.

A transformative psychedelic experience often includes the loss of a sense of a separate ego and the emergence of unity consciousness. At its best, Jungian analytic work brings one into the heart of an *intra-connected,* relational, awe-embracing (Siegal, 2022) field that challenges the myth of the separate self. This chapter is an exploration of what I am calling *sharing in the field*—a paradigm that challenges the Newtonian view of a solo self, leading one into a shared, co-created energetic field of consciousness.

What does it mean to live the *extensive self*—to free the individual from the prison of their own subjectivity? How do we escape the trap of the known self to reside in full, alive presence, while awakening the soul for the purpose of deepening and expanding a connection to those we love, our society, the natural world, the source of all being, and the great unfathomable mystery? In this state of primordial being, beyond the personal self and its stories, the *mundus imaginalis* (Corbin, 1998) is awakened, taking the individual beyond *imagination,* as commonly cited, to *an imaginal dimension beyond all our constraints and fictions.*

The first lesson on my journey beyond the constraints of consensus reality, toward a more expansive *cosmic consciousness* (Bucke, 1991), emerged with the plant teacher *Yagé,* Ayahuasca vine as prepared in the *Secoya* tradition (Weisberger, 2013), in the Amazonian jungle accompanied by the elders of the Siekopai Nation of Ecuador. As I deepened my relationship with the spirits of the medicine, I was gifted with a vision of what I, as a seemingly separate individual, would call *my thoughts,* floating in a water bottle belonging to a fellow participant. This paradigm-shattering vision was shocking. As I pondered the improbability of my personal thoughts contained in a bottle I didn't even own, a realization emerged. *Oh, none of this belongs to us.* I may bottle up my thoughts, like water, into a separate mind and call it *my idea* but that is illusory. Thoughts may be more like water in the vast ocean, flowing between continents, and so what I call *mine* and *yours* ultimately all belongs to the vast cosmic sea.

In the 1999 film, *The Matrix*, the image of taking the *red pill* versus the *blue pill* represents a choice between the willingness to learn a potentially unsettling truth by taking the *red pill* or remaining in the familiarity of consensus reality by ingesting the *blue pill*. My paradigm-shattering awakening to the realization that thoughts do not live inside one isolated, finite being was analogous to taking the *red pill*, thus waking me up to the unbearable weight of deep truths and the limitations of a constructed reality.

My ongoing work exploring the energetics of psychedelic medicines has suggested that, in the language of quantum mechanics, I needed to become more wave than particle. Whereas a particle is a finite entity, waves are boundaryless oscillations that spread out, transporting energy from one place to another. The image of wave-particle duality speaks to the call to rest in possibility while tolerating living on the knife edge of nonsense, or even madness—a frontier, where thoughts and emotions do not reside inside one body but rather permeate the atmosphere like weather.

Jung describes his encounter with the edges of madness in *The Red Book* (2009), wherein he tells the story of facing his own demons as they emerged from the shadows. Jung's surrender to an autonomous process, which ultimately revealed a deeper level of objective reality, calls to mind the sacrifices demanded of the initiand to engage fully in a deep psychedelic process. Through a dissolving of boundaries and shedding the protective cloak of normality, sacred wounds and gifts are exposed, opening one into a deeper and more fundamental order of reality, where space and time are no longer the dominant factors; to a dimension beyond surface phenomena; to a place where synchronicity, uncanny knowing, and mystery resides.

Despite his own experience of going to the edge of madness, Jung was profoundly mistrustful of psychedelics and opening to the "pure gifts of the Gods" (2015, p. 173). During what has been called a *psychedelic renaissance* with psychedelic-enhanced psychotherapy being gradually integrated into Jungian analysis, we are called as practitioners to face into a myriad of complexities. Indigenous cultures have deep and complex root structures in place informing their relationship with sacred plants and medicines, whereas for many Westerners there is no such anchoring tradition. The modern world has veered toward Cartesian dualistic principles, ostensibly forgetting the non-dual sacred practices that lie at the ancient roots of Western civilization. My clinical approach of working energetically with psychedelic medicines is an attempt at elucidating a new, yet ancient paradigm of healing within my own Irish Celtic cultural lineage.

There is a Hebrew phrase that has become a guiding mantra in this exploration. I find myself repeating the English translation: *The old shall be made new and the new sacred*, as I attempt to re-create a more alive and sacramental way of working with these medicines. How do I reinfuse numen back into my practice, allowing for a rebirth of the primordially ancient in the new?

What I am reaching toward is a mystical worldview that not only the ancient Greeks described in the Orphic tradition and Eleusinian mysteries, but that breathes through my Celtic pagan bloodline. The art of working energetically with psychedelics is informed by ancient Western traditions of inspired prophecy and enchantment. This is not Hippocratic medicine, but an ancient shamanic world, not of rational thought but of ecstasy and expanded states of consciousness, incantation, and deliberate, repetitive use of words, vibration, and sound; the ritualized art of stillness and meditation. Through the practice of incubation in dark places, the initiand deliberately accesses the realm of dreams and visions (Kingsley, 2018, 2020). This is a world in which "everything breathes together" (Plotinus, as cited in Tarnas, 2006, p. 77), an "interconnected participatory universe" in which there is no objective reality out there, independent of an observer (Levy, 2018).

Introduction to the Work

The work with my patient Ilana is an attempt at sharing in the energy field the potential to awaken a mysterious, yet potent *inner healing intelligence* that has been forgotten. In Jungian language this could be called the wisdom of the Self, though I hesitate to do so, for this word, like many sacred names, has lost its potency through overuse, becoming a shorthand for something too known. Instead, I turn to the poetics of Wallace Stevens (1937, p. 61) when he implores in *The Man with the Blue Guitar*:

> *Throw away the lights, the definitions,*
> *And say of what you see in the dark*
>
> *That it is this or that it is that,*
> *But do not use the rotted names.*

Our work represents a move away from familiar definitions, *rotted names*, and the security of a material worldview. This paradigm shift nudges us toward an energetic cosmos, while weaving ancient shamanic and visionary practices into a contemporary model, pointing to an underlying reality that is neither mental nor material, toward what Jung called the *unus mundus* (one world), or in more contemporary language, the unified field of consciousness.

In an expanded state of consciousness, is it possible to access the psychic energy of psychedelics, particularly the empathogen MDMA and the entheogen psilocybin without the patient taking the actual material substance?[1] Here, I explore this question through a description of a new chapter in a 14-year, twice a week analysis, in which an iconoclastic paradigm emerged out of a confluence of tragedy and creativity.

Ilana is in her forties and was born with multiple congenital anomalies. At birth she was presumed to be completely blind and deaf, though over time it was evident that she was, in fact, partially sighted. From birth until the present, Ilana had undergone a seemingly endless series of surgeries and painful medical procedures to repair countless structural anomalies—thus contributing to a fragmented identity formed through a medical lens.

Ilana is often met with the assumption that she is cognitively impaired because of her physical appearance. She describes feeling like a head, containing an intelligent mind and alive spirit, with nothing below. She hates her body, for in her words, "*It's just a mass of problems. I feel like my body continually betrays me. Why should I care about it?*"

For all the work we have done over the years, residual symptoms of anxiety persisted. I understood her desire for a fuller way of metabolizing the overwhelming trauma locked away in her body, spilling out whenever she needed another surgery. Her life often felt like one medical problem arising after another, with each procedure stirring flashbacks of being pinned down and the resultant feeling of being trapped and unable to see or hear what was happening.

The following events set us on this uncharted path of working energetically with psychedelic medicines. During the initial surge of Covid-19, Ilana was shaken to her core by several losses in her family circle. Then the unimaginable happened. After a lifetime of surgeries to save her remaining vision, she lost all sight and was now completely blind. Her emotional state had been challenged further by the development of a rare neurological syndrome, which produced visual and auditory hallucinations, contributing to a feeling of being unsafe in the world.

All these losses transpired as we were in a pandemic, with the phone as our only source of connection. As Ilana's vision was declining quickly, she pleaded to be seen in person, while she had some sight left. To fortify her recall, Ilana would stare at an enlarged photo of me on the computer screen, trying to memorize my face before all vision disappeared. It was clear that I needed to make an exception to see her in person. The phrase *extraordinary times call for extraordinary measures* resonated, even though I lacked a clear idea of what I was being called to do. I knew that our creative aliveness required something more far-reaching and that my own imagination needed to be set free from old paradigms and conventions.

Ilana expressed interest in MDMA as a treatment for her severe anxiety and intractable symptoms of PTSD, from medical trauma that left her feeling *"like a rare medical specimen, repeatedly poked and prodded."* She desperately hoped this breakthrough treatment would be available for her. So, it was sobering to inform Ilana that her complex medical history and long list of medications disqualified her from applying to any of the clinical trials and prohibited the safe use of any psychedelic substance.

Having completed the MAPS (Multidisciplinary Association for Psychedelic Studies) MDMA Therapy Training Program and gaining first-hand experience of what this treatment has to offer, I hoped Ilana could have the opportunity to awaken her own inner healing intelligence. During this period, I woke many mornings with the same dream, a voice, almost a command stating, *Reinfuse numen into matter! Reinfuse numen into matter!* It was insistent and so I listened deeply. I sensed that my words, practices, and ways of relating had become dead through mindless repetition; they needed to be reinfused with fresh sparks of divine aliveness.

It is a well-known fact that "plasticity has been documented at every stage of life. Habit impedes us as we age as much as any change in innate capacity" (Power, 2021, p 115). The work with Ilana was stuck in old habits and tired analytic rituals. A quote inspired by the work of psychoanalyst Paul Russell (Teicholz et al., 1998) emerged and became another guiding mantra, *"When we repeat, we cease to live."* Perhaps the analysis and our relationship were not fully alive? We were repeating. But where was the enchanted repetition of poetry and song, of sacred ritual?

What is the knocking at the door in the night? In my countertransference, I had been struggling with a feeling of irritation, igniting an even more shameful inner response. *How could I be so cold and unfeeling after all she had been through*? Over time, my irritation has become one of my wisest teachers, informing me that a hidden truth has not yet been brought to consciousness. Was my anger and irritation telling me that there was a door to a deeper layer of feeling that we needed to go through?

Donald Kalsched (2013) has written extensively on trauma as an injury to the capacity to feel. Trauma survivors like Ilana have been subject to circumstances that stir feelings beyond what the ego can metabolize, so they've had to dissociate. Dissociation is something the psyche does to protect us, to safeguard something sacred and imperishable about the human spirit by splitting off vulnerable parts into the inner world and protecting them there with defenses. These splintered-off islands of unbearable truth protect the integrity and stability of the known self and ultimately the soul; though with so much locked away, they ultimately keep us living a constricted life.

As Ilana's suffering was so overwhelming, the capacity to face into, truly bear, and integrate the full extent of her losses was blocked. Her self-perception was then formed in this limited way. Central to

Jung's view, individuation is an instinctual, archetypal pull toward truth, a naturally unfolding force urging us to live the fullness of who we are (Williams, 2017). This unveiling, moving us toward new potential, is hindered without an acknowledgment and lived relationship to the sealed-off aspects of the personality. My irritation arose whenever I arrived at a locked door. This door is the protective layer of defenses that guards the vulnerable, unmetabolized experiences that have never seen the light of day. I felt profound sympathy for all Ilana had to go through, but genuine empathy was harder to locate in those moments, and I knew that the block to true feeling flowing again would be found in the space between us and by empathically facing into any silenced parts of the Self—both hers and mine.

Having been the recipient of so much aggression, with her body and sense of self repeatedly assailed, Ilana found it challenging to acknowledge her own dissociated anger and aggression. She desperately needed the help of others and could not afford to alienate her support structure, and so those more threatening emotions that could never be expressed went underground. To move forward with the energy field open for sharing, these locked away emotions needed to be more consciously expressed, clearing the field for the next stage of our work.

I wanted to share with Ilana, not only the best of what has emerged in the research with psychedelics, but also the magic and mystery alive in these practices—the sacramental nature of what is possible in a vibrantly alive process. How could I reinfuse numen into an analysis that had become drained of spirit as I sat in my chair and listened? Native Americans and other Indigenous peoples have an alive culture that honors sacramental mysteries, but where was it in my own culture, in my Celtic soul?

After facing into the reality that she was unable to work with the substance of MDMA, I said, "*Well if you really want to work with MDMA, we can start right now!*" I shared my belief that the material substance of the medicine was not essential—that there was an energetic field constellated around these medicines and we could work with that. I let Ilana know that I would work with her in the same way I would with a patient on MDMA, but without her taking the material substance.

Ilana's whole life had been ruled by a reductionistic medical model that focused on repairing parts of her body at the expense of a sense of being a whole person. We needed to restore a sense of underlying wholeness. Jung's one-time patient, collaborator, and quantum physicist, Wolfgang Pauli, saw this underlying wholeness to the universe—*unus mundus* (one world)—alive in synchronicities where matter, soul or psyche, and meaning come together in a surprising way.

I decided to intuitively create a paradigm that worked for both Ilana and me. We were going to work together, as interacting conscious agents in a co-created field—acting more wave-like than particle-like.

I drew from what I knew best—my own deep dive with these medicines, which was a radically transformative experience of waking up from a long, deep sleep into a latent potential that I believe is in each of us to heal ourselves and our bodies. I was able to rewrite my own story of debilitating autoimmune, gastrointestinal, and neurological symptoms. The work with sacred medicines opened me to states of consciousness that over time allowed me to move beyond each of these limitations and to continue to live symptom free. In an early journey, a commanding voice shouted repeatedly, "Wake up! Wake up to your f...ing life, Susan! If you don't do what you came here to do, you will get sick!"

I knew that I had to step up more fully, to inhabit a larger destiny, but also to open to any hidden areas in myself, facing all the survival adaptations that protect our vulnerability and block access to the flow of grace into our lives. How could I open the field and reinfuse the sacred back into matter, while helping Ilana do the same?

Despite a pandemic, Ilana and I agreed to meet in my consulting room. She was having episodes of crippling panic. Recurring nightmares of tsunamis or surgical procedures being performed against her will filled her nights. In the dream state, Ilana would attempt to kill herself to wake up. These dreams left me wondering: what part of her and our way of working needed to die, for her and us to wake up to a fuller self and into a reality that could hold so much complexity and hardship?

Ilana had no real relationship with her body and so we began there. For her psyche, it had been a matter of surviving in pieces, but now was the time for an encounter with all that had been locked away, opening the door to a deeper integration of these unbearably painful experiences.

One of the gifts of working with the empathogen MDMA in psychotherapy is that the elevation of oxytocin and release of serotonin, norepinephrine, and dopamine allow traumatic memories, which would otherwise be overwhelming and flood the psyche, to be experienced in a deep bodily sense with compassion and enough perspective to have the experience and survive it (Mithoefer et al., 2010). A reduction in fear, with decreased amygdala activation, opens a window, a rare moment in time for the retrieval of split-off memories to be integrated into the cells of the body and mind. I went into this experience with Ilana with a sense of knowing that all of this was available to her, to us, even if she was not taking the material substance.

As the psychoanalyst and psychedelic therapist, I gave myself complete creative freedom to play, to make it up as I went along, drawing on years of working with autistic children, where I would try anything to make contact, knowing that they wouldn't judge me if I looked ridiculous in the process. I invoked the spirit of MDMA, drawing on my own deep inner knowing and respect for this medicine's potential to bring one into a radically new experience of the body—free and full of compassion for all it has been through, thus allowing one to rewrite old stories stored in their cells through the development of new neural pathways (De Vos et al., 2021).

In terms of set and setting, we altered our schedule to include a longer medicine session each week, with an integration hour later in the week. We began with dancing, movement, yoga, and guided meditations. Lying on the floor, bathed in evocative music, Ilana was able to move beyond her defenses and finally got a taste of coming home to a somatic sense of safety and peace.

To contact and then share the energetic signature of MDMA, without either one of us taking the material substance, I allowed myself to tune in and intuitively become a vibrational match to this medicine—sharing with Ilana the sensations of MDMA coming on as I re-experienced them in my own body. I reminded Ilana, as I would a patient on the physical substance that she could not do this wrong and suggested that she invite the medicine in. I offered flight instructions: *There is nothing you need to do or fix here. Trust the medicine, trust the process, and let go. If you come across something scary, go toward it. Remember, you are supported*

After 12 minutes of silence, she speaks:

Ilana: I feel scared, someone is going to break in and try to hurt me. Where are you?

Susan: (moving closer) I'm right here with you. This room has double doors that are both locked, and I am here to make sure you are safe. Your dog Teddy is here too. Can you let this scared feeling move through you?

Ilana: (in a pleading voice) Don't let any one touch me!

Susan: I'm protecting you! I will not allow anyone to touch you.

Ilana: (visibly soothed) I want to feel safe and healed in my body.

Susan: Ilana, let's say that as an invocation.

Ilana: (repeating the same words but this time as invocation, as incantation) I am open to feeling safe and healed in my body. I am open to feeling whole and being in charge. I am open to feeling whole and safe.

Susan: Ilana, what does your body need to hear right now?

Ilana: That I'm whole and safe even when I'm touched. People don't intend to hurt me. The doctors and nurses were trying to help me. I can provide the best love for myself. I can trust that I know what I need. I am open to feeling healed. My body is whole. I can let down my guard and trust.

Susan: Ilana, let your body feel the vibration of those words. Really feel the vibrational signature of each word and let it move through your body.

As the session was soon ending, Ilana slowly got off the floor and back into her seat. Taking time to settle, as she was still feeling dizzy.

Ilana: I was feeling so relaxed, yet also feeling like people were touching me. I had this odd sensation of hands all over me. All the nurses and doctors were touching me. During procedures they would use my body as a table. They don't see that I'm a person. But then I imagined that I was standing in water, remembering how water is where I feel the happiest. The medicine helped me shift from the sensations of being touched to a place where I am most comfortable.

As the session ends, Ilana remarks, *"It was so helpful to be reminded that I was on medicine. I loved when you said, 'Let the medicine help you.' I love lying on the floor and feeling so grounded."*

Integration and Further Reflections

In our follow-up integration session later that week, Ilana commented on her experience of this new way of working. *"I felt a bit dizzy and out of it all day, like I literally took the medicine. Is that possible?"* I affirm that this is a common experience with this medicine, for in my view, we are working with MDMA. The psychedelic-enhanced psychotherapy sessions are opening Ilana to expanded states of consciousness that are not a metaphor or an *as if* experience, but rather a living psychic reality, an ontological reality of its own.

Throughout this exploration, I have drawn not only from my analytic and psychedelic trainings but more deeply from the buried wisdom of my own ancestors. Fódhla, one of the names for Dreamtime Ireland, is not a separate world, for "the otherworld is a way of seeing this world, it is a way of being in this world." (Moriarty, 1999, p. 6). While I am no longer a practicing Catholic, Irish Catholicism, with its pagan, shamanic influences, vibrates in the cells of my body. I grew up seeped in the experience of the sacrament of the Mass as a transmutation, a transubstantiation, a mystery. In the Catholic Mass, Communion is not a metaphor. It is the body and blood of Christ and considered a living reality. Yet the ancient Irish Celtic roots, which I call upon in this work, run much deeper than the Catholic Mass. What I beckon is primordial, eternal, feminine, and watery—an indwelling presence able to share her gifts of the heart, alchemizing the pain of those who suffer.

Ilana reflects on the openness that is emerging. *"It's amazing, but throughout the week, I can hear your voice and I start to feel relaxed again. There really is something about your voice in these sessions. I know this sounds weird, but could you record a voice memo for me of you speaking some of the phrases you use."*

As we discuss this request, I am reminded that just as MDMA moves freely in the energetic, vibrational field, so does the voice. Incantation is an alive, flowing process, an oral tradition that is drained

350

of numen when captured or pinned down. I knew that the recording could not replicate the original experience. For *when we repeat, we cease to live.* Yet in a wave-like state of surrender and flow, the sacred is reinfused into matter .

W.S. Merwin in, *One of the Butterflies,* illuminates the illusory desire to bottle our pleasurable experiences.

> *...and it seems I cherish*
> *only now a joy I was not aware of*
> *when it was here although it remains*
> *out of reach and will not be caught or named*
> *or called back and if I could make it stay*
> *as I want to it would turn into pain*
> –(W.S. Merwin, *The Shadow of Sirius*: Copper Canyon Press)

In modern language, I have wondered whether this energetic process could be viewed as a form of *limbic resonance* (Lewis et al., 2007), of entraining Ilana's brain to MDMA, to a state of ecstasy? This creative right brain to right brain process is shared in the energetic field between two interacting, attuned conscious agents, aligning with morphic memory and resonance in the field (R. Sheldrake, 2009). Through sharing my access to these dimensions in the field, was Ilana learning something about the state of ecstasy, of compassion for herself, her body and all it had gone through? Perhaps "well-being is like a virus. One self-assured person at home in this world can infect dozens of other" (Powers, 2021, p. 180).

Going Forward: The Energetics of Psilocybin

> *Send me out into another life*
> *lord because this one is growing faint*
> *I do not think it goes all the way.*
> (W.S. Merwin, *Words from a Totem Animal*, 1969)

Once again, we had come to the end of a road. Working energetically with MDMA had allowed the processing of many painful, traumatic memories, opening a door for Ilana to a flow of oxytocin and love for herself, her body, and all that she had been through. As we passed "through the agonies of emergent consciousness" (Gebser, 1986, p. 103), deeper questions of meaning arose. As the protective defences softened, Ilana no longer needed to profess being strong, optimistic, or convince me that she was "trying hard." Despite all the gains, she began to reflect more honestly on the fuller meaning of her life, questioning whether she wanted to continue to live in such a state. Was there any pleasure or enjoyment left in life without vision? Everything was so hard.

While Ilana loved the MDMA sessions, in particular the sensations of deep relaxation and acceptance in her body, I intuited that we were beginning to repeat and that another *strange angel* was knocking at our door. I could feel my creative juices abating, and some irritation returning. Was it time for something new? Existential questions of meaning—such as *Why me? Why would a loving God create me this way? Why should one person have to deal with so much? It isn't fair!*—all required an expanded view of meaning and wholeness. From a personal, subjective point of view there are no satisfactory answers to these profound inquiries. We needed to engage in a spiritual process that could uncover a deeper layer of objective, cosmic reality.

Trauma may shatter us, but it also may crack us open, creating an opportunity for the soul and its evolutionary purpose to reveal itself. To descend further, I called upon the spirit of psilocybin for guidance. Psilocybin, the psychedelic substance in magic mushrooms, has been well-documented in studies at Johns Hopkins University to ease existential anxiety in people with life-threatening illness. Most participants in these studies rated the experience to be among the top five most personally meaningful and spiritually significant of their lives (Griffiths et al., 2022). I wanted Ilana to have a glimpse into an expanded dimension of consciousness and meaning beyond all the personal hardships and limitations of space-time reality.

Psychedelics like psilocybin can defamiliarize the familiar, opening awareness to states of consciousness that seriously question modern-day emphasis on physical matter, reorientating the initiand toward the invisible, energetic dimensions of reality. Yet, how can Ilana live a full life between these two worlds? This dance between transcendence and immanence represents a difficult marriage: between the world of trauma, with unbearable pain and suffering, and the realm of the numinous. How does she manage to live a full life between these two worlds and how is this possible, without either world used as an escape from the other? If, as ancient wisdom teaches, the individual and cosmic soul are one, then the real potential in psychedelic-enhanced psychotherapy lies in a bridging of transcendence with immanence, a relinking of wave and particle, of spirit and matter, a remembering of our undivided wholeness.

Introducing a new medicine into the analytic container requires long preparation. Although we both knew that this was the right path forward, how to proceed was uncertain. Again, this would require stepping out onto the edge of the unknown—to invite this medicine into our field and to learn together how to receive its wisdom without either one of us ingesting the material substance. This phase represents another shift away from a medical model of *using* medicines, toward relating to them, honoring their sacred knowledge. This relational cosmology recognizes the plants as intelligent entities, living conscious beings—and that *right relationship* with the plants, other beings, ourselves, and the planet is integral to health and healing.

Since going completely blind, Ilana was struggling with the visual, auditory, and tactile hallucinations brought on by her neurological syndrome. Rather than viewing the hallucinations as yet another disturbing symptom to be treated or gotten rid of, we have decided to work with the messages coming through the visionary and sensory experiences, as if on the actual substance of psilocybin.

As we begin to recover the sacred in her painful life, we are also reclaiming other lost gifts. *Songlines* of my ancestors, have emerged, compelling me to reach down to the *root-voice*, to learn its sounds and melodies, to guide us on this unfamiliar journey. Dreamtime is often thought of as an Australian Aboriginal phenomenon, though there is an *Irish Dreamtime* and its *Celtic songline* teaches that "out of a healed past a healed present will grow" (Moriarity, 1999, p. viii). This long-forgotten memory of how we heal, that flows through "*not I, not I, but the wind that blows through me*" is what I aspire to share with Ilana in the energetic field (Lawrence, 1994, p. 195).

Conclusion

We carry our ancestors molecularly and suffer without adequate sacred ritual to link, guide, and liberate us through eternal time. In the words of James Baldwin: *"People are trapped in history and history is trapped in them"* (Baldwin, 1998 p. 294).

I offer this chapter as an *aisling*, a Gaelic word that means dream-vision, a poem of the dispossessed who are waiting for the feminine healing waters to flow again (Moriarty, 1999, p. viii). I have thought of the work with Ilana as representing the end of a dualistic medical model focused on fixing broken body parts. The end of surviving in pieces. The vision of my thoughts floating in another's water bottle suggested that the time has come for facing into the illusion of separateness. To shift from *me* to *we*. As I drop into the depth of my own experience of healing through sacred medicine and Ilana willingly meets me in a resonant state, we are no longer bottled up in separate minds, but vibrate together in a state of oneness. If the universe is a sacred, single unbroken whole, then there is no solo self. If we are all aspects of one living being, my work then is not to fix you, but rather, to locate and heal those wounds in myself and to share the gifts and capacities of that healing in the field. By admitting the strange angels, Ilana and I find ourselves in an inner sanctuary, where identity is not the same as tragic biography, a place where she is made whole once again, where both she and I are made whole and full in this Great Reciprocity.

References

Baldwin, J. (1998). *James Baldwin: Collected essays (LoA #98): Notes of a native son / Nobody knows my name / The fire next time / No name in the street / The devil finds work*. Library of America.

Bucke, R.M. (1991). *Cosmic consciousness: A study in the evolution of the human mind*. Penguin Books.

Corbin, H. (1998). *Alone with the alone: Creative imagination in the Ṣūfism of Ibn ʿArabī*. Princeton University Press.

De Vos, C.M.H., Mason, N.L., & Kuypers, K.P.C. (2021). Psychedelics and neuroplasticity: A systematic review unraveling the biological underpinnings of psychedelics. *Frontiers in Psychiatry, 12*.

Gebser, J. (1986). *The ever-present origin* (N. Barstad & A. Mickunas, Trans.). Ohio University Press.

Griffiths, R.R., Sweeney, M.G., Nayak, S., Hurwitz, E., Mitchell, L.N., & Swift, T. (2022). Comparison of psychedelic and near-death or other non-ordinary experiences in changing attitudes about death and dying. *PLOS ONE, 17*(8), e0271926.

Jung, C.G. (1977). *C.G. Jung speaking* (W. McGuire & R.F.C. Hull, Eds.). Princeton University Press.

Jung, C.G. (2015). *Letters of C.G. Jung: Vol 2, 1951–1961* (Gerhard Adler & Aniela Jaffé, Eds.). Routledge.

Kalsched, D. (2013). *Trauma and the soul: A psycho-spiritual approach to human development and Its Interruption*. Routledge.

Kingsley, P. (2018). *Catafalque (2-volume set): Carl Jung and the end of humanity*. Catafalque Press.

Kingsley, P. (2020). *REALITY*. Catafalque Press.

Lawrence, D.H. (1994). *The complete poems of D.H. Lawrence*. Wordsworth Editions.

Levy, P. (2018). *The quantum revelation: A radical synthesis of science and spirituality*. Select Books.

Lewis, T., Amini, F., & Lannon, R. (2007). *A general theory of love*. Random House of Canada.

Merwin, W.S. (1969, January). Words from a totem animal. *The Atlantic*. https://www.theatlantic.com/magazine/archive/1969/01/words-from-a-totem-animal/660904/ (Last Accessed 7/8/23).

Merwin, W.S. (2009) *The Shadow of Sirius*. (n.d.). Copper Canyon Press.

Mithoefer, M.C., Wagner, M.C., Mithoefer, A.T., Jerome, L., & Doblin, R. (2010). The safety and efficacy of ±3,4-methyl-enedioxymethamphetamine-assisted psychotherapy in subjects with chronic, treatment-resistant posttraumatic stress disorder: The first randomized controlled pilot study. *Journal of Psychopharmacology, 25*(4), 439–452.

Moriarty, J. (1999). *Dreamtime*. The Lilliput Press.

Powers, R. (2021). *Bewilderment: A novel*. W. W. Norton & Co.

Sheldrake, M. (2021). *Entangled life: How fungi make our worlds, change our minds & shape our futures*. Random House Trade Paperbacks.

Sheldrake, R. (2009). *Morphic resonance: The nature of formative causation*. Park Street Press.

Siegel, D.J., MD. (2022). *Intraconnected: MWe (Me + We) as the integration of self, identity, and belonging*. National Geographic Books.

Stevens, W. (1937, May). The man with the blue guitar. *Poetry, L*(ii), 61.

Tarnas, R. (2006). *Cosmos and psyche: Intimations of a new worldview*. Penguin.

Teicholz, J.G., Kriegman, D.H., & Fairfield, S. (Eds.). (1998). *Trauma, repetition, and affect regulation: The work of Paul Russell*. Other Press.

Weisberger, J.M. (2013). *Rainforest medicine: Preserving indigenous science and biodiversity in the Upper Amazon*. North Atlantic Books.

Williams, S.G. (2017). The unbearable weight of truth: Carrie in *Homeland. Jung Journal: Culture & Psyche, 11*(3), 26–42.

Williams, S.G. (2018). Awakening to inter-subjectivity: Working with autism spectrum disorders. In A. Punnett (Ed.), *Jungian child analysis* (pp. 157–182). Fisher King Press.

Endnotes

[1] *Empathogens* or *entactogens* are a class of psychoactive substances that produce experiences of emotional communion, oneness, relatedness, emotional openness—that is, empathy or sympathy—as particularly observed and reported for experiences with 3,4-methylenedioxymethamphetamine (MDMA). MDMA is also popularly known as Ecstasy or Molly. An *entheogen* is a psychoactive, hallucinogenic substance or preparation (such as psilocybin or ayahuasca) especially when derived from plants or fungi and used in religious, spiritual, or ritualistic contexts.

The Combination Method: Use of Ketamine as an Adjunct to Analytic Treatment

Linda Carter and I. Joseph McFadden

Over the past three years, we have met weekly to discuss analytically oriented treatment in conjunction with infusions of ketamine, administered by a physician apart from the clinical hour. In this chapter, we offer a brief overview of the history and pharmacological actions of ketamine. Case material provides grounding for the theoretical ideas that we have co-constructed as collaborating peer supervisors. Remarkable is the evident improvement in depressive and dissociative symptoms, along with dramatic diminishment in suicidal ideation previously unrelieved by psychotherapy and/or antidepressant trials. For some, these improvements are apparent even after the first infusion. Ketamine appears to open portals into unconscious healthy aspects that have been foreclosed upon by what we call the "trauma complex" amongst those suffering under the enormous duress of protracted depression, bipolar disorder and post-traumatic stress disorder. The synthesizing effects of the ketamine/ analysis combination (hereafter referred to as the *combination method*) has extended the durability with our patients, very much in keeping with Jungian notions of integration moving toward an emergent sense of Self, hard won.

Current literature and research have not yet addressed the possibilities of what long-term analytical treatment may offer in extending the durability of ketamine, a well-known problem with this agent. For example, ketamine has been used in major teaching hospital emergency rooms to treat acute suicidal thinking; however, relief of this symptom may last only two to four weeks, and with limited follow-up resources, patients then present again for urgent intervention. The combination method has been effective in expanding the durability with our limited number of patients.

To demonstrate the synergistic value of the ketamine/analytic approach, we will use the case study method of research. Basic training and knowledge of ketamine's pharmacokinetics, potential side effects and limits, along with benefits, is essential for practitioners interested in a combination model such as what we have been developing. Ketamine assisted therapy (KAT) provided by practitioners during and after ketamine administration is not what we are putting forward. Our goal is to synthesize pharmacological understanding with analytic process and reflect on outcomes.

There are many pathways into the unconscious and we will address how ketamine helps to expand what Siegel calls the "window of tolerance," a banded state of regulation between hyper- and hypo-arousal (2020). Entering a regulated state within the window of tolerance can be difficult for those plagued by unrelenting emotional surges characterized by fluctuating amplitudes of fight/flight and/or freezing. As a result, psychoanalytic process is compromised in major ways. To work through past overwhelming, embodied memories, the analyst and patient must become aware of what Ogden (2006) (drawing from the work of Wilbarger and Wilbarger (1997)) describes as an "optimal arousal zone," attending to the need for sensitive titration of small amounts of past distress in order to avoid re-traumatization. Ketamine's regulating influence helps open space for therapeutic engagement not previously accessible.

Central Hypothesis

In trying to understand why a dissociative agent assists those suffering dissociation, we hypothesize that ketamine may "anesthetize" what we designate as the *trauma complex,* by calming the nervous system so work can be done to expand alternative self-state experiences, shore up ego capacities, strengthen reflective function, and importantly, restore a sense of meaning and vitality. From our view, active imagination is not possible during an infusion but can be employed within the analytic container afterward as a valuable method that allows for integration of the ketamine experience as well as integration of parts not previously accessible for treatment.

Ketamine Pharmacology

History

For a succinct review of ketamine pharmacology, we have drawn from a review by Zanos et al., (2018). Ketamine is a derivative of phenylcyclohexylamine (Adams et al., 1978) that first became available for human use in 1970 as a rapid acting intravenous anesthetic (Dundee et al., 1970). It was derived from phencyclidine (known as PCP or on the streets as "Angel Dust"), in order to lessen serious side effects typically brought on by hallucinogenic mental states described as psychomimetic (mimicking psychosis) and psychodysleptic (meaning psychedelic effects involving dissociation, depersonalization, vivid dreams, and hallucinations "sometimes involving outer space"[1] (Domino et al., 1965; Domino, 2010; Mion, 2017). Production of PCP was stopped in 1968 due to side effects and abuse potential, but research on its derivative ketamine, thought to be safer than PCP, persisted with first clinical studies published in 1965 (Mion & Villevieille, 2013).

Anesthetic, Psychological, Anti-inflammatory and Analgesic Effects

The primary anesthetic effects of ketamine include dissociation, catalepsy, pain relief, and unconsciousness, with cardiovascular and respiratory stability when used as a general anesthetic (Kohtala, 2012; White, 1982; Zanos et al., 2018). Of importance for therapists is ketamine's non-anesthetic properties showing psychological ramifications apparent in significant abatement of depressive symptoms. Ketamine can be a substantial adjunct to psychotherapy because it has significant effects on treatment resistant depression (Zanos et al., 2018; Zarate et al., 2006) and relieves symptoms of PTSD (Liriano et al., 2019). In addition, it provides pain relief and anti-inflammatory effects (Loix et al., 2011; Nikkheslat, 2021). Inflammation has been shown to be a part of treatment-resistant depressive syndromes (Lee & Guiliani, 2019). Pain and depression are often comorbid conditions that have similar underlying neurological connections (Bonilla-Jaime et al., 2022).

Neuroplasticity, Synaptogenesis and Rapid Antidepressant Action

Although the exact mechanisms of ketamine's impact on depressive symptom relief remain elusive (Kohalta, 2021), animal models have shown that this agent produces robust markers of neuroplasticity in depression-relevant brain regions. It increases the number, function and plasticity of synapses that have been diminished due to stress and depression; research using neuroimaging may help to further specify the intricacies of ketamine's influence on human brain pathology, function and repair (Kopelman et al., 2023). In concurrence, Wu et al. (2021) propose that the biological basis for ketamine's *rapid therapeutic action*, may have to do with this seeming ability to promote "synaptogenesis in brain regions such as the medial frontal cortex and hippocampus, countering the dendritic atrophy and synapse loss associated with chronic stress and depression." In other words, such influences may facilitate adaptive rewiring of damaged and pathological neurocircuitry (Collo, 2018). This is highly relevant as the increase in number of synapses and their greater flexibility, along with complex rewiring induced by ketamine, may also relate to greater emotional and cognitive flexibility and connectivity in psychotherapy.

Glutamate Systems

Of further note from the scientific literature, major depressive disorder has been associated with glutamate, the principal excitatory neurotransmitter in the brain and glutamatergic mechanisms play a significant role in nearly all key functions affected by depressed states (Khoodoruth et al., 2022). Biologically, ketamine's ability to affect glutamate results in a cascade of interactions leading to increased neurogenesis and neuroplasticity that ultimately resets the brain to a healthier state (Ko, 2019). The relationship between glutamate and ketamine is of consequence in appreciating the rapid alleviation of depression for responders within 24 hours after administration (Dutta et al., 2015). Ketamine's actions on glutamate systems are different from currently prescribed antidepressants intended to specifically target the serotonin and norepinephrine systems, which take much longer for symptom relief and are ineffective for many people (Khoordoruth et al., 2022; Singh & Gottlib, 2014). In addition to ketamine's influence on glutamatergic systems, ketamine also influences the default mode network (DMN), another brain system that requires some consideration.

Default Mode Network (DMN) and Task Positive Network (TPN)]

A brief review of the biology and function of the DMN and how ketamine may interact with this network to relieve treatment resistant depression is summarized in the following. In brief, the DMN is a large-scale, associational cortical network linked with internal mentation, known for increased activity when externally oriented task performance is not required (Shofty et al., 2022). The DMN was studied by Raichle, et al. who published their results in 2007. They used positron emission tomography scans (PET) to confirm that "the frontal lobe is most active when a person is not doing anything," labeling this system the "DMN, comprising the medial fronto-parietal cortex, the posterior cingulate gyrus, the precuneus, and the angular gyrus" (Nasrallah, 2023). This interwoven network has many functions and the following offer some of the various descriptions in lay terms: "daydreaming," "autopilot," "mind-wandering," "self-reflection," the "neurological basis of the self," and the "seat of literary creativity" (Nasrallah, 2023). The DMN is inversely related to another brain network, the "attention network" also known as the "task positive network" (TPN); The TPN is aroused during activities such as text messaging, playing video games or continuously interacting with social media, while the DMN activity declines (Nasrallah, 2023).

It has been found that those who are struggling with depression and PTSD have high levels of DMN activity at resting states that have been associated with maladaptive rumination (Hamilton, et al., 2011; 2015) and negative internal preoccupations. With evidence accumulated from a variety of studies, Gatusso et al. (2023) see associations between the ability of psychedelics to reduce functional connectivity within the DMN and increase connectivity to other networks, ultimately culminating in positive therapeutic outcomes. In other words, when administered in doses that alter consciousness, ketamine decreases the connectivity within the DMN, with subsequent calming of relentless depressive thoughts and feelings; further, it increases between-network connectivity (Gatusso et al., 2023). As a result, there seems to be a decrease in the segregation of brain regions; it follows then, that a less segregated, modular brain shifts to a more interconnected global network, potentially leading to sensations of interconnection and wholeness not previously possible due to depression, possibly inflammation, etc. This decrease in inter-network segregation is not present with selective serotonin reuptake inhibitors, stimulants, sedatives or MDMA antidepressants (Gatusso, 2023). The influence of ketamine on the DMN related to numinous experiences of oneness and mystical connections to the universe will be explored later in the paper.

Second Set of Hypotheses: Bringing Together Neuroscience and Clinical Applications within the Combination Method

We hypothesize that both the biological and functional brain changes stimulated by ketamine infusions resonate with an increase in connections within the analytic relationship. The research findings and hypotheses noted above have resonated with our observations of four patients within the combination method context. We have witnessed post-infusion manifestations including increased flexibility, movement and interaction with internal figures and images (via active imagination), as well as expansion of interpersonal relatedness and capacity for reflection. Ketamine has significantly helped relativize constricting trauma complexes so that opportunities for alternative self-state aspects can emerge. It seems to offer neurobiological glue for people who struggle with fragmentation and lays the ground for relational interactions. In resonance, Siegel offers a valuable thought: cohesion in the moment, if repeated, promotes coherency of self over time (2020, p. 84), very helpful for patients and fortifying for those of us working with them.

In addition, we might wonder if the confluence of ketamine's ability to calm an affectively dysregulated nervous system and reduce depressive rumination may allow space for creative daydreaming and imagination that enhance play within one's own mind. Shofty et al.

(2022) propose that interactions between the DMN and areas such as the salience and executive networks, together may underlie creative thinking. This makes sense, given that creative thinking necessitates integration of multimodal information and seemingly unrelated thought processes in conjunction with introspective capacities that characterize the DMN, such as its ability to mediate spontaneous cognition, or the stream of consciousness, as well as its capacity for flexible retrieval of memories and generation of ideas (Shofty et al., 2022). It seems likely that if the DMN is loaded with disturbing anxieties, it is not in a resting state open for healthy arousal and therefore, not available for internal interconnections and subsequent creative manifestations.

Side Effects and Potential Problems

Ketamine has physiological actions on the sympathetic nervous system and can produce palpitations, tachycardia, and hypertension when used for the treatment of depression. Most of the side effects of ketamine are dose dependent, transient, and are usually self-resolving (Zanos et al., 2018). However, urinary and bladder problems (now known as ketamine-induced cystitis) have been reported, especially by those who dose at home or buy ketamine on the streets for recreational purposes (Anderson et al., 2022; Srirangam & Mercer, 2012). Chronic users may undergo frequent cognitive disturbances, as well as frontal white matter abnormalities (Mion & Villevieille, 2013).

In 1999, pharmaceutical ketamine became a Schedule III controlled substance under the Controlled Substances Act, however "according to recent national survey, non-medical misuse is still relatively low, as 0.7% of the US population uses ketamine illegally" (Geoffrion & Thomas, 2022). Nemerov (2018) citing Schak et al. (2016) states that "ketamine remains a significant drug of abuse in the US and elsewhere." Nemeroff (2018) goes on to articulate concerns about the use of ketamine: limited randomized control studies; lack of regulation and oversight of ketamine clinics that may not comply with minimum recommendations from the APA task force consensus report; limited durability; and limitations of the current ketamine data base. The long-term effects of ongoing use of ketamine have yet to be determined. Gerard Sanacora, from the Yale School of Medicine emphasizes his biggest concern about ketamine treatment: "It is critical for it to be a part of a comprehensive mental health plan, not in isolation" (as cited in Backman 2023). A clinical anecdote of concern: with ongoing infusions, one of our patients developed numbness in finger tips, toes, tongue, and lips that has not abated, although it had done so after several previous infusions. He was evaluated by a neurologist who could not give a clear diagnosis. No other reports of this problem in relation to ketamine have surfaced in the literature *to date.*

Clinical Case I: Joe McFadden

We have observed that the addition of ketamine markedly and rapidly (within hours) improves depressive symptoms previously unrelieved by either psychotherapy and/or use of antidepressant medication. A major additional effect has been an ability to view well known historical trauma material from a new perspective. The ketamine experiences appeared to facilitate work we had done with patients from the perspective of Schwartz on Internal Family Systems Therapy (1997), similar to active imagination. Each of the analytic patients had been on a combination of antidepressants, mood stabilizers, and/or third generation neuroleptics. Each continued to suffer from ongoing high levels of depression, anxiety, and problematic interpersonal relationships. An understanding of their traumatic backgrounds, and their impact on current functioning, had done little to relieve these symptoms. Negative self-attributions and self-blaming continued prominently. Thus, a series of weekly ketamine infusions were instituted. During or following these infusions there were described differing states of consciousness, if not overt psychedelic trips.

Mrs. C., an attorney, married with three adult children, presented with a history of life-long depression. She dated the onset of her depression to age seven when her father abandoned her, her mother and two siblings. Her mother was depressed, paranoid, and an alcoholic, and was verbally, emotionally, physically, and sexually abusive to her. Within a year or so of her father leaving, Mrs. C. recognized that she was essentially totally on her own with no adult upon whom she could depend. Her relationships with both her mother and siblings were stormy. Her high I.Q. and academic performance resulted in major jealousy and aggression from her siblings but provided at least a partial escape from the family dynamics. To try to be freer from her family of origin, she married while still in college. She worked professionally for a number of years. After the birth of her third child, she became quite depressed and required electroconvulsive therapy. Concomitant with her depression, she suffered from several different medical problems: asthma, irritable bowel syndrome, and migraine headaches. She also suffered from recurrent nightmares relating to her early childhood traumas, and her now deceased mother returning. Repeated depressive spirals regularly resulted from her husband's angry, accusing, abusive behaviors.

We began three times per week analytic therapy on the couch. In the ensuing months her depression lifted but was not absent. The frequency of her nightmares involving her mother, previously quite frequent, decreased. Her somatic symptoms, particularly the migraine headaches, were unimproved, as was her relationship with her husband. The continued regular stressful interactions with her husband constituted ongoing re-traumatization. Much of the therapy was an attempt to look realistically at that relationship. Her self-blame for the problematic marriage fluctuated but continued as a major issue. About 18 months into the analysis, I broached the subject of a trial of ketamine. Her level of depression and somatic issues were of such severity that they were interfering with her ability to fulfill professional responsibilities, and any realistic attempt to make a life for herself outside the marriage.

With the addition of ketamine, there was a rapid lifting of the depressive mood. More slowly, but noticeably, the ongoing attempts at examining the marital conflicts shifted. Mrs. C. ceased negating her understanding about her husband's part in their difficulties. She even began to accept that some of her own negative behaviors could be understood from the perspective of that with which she had to contend. She became able to have brief internal conversations with younger child parts in my presence. I never made any attempt directly to communicate with the inner parts but did at times suggest ideas or make comments that she might consider making to those internal parts. Sufficient improvement resulted in ending the ketamine infusions after seven months.

Several months later, Mrs. C. was confronted with another major stress and loss. She became more depressed than at any time since I had been working with her. A decision was made to resume the ketamine. We met within two hours following her second ketamine treatment of this series. She was able to describe her first clear experience of a visually altered state of consciousness, one in which she saw herself as dead, a brick being placed in a wall, and saw the total waste and futility of her life. In a synchronistic experience during this session, she received a text telling her of the death of a close friend. Her immediate response was one of the usual self-recrimination and sense of worthlessness. However, drawing on her past history of trauma and losses, we were able to consider her inappropriate response to this new loss, and to make linkages to many earlier losses that previously were not possible for her to process. Imagery arising from the ketamine session was understood as representing the need for old ways of identifying and thinking to be allowed to die. While this seemed important, over a period of time, it became clear that Mrs. C. had encased herself in a mummified numbness and went about her life denying any emotional significance to any stress. The focus of our work shifted even more to the split, dissociated somatosensory aspects of her life and experiences. She discussed, and even tacitly accepted this exploration, but nothing changed. She continued the ketamine infusions on a monthly basis.

Several months elapsed when she reported her first bad ketamine trip in which she experienced herself on a submarine, dropping to the bottom of the ocean to imminent death. She was terrified, began thrashing about so strongly that the nurse anesthetist entered the treatment room. They established some communication and discontinued the infusion. So disturbed were both Mrs. C and the anesthetist that the attending physician was summoned, and he prescribed that future doses of ketamine should be reduced.

Contrary to their opinion, I heard of an intense sensory/emotional experience, without the consuming numbness, and emphasized the importance of having those feelings and sensations. To me, it was important that she had had an intense experience at all. We then worked on finding some positive experience from the past, one that could serve as a containing, grounding, somewhat secure, base-like memory that could counter the negative thoughts and feelings that dominated her inner world. That it would have a positive sensory component seemed critical to me. This was not easy, but we had some success. It did appear that the ketamine assisted in her ability to develop both imagery and a narrative of an anchor from the past.

There followed a remarkable improvement. Her physical appearance changed. She went from a wooden, nondescript woman, to one who started appearing lively and thoughtful about her appearance. Not only did her mood improve dramatically, but there was a major lessening of her somatic symptoms. Her need for medications previously prescribed to be taken as needed for her medical symptoms almost disappeared. She also became appropriately reactive and engaged with issues with her children.

Several weeks later, she brought another dream, a nightmare of her deceased mother. She and several other women dressed in black were trying to kill Mrs. C. She fought back, escaped, and awoke. She reported the dream feeling confused. Nothing bad had happened the day before. In fact, she had a rather pleasant and rewarding day at work and at home. I suggested that this negative mother dream had come to represent the dissociative-splitting structure in her psyche. Her positive changes and experiences now threatened this dissociative structure, as described similarly by Bromberg (2011) in *Shadow of the Tsunami*. Her being sensorially alive was now the dream stimulus. After considerable silence, she stated that this felt right. Her ensuing clinical course, emotional and physical, has continued stable and improved.

Discussion

In essence, Mrs. C., a survivor of severe developmental and ongoing marital trauma extensively used body-mind dissociation as a regular coping mechanism. There was an ongoing deficit in her ability to alpha-process (Bion, 1962), or use sensory or emotional stimuli in the development of symbols, thoughts, or narratives. Instead, in her detached state, she was victim to unchanging self-derogations, predictions of failure and loss, and psychic fragmentation that flooded her psyche. Beta elements, described by Bion (1962) as the consequence of impairment of alpha-processing, played havoc with her psyche-soma. The transcendent function could not take place. Mind-body dissociation severely interfered with her perception of reality and her ability to use that reality in adapting to life and its stresses. The addition of ketamine, as part of the ongoing analytic, containing relationship, assisted in some resetting of her psychic functions. She could then allow thoughts from the analyst to circulate without destroying them or her own awareness of that which she experienced. She could allow herself to know sensory and emotional reality, and use it in adapting to life.

Clinical Case II: Linda Carter

Context: Jungian Perspectives, Trauma and the Essential Value of Play

The fundamental archetypal underpinnings of this paper have to do with fragmentation/integration and contraction/expansion. With these core abstract concepts in mind, I will offer case material along with theoretical perspectives as to how and why ketamine can be an enormously helpful adjunct: the context is the therapeutic dyad with a *well-established attachment relationship* developed over time, in part, via "disruption" and valuable moments of "repair," (Beebe and Lachmann, 2002) not readily available in the patient's family of origin. The ongoing nature of the depth-oriented analytic container provided by the combination method is in contrast to counseling offered to patients by those who administer, sit with or provide brief follow-up sessions with a focus on symptom relief and the journey experience itself. We see ketamine as an intervention that ameliorates profound suffering, provides a re-set and opens portals into self-state experiences previously constricted by trauma, depression, or bipolar disorder as it creates space for expansion and unfolding of the personality. Our interest is not in ketamine per se but as an aid to look both at retrospective issues limiting our patients' full functioning as well as on prospective possibilities for an unfolding future. The analytic dyad emerges from within concentric circles or fields of influence in which we are always and forever embedded, ranging from neuronal connections to reverberations with the stars above and the Infinite as it surrounds us. Specifically, the combination method seems to clear free and open space for play, imagination, and for the recontextualizing of an individual's self-state experiences within an expanding field that can be considered as an influencing entity in and of itself.

Traumatized people have great difficulty with free play, an essential aspect of life that is diminishing globally for children and adults to the detriment of all (Carter, 2022; Yogman, et al., 2018). Access to open play space is limited by anxieties related to safety evident in hyper-focused attention and vigilance fueled by affect dysregulation, preventing creativity internally and in the field. Many patients experience "the dog chasing its tail complex" with a compulsive press for return to traumatic memories. Entrenched internalized interaction patterns, usually outside conscious awareness within the implicit, non-conscious domain, play out through circular iterations that reinforce dominating pathological neural pathways.

Given such circumstances, the imaginal field has collapsed under the weight of excruciating partial memories and bodily sensations. Ketamine seems to breath air into a flattened system, a world of either black or white, one of deadness lacking in vitality. The process of dissolution of the trauma and ego complexes during ketamine journeys, along with suspension of thick defenses, together allow distance from the extremes of intense and fluctuating emotions; it becomes possible to enter a field of pleasant chaos, very different in nature from the disintegrating chaos that goes along with affect dysregulation. With subsequent symptom relief and a nervous system not so easily triggered, play, paradox and ultimately symbol formation become possible within the analytic container. Free play, of necessity, requires open space and a certain amount of unpredictability and chaos therein, leading to creativity and the beginnings of vitality. *Free play, chaos, imagination, and creativity go together.*

The ketamine journey itself induces a restful dream-like state, similar in some ways to what can be known within the transitional space described by Winnicott (1971). It seems to be one of usually agreeable chaos with morphing colors, shapes, and images but most often, without words, cognitive thoughts, or a specific narrative coherence. In fact, it has been reported that trying to remember what is seen in the journey by employing ego consciousness or cognitive processing, disrupts and sidetracks the unfolding immersion. Interestingly, following a tour through a ketamine world where the patient is an observer of moving, changing visual presences, patients report a sense of cohesion and stability not felt moments prior to the infusion. With protection from the trauma complex now anesthetized, the patient is in a relaxed state similar to that of REM sleep (and that has been shown to be similar to the relaxed state in free -play (Carter, 2022[2]); the field is open for visitors, both as helpers as well as those who are troubled but who are now able to dialogue with the analyst. Such new elements, perhaps not fully formulated as complexes, can be felt as body sensations exerting energies that further expand the field of influence.

From an alchemical angle, through the operation of *solutio*, what has been fixed is dissolved, allowing for awareness of an expanded surround and a loosening of tension so that engagement in options leading ultimately to reconfiguration is possible. Along the lines of Schwartz's Internal Family Systems (1997), various parts are invited to the table for conversation thus relativizing the disempowered trauma complex. As a result, with support and relational attention, scaffolding can be constructed around the black hole of trauma that is never completely eradicated but that can be better contained, thereby allowing creative space for a more cohesive life narrative to be written.

Arthur's Journeys, Dreams, Imaginings and Memories

In this section, I will describe the experiences of immersion in open space and the numinous as described by a long-term patient, along with subsequent changes in capacity for connectedness and free play.

Arthur is a successful, professional man in late middle age who has been involved in analysis multiple times a week over many years for treatment of depression, historical family trauma, and for ongoing severe crises with an ill family member. Due to a confluence of life changes, he fell into a black depression with the re-emergence of dominant trauma complexes. His new psychiatrist recommended ketamine.

Weighed down by psychomotor retardation, Arthur was barely able to walk in the door for the first treatment but hopeful about this intervention within the relational context of his doctor's care and ongoing analysis with me. He consistently described meaningful altered states of consciousness, with only one that was anxiety provoking and frightening. On this occasion, his doctor was not able to attend the infusion and was unexpectedly replaced by an unknown practitioner in a different room. His psychiatrist's presence had provided a necessary secure base, important when in states of partial paralysis and dissolution of mental structures.

Set and Setting

The usual setting was a home-like room, not a sterile hospital environment. Lights were dimmed, scented candles lit, and Chagall prints were within the visual field of the soft leather couch where the patient laid supine under a weighted blanket. Similar to this careful attention to the milieu provided by Arthur's physician, Muscat and colleagues (2023) who offer an integrative approach, emphasize the importance of a physical surrounding that invites focus of attention on inner states. The visual, auditory, and sensate distortions that emerge at doses lower than those causing anesthesia, allowing for therapeutic benefits, can be felt as disturbing to some but can be mitigated and managed, by creating a neutral or positive atmosphere. For example, music can be an important component in maintaining a positive emotional tone (Muscat et al., 2023).

Arthur described the containing presence of his doctor and the cocoon-like surround as inviting, enhanced by Chopin's *Nocturne Op. 9. No. 2* that offered auditory continuity. Other pieces were felt to be too disruptive. The rhythmic and tonal familiarity as well as the beauty of this music without lyrics, deepened and supported the process of emotional quietude where visual, imagistic, and auditory experiences were part of an unfolding surround where language was not predominant.

Immersion: Belonging within the *Unus Mundus*

Within minutes of the intramuscular injection, the anesthetic effects took hold, dampening body movement that limited the possibility of speech. Embedded within an unknown but fascinating world that seemed archetypal in nature rather than personal, Arthur felt as if he were an observer on a guided tour, not of his own determining. He watched as morphing shapes, colors, seemingly biological forms, sculptures, and faces moved through. Often, arial views as if from a plane, gave perspective on large expanses of earth and water below. From conscious memory, he had never before witnessed what was revealed to him during these rides through uncharted lands.

The specifics of what actually was witnessed during the trips was not necessary; of utmost value was the overall sense of "belonging" (to be differentiated from attachment which is more dyadic in nature) where he felt his very being was woven into the fabric of something much larger, universal. These descriptions seem similar to neuroscientist Daniel Siegel's view of the mind as "non-local" and not simply "enskulled" (2020, p. 8). Siegel's idea that the system of mind is both embodied and relational, within and between, and that we all are embedded within "mind" feels quite resonant with Jung's prescient notions about the collective unconscious and rhizomatic interconnections through the *unus mundus*. The psyche is both individual/internal and all-encompassing as it surrounds us; the Jungian Self is, simultaneously, the center and the circumference.

Opening to the Depths: Religious Function of the Psyche

Reflecting on his ketamine excursions, Arthur felt a resonance with Jung's stories of confrontation with ghostly ancestors in 1916 (1916/2009) that opened to both the fascinating and terrifying presence of the Infinite. He could appreciate Jung's attempts to cope with anxieties of dissipation into an all-encompassing cosmos through the grounding and containing physical actions of creating organizing structures, including drawing his first mandala, *Systema Munditotius* and writing *Seven Sermons to the Dead*, a brief text that Jung saw as fundamental to all of his future explorations (1916). It is as if Jung entered trance states allowing for engagement with deep layers of the unconscious without the infusion of a chemical agent. Similarly, Arthur was fascinated by the expanse opened to him outside conscious volition and felt gratitude for the biological healing effects of ketamine on symptoms, as well as gratitude for renewal of his spiritual essence. Ketamine opened a portal into alternative worlds and an emergent presence of a multiplicity of selves. He connected to a depth of *knowing*: not just personal knowing, but a knowing awareness and a sense of being and belonging within a mystical universal context, not easy to articulate in words.

Infinity

Although active imagination or seeking symbolic significance during his internal immersions could not take place, interactions with emergent dream figures and with the analyst were freed up in the aftermath, along with significant memories never before shared analytically. Such was the case when Arthur recalled the following: During nursery school nap time as a four-year old, he looked up to see a picture of Jesus with the little children. He asked his elderly teacher, "If God, Joseph and Mary were Jesus's parents, who were God's parents?" The dumbfounded lady deferred to their pastor who was soon to come through on daily rounds. On arrival, the kindly man knelt and responded in an amazingly sophisticated way: "God is infinity, like all the stars in the sky. There are stars and behind the stars are more stars and more stars...." Awestruck, Arthur spent the rest of naptime and, indeed, the rest of his lifetime pondering the picture of stars beyond stars, beyond stars...

Witch Dream: What if the Tether Breaks?

A dream, also never before discussed prior to ketamine emerged: as a slightly older child, about seven or eight, he dreamt of a wicked witch who cast a spell whereby he could only walk forward. A terrifying realization was awakened: he would not ever return to his home and his mother's care. This memory correlated with dawning consciousness at that time of his mother's inability/unwillingness to protect him from his father's abusive behavior. He amplified emotions felt as a child in the present analytic moment through the image of a single astronaut tethered to a spaceship with the earth far away in the background. *What if the tether breaks?*

Despite the intensity of emotion, the field had become vibrant and alive, quite different from the sense of stuckness that had previously prevailed. The process of raveling and unraveling the emotional threads related to the image of an untethered astronaut could commence with caution and in small increments over time. A felt resonance between Arthur and myself emerged as I was drawn in by the somatic countertransference that gripped me at multiple levels: body, mind and soul. At first, he expressed overwhelming fears of utter abandonment that seemed at the core of his lifelong struggles with depression and PTSD, but given our substantial history, companionship came forth mediating what had previously been kept at a distance as an "unthought known" (Bollas 2018). Eventually, cognitive understanding and reflection could be paired with emotions, mediated and then dissipated within a regulating safe-enough context of collaboration, so that he was not alone with powerful, archetypal forces.

Arthur, like Jung in some ways, encountered both the fascination and terror of the awesome and numinous qualities of the Infinite that came into play with ketamine. Memories ignited archetypal energies in the present moment, taking shape and form such as the untethered astronaut so that metabolization at the human level could become a shared analytic process. Ketamine opened a portal for the emergence of a reverberating, multi-layered field of influence, now possible because their shared, co-created, ego-supportive companionship could hold this formidable memory. Collaborative insights evolved from synaptic connections leading to relational connections and ultimately to an expansion of the Self and remembrance of soul as it exists within and between.

Crossing into Death During Infusions

One final anecdote from Arthur, regarding the numinous qualities of ketamine, has to do with two separate occasions when he experienced himself "not as dying but as dead." As reported, this was not at all frightening but reassuring as he simply "crossed over" into another reality, not better or worse, not clearly defined but an easy shift into a state of being within the Infinite. The word *dead* and the letters therein made absolutely no sense and were not needed as they held no significance when transitioning to a world beyond. Arthur felt a persistent sense of deep peace subsequent to his "knowing" encounters with the ineffable.

Ketamine, Numinosity and Science

Scientists, such as Gatusso et al. (2023) and others (Letheby and Gerrans, 2017; Mason et al., 2020), acknowledge that psychedelics induce meaningful, mystical experiences and ego dissolution, as well as a relaxation of subject-object distinctions during which the borders and constraints of the self dissolve. Ego dissolution is considered as central for unitive, mystical states and oneness with nature that may be therapeutic because "an individual's cognitive attributions and affect are viewed with greater distance and objectivity" (Gatusso et al., 2023). Decreased precision with previously held beliefs lends to revision of self and the world (Stoliker and colleagues, 2022, cited in Gatusso et al., 2023). Neurobiological interactions set in motion by ketamine's ability to increase interconnectivity between the DMN and other systems, in addition to its ability for decreasing brain segregation with shifts to a more global network, as noted, may open to "oceanic feelings"[3] and a sense of oneness described as a significant element of psychedelic treatment. The combination of systemic shifts along with ego dissolution (and from our view, dissolution of the trauma complex), may allow the brain/mind greater access to an expanded repertoire of meta-stable sub-states allowing for increased flexibility (Gatusso et al., 2023). This is of interest to us as analysts who have witnessed the emergence of healthy self-state complexes, following ketamine infusions. Review of the literature in conjunction with our clinical observations, point to the need for further study of psychedelics, ketamine and the DMN as potentially central in widening our appreciation of neural, relational and spiritual correspondences that resonate in circular fashion from synaptic connections to the Infinite as mutually influential.

Conclusion

In keeping with Complex Adaptive Systems (CAS) and theories of emergence, we all are always and forever embedded within concentric circles of influence, or ever expanding or contracting fields of influence from neuronal interactions to the "low-pitch hum of gravitational waves reverberating across the universe" that scientists see as "the collective echo of pairs of supermassive black holes" that are metaphorically described as a "choir or an orchestra" (Miller, 2023). We are influenced by the stars above as well as by synaptic connections, or lack thereof. The humming of galaxies is outside conscious awareness as are early memories stored as body sensations. (Is it possible that during the ketamine journey, patients enter not only their personal vibrations but the vibrations of the universe, as well?) In addition, implicit non-verbal communication is also usually outside conscious awareness but according to Daniel Stern et al. (1998) this domain shapes explicit verbal interactions. These are field phenomena that impact all of life, not only human life, and that are sometimes made manifest and visible but more often are invisible, powerfully holding sway over interactions from the microcosm to the macrocosm and back again. *The point here is that ketamine not only makes relationships within and without more possible, it also disrupts and shifts the field itself.*

For those struggling with severe depression, unremitting trauma and other psychiatric maladies, ketamine combined with ongoing depth-oriented psychotherapy seems to calm the overall nervous system, thus opening portals of experience for recontextualizing suffering within an expanded sense of self from synapses to the stars above. The field itself reconfigures from one constricted with little movement to one that has increased flexibility for engagement as an open space for play and paradox, and that invites the taking in of new information and revision of perspective, leading to expansion of creativity and complexity over time.

References

Adams, J.D. Jr, Aaille, T.A., Trevor, A.J., Castgnoli, N., Jr., (1981). Studies on the biotransformation of ketamine: 1-Identification of metabolites produced in vitro from rat liver microsomal preparations. *Biomedical Mass Spectrometry, 8*(11). 731-756.

Anderson D.J., Zhou J., Cao, D., McDonald. M., Guenther, M., Hasoon, J., Viswanath, O., Kaye, A.D. & Urits, I. (2022). Ketamine-induced cystitis: A comprehensive review of the urologic effects of this psychoactive drug. *Health Psychology Research, 10*(3).

Backman, I. (2023). Ketamine: Handle with care. Yale School of Medicine. https://medicine.yale.edu/news-article/ketamine-handle-with-care/ (Last accessed: 15 July, 2023).

Beebe, B. & Lachmann, F. (2002). *Infant research and adult treatment: Co-constructing interactions*. The Analytic Press.

Bion, W.R., (1962). *Learning from experience*. Karnac Books.

Bollas, C. (2018). The shadow of the object: psychoanalysis of the unthought known. Routledge.

Bonilla-Jaime, H., Sanchez-Salcedo, J.A., Estevez-Cabrere, M.M., Molina-Jimenez, T., Cortes-Altamirano, J.L. & Alfaro-Rodriguez, A. (2022). Depression and pain: Use of antidepressants.*Current Neuropharmacology, 20*(2), 384-402.

Bromberg, P.M., (2011). *Shadow of the tsunami and the growth of the relational mind.* Taylor and Francis Group.

Carhart, R.L., Leech, R., Hellyer, P.J., Shanahan, M., Feilding, A., Tagliazucchi, E. Chiavalvo, D.R. & Nutt, D. (2014). The entropic brain: A theory of conscious states informed. *Frontiers in human neuroscience.* https://www.frontiersin.org/articles/10.3389/fnhum.2014.00020/full (Last accessed: 15 July, 2023).

Carter, L. (2022). The flux and flow of free play and paradox. *Journal of Analytical Psychology, 67 (4),* 1045-1069.

Carter, L. (2023). Going the full circle: Pattern resonance from microcosmic interactions to macrocosmic amplifications. In M. Stein (Ed.), *Jung's Red Book for our time (Volume V),* 223-252. Chiron.

Collo, G. & Merlo Pich E. (2018). Ketamine enhances structural plasticity in human dopaminergic neurons: possible relevance for treatment-resistant depression. *Neural Regeneration Research, 13*(4), 645-646.

Domino, E.F., Chodoff, P. & Corssen, G. (1965). Pharmacologic effects of CI-581, a new dissociative anesthetic, in man. *Clinical Pharmacology & Therapeutics, 6,* 279–291.

Domino, E.F. (2010). Taming the ketamine tiger. *Anesthesiology,* 113, 678-686.

Dundee, J.W., Knox, J.W., Black, G.W., Moore, J., Pandit, S.K., Bovill, J., Clarke, R.S., Love, S.H., Elliott, J., & Coppel, D.L. (1970). Ketamine as an induction agent in anaesthetics. *Lancet. 27,* 1370-1371.

Dutta, A., McKie, S. & Deakin, J.F.W. (2015). Ketamine and other potential glutamate antidepressants. *Psychiatry Research, 225*(1-2), 1-13.

Gattuso, J.J., Perkins, D., Ruffell, S., Lawrence, A.J., Hoyer, D., Jacobson, L.H., Timmermann, C., Castle, D., Rossell, S.L., Downey, L.A., Broc, A.P., Galvão Coelho, N.L., Nutt, D., & Sarris, J. (2023). Default mode network modulation by psychedelics: A systematic review. *International Journal of Neuropsychopharmacology, 26,* 155-188.

Geoffrion, L. & Thomas, S. (2022). Ketamine abuse: Addiction, effects, and treatment. *American Addiction Centers.* https://americanaddictioncenters.org/ketamine-abuse (Last Accessed: 15 July, 2023.

Hamilton, J.P., Furman, D.J., Chang, C., Thomason, M.E., Dennis, E. & Gotlib, I.H. (2011). Default-mode and task-positive network activity in major depressive disorder: Implications for adaptive and maladaptive rumination. *Biological Psychiatry, 70*(4), 327-333.

Hamilton, J.P., Farmer, M., Fogelman, P., & Gotlib, I.H. (2015). Depressive rumination, the default-mode network, and the dark matter of clinical neuroscience. *Biological Psychiatry, 78*(4), 224-230.

Jung, C.G. (2016/2009). *Seven Sermons to the Dead, The Red Book.* Norton.

Khoodoruth, M.A.S., Estudillo-Guerra, M.A., Pacheco-Barrios, K., Nyundo, A., Chapa-Koloffon, G. & Quanes, S. (2022). Gluta-matergic system in depression and its role in neuromodulatory techniques optimization, *Frontiers in Psychiatry*, 13.

Khorramzadeh, E. & Lotfy, A.O. (1973). The use of ketamine in psychiatry. *Psychosomatics, 14*(6) 344-346.

Ko, S. (2019). A beginners' guide, chronic pain, ketamine. https://www.resetketamine.com/blog/2019/7/29/a-beginners-guide-to-ketamine-infusions (Last Accessed 14 July, 2023).

Kohtala S. (2021). Ketamine-50 years in use: From anesthesia to rapid antidepressant effects and neurobiological mechanisms. *Pharmacological Reports, 73*(2), 323-345.

Kopelman, J., Keller, T.A., Panny, B., Griffo, A., Degutis, M., Spotts, C., Cruz, N., Bell, E., Do-Nguyen, K., Wallace, M.L., Mathew, S.J., Howland, R.H. & Price, R.B. (2023). Rapid neuroplasticity changes and response to intravenous ketamine: A randomized controlled trial in treatment-resistant depression. *Translational Psychiatry, 13*(159), 1-9.

Letheby, C. & Gerrans, P. (2017). Self unbound: Ego dissolution in psychedelic experience. *Neuroscience of Consciousness*, 2017(1).

Lee, C-H. & Giuliani, F. (2019). The role of inflammation in depression and fatigue. *Frontiers in Immunology, 10*,1696, 1-12.

Liriano F., Hatten, C. & Schwartz, T.L. (2019). Ketamine as treatment for post-traumatic stress disorder: A review. *Drugs in Context,* 8;8:212305.

Loix S., De Kock, M., & Henin, P. (2011). The anti-inflammatory effects of ketamine: State of the art. *Acta Anaesthesiologica Belgica., 62*(1), 47-58.

Mason, N.L., Kuypers, K.P.C., Müller, F., Reckweg, J., Tse, D.H.Y., Toennes, S.W., Hutten, N.R.P.W., Jansen, J.F.A., Stiers, P., Feilding, A. & Ramaekers, J.G. (2020). Me, myself, bye: Regional alterations in glutamate and the experience of ego dissolution with psilocybin. *Neuropsychopharmacology, 45*(12), 2003-2011.

McNamera, D. (2021). REM sleep, the default mode network, and behavioral modernity. *Psychology Today.*

Miller, K. June 23, 2023. The cosmos is thrumming with gravitational waves, astronomers find. *New York Times.*

Mion, G. (2017). History of anaesthesia: The ketamine story – past, present and future. *European Journal of Anaesthesiology, 34*((9), 571-575.

Mion, G. & Villevieille, T. (2013). Ketamine pharmacology: An update (pharmacodynamics and molecular aspects, recent findings). *CNS Neuroscience & Therapeutics, 19*(6), 370-380.

Muscat, S., Hartelius, G., Crouch, C.R. & Morin, K.W. (2021). An integrative approach to ketamine therapy may enhance multiple dimensions of efficacy: Improving therapeutic outcomes with treatment resistant depression. *Frontiers of Psychiatry*, 12.

Nasrallah, H.A. (2023). Is the contemporary mental health crisis among youth due to DMN disruption? *Current Psychiatry, 22*(6), 10-11, 21.

Nemerov, C.B. (2018). Ketamine Quo Vadis? *American Journal of Psychiatry.* 175(4), 297-299.

Nikkheslat, N. (2021). Targeting inflammation in depression: Ketamine as an anti-inflammatory antidepressant in psychiatric emergency, *Brain, Behavior, & Immunity Health*, 18.

Raichle, R.E. & Snyder, A.Z. (2007). A default mode of brain function: A brief history of an evolving idea. *Neuroimage, 37*(4),1083-1099.

Ogden, P., Minton, K., Pain, C., Siegel, D. van der Kolk, B. (Forward). (2006*). Trauma and the body: A sensorimotor approach to psychotherapy (Norton Series on Interpersonal Neurobiology) 1st Edition.* W. W. Norton & Company.

Schak K.M., Vande Voort, J.L., Johnson, E.K., Kung, S., Leung, J.G., Rasmussen, K.G., Palmer, B.A. & Frye, M.A. (2016). Potential risks of poorly monitored ketamine use in depression treatment. *American Journal of Psychiatry, 173*(3), 215-218.

Schwartz, R.C. (1997). *Internal Family Systems Therapy (The Guilford Family Therapy Series) First Edition.* The Guildford Press.

Shofty, B., Gonen, T., Bergmann, E., Mayseless, N., Korn, A., Shamay-Tsoory, S., Grossman, R., Jalon, I., Kahn, I. & Ram, Z. (2022) The default mode network is causally linked to creative thinking. *Molecular Psychiatry, 27,* 1848-1854.

Siegel, D. (1999). *The Developing Mind.* The Guilford Press.

Siegel, D. (2020). *The Developing Mind, Third Edition.* The Guilford Press.

Singh, M.K. & Gotlib I.H. (2014). The neuroscience of depression: Implications for assessment and intervention. *Behavior Research Therapy, 62,* 60-73.

Srirangam, S., & Mercer, J. (2012). Ketamine bladder syndrome: An important differential diagnosis when assessing a patient with persistent lower urinary tract symptoms. *British Medical Journal,* 2012.

Stoliker, D. Egan, G.F., Friston, K.J., & Razi, A. (2022). Neural mechanisms and psychology of psychedelic ego dissolution. *Pharmacological Reviews, 74*(4), 876-917.

White, P.F., Way, W.L. & Trevor, A.J. (1982) Ketamine--its pharmacology and therapeutic uses. *Anesthesiology.* 56(2), 119-136. *https://api. semanticscholar.org/CorpusID:45920011*

Wilbarger, P. & Wilbarger, J. (1997). *Sensory defensiveness and related social emotional and neurological problems.* Van Nuys.

Winnicott, D.W. (1971) *Playing and Reality.* Routledge.

Yogman M., Garner, A. & Hutchinson J. et al. (2018). AAP Committee on Psychosocial Aspects of Child and Family Health, AAP Council on Communications and Media. The power of play: a pediatric role in enhancing development in young children. *Pediatrics, 142*(3), 2018-2058.

Zanos, P., Moaddel, R., Morris, P.J., Riggs, L.M., Highland, J.N., Georgiou, P., Pereira, E.F.R., Albuquerque, E.X., Thomas, C.J., Zarate, C.A. & Gould, T.D. (2018). Ketamine and ketamine metabolite pharmacology: Insights into therapeutic mechanisms. *Pharmacological Reviews*, *70*(3), 621-660.

Zarate, C.A., Jr, Singh, J.B., Carlson, P.J., Brutsche, N.E., Amel, I.R., Luckenbaugh, D.A., Charney, D.S. & Manji, H.K. (2006). A randomized trial of an N-methyl-D-aspartate antagonist in treatment-resistant major depression. *Arch Gen Psychiatry*, *63*(8), 856-864.

Endnotes

[1] Through their early ketamine studies during 1964, Corssen (anesthesiologist) and Domino (neuropharmacologist who coined the term "dissociative anesthesia") noted that patients receiving this agent experienced "feelings of floating in outer space and having no feelings in the limbs" (Domino 1965/2010). See Carter's clinical case where an untethered astronaut drifting in "outer space" is a relevant symbolic component.

[2] See Carhart et al. (2014) who propose a new theory of conscious states that incorporates principles from physics, neurobiology, and psychoanalysis (including Jung). They define two fundamentally different styles of cognition: primary consciousness is a pre-ego, regressive style of cognition, qualitatively different from secondary consciousness, dominant during waking states. Primary states are evident in psychedelic experiences, REM sleep, onset of psychosis, and the dreamy state of temporal lobe epilepsy (pp. 6-7). Based in CAS, these findings and propositions are resonant with Jung's early ideas about the many layers of the conscious/unconscious. In addition, McNamera notes that brain structures activated and deactivated during REM overlap with the DMN: "It is as if REM neurobiology produces dreams when the individual is asleep and daydreams when the individual is awake" (2021).

[3] See Carter 2022 on Freud's admission that he was unable to experience the "oceanic feeling" described by his friend, the pacifist scholar of Indian mysticism and Nobel Prize winning poet Romaine Rolland. It seems that Ferenczi and Jung had access to these sources beyond the personal. *The Red Book* gives evidence of this capacity in Jung.

Index

Printed in the USA
CPSIA information can be obtained
at www.ICGtesting.com
LVHW091527201123
764189LV00002B/3